clean cuisine
COOKBOOK

130+ Anti-Inflammatory Recipes to Heal Your Gut, Treat Autoimmune Conditions, and Optimize Your Health

Ivy Ingram Larson & Andrew Larson, MD

VICTORY BELT PUBLISHING
Las Vegas

To Ivy's dad, Norman Ingram, who taught her that she could do anything,
but that nothing worth having would ever come easy.
You were right, Dad. I love you.

First Published in 2019 by Victory Belt Publishing Inc.

ISBN-13: 978-1-628602-93-7

The information included in this book is for educational purposes only. It is not intended or implied to be a substitute for professional medical advice. The reader should always consult his or her healthcare provider to determine the appropriateness of the information for his or her own situation or if he or she has any questions regarding a medical condition or treatment plan. Reading the information in this book does not constitute a patient-physician relationship.

The author/owner claims no responsibility to any person or entity for any liability, loss, or damage caused or alleged to be caused directly or indirectly as a result of the use, application, or interpretation of the information presented herein.

Food styling and food photography by Gail Ingram
Front and back cover photos by Debby Gans
Front cover and back cover styling by Gail Ingram
Cover design by Erin Lodeesen
People photos by Debby Gans and David Scarola
Interior design by Yordan Terziev and Boryana Yordanova

Printed in Canada
TC 0118

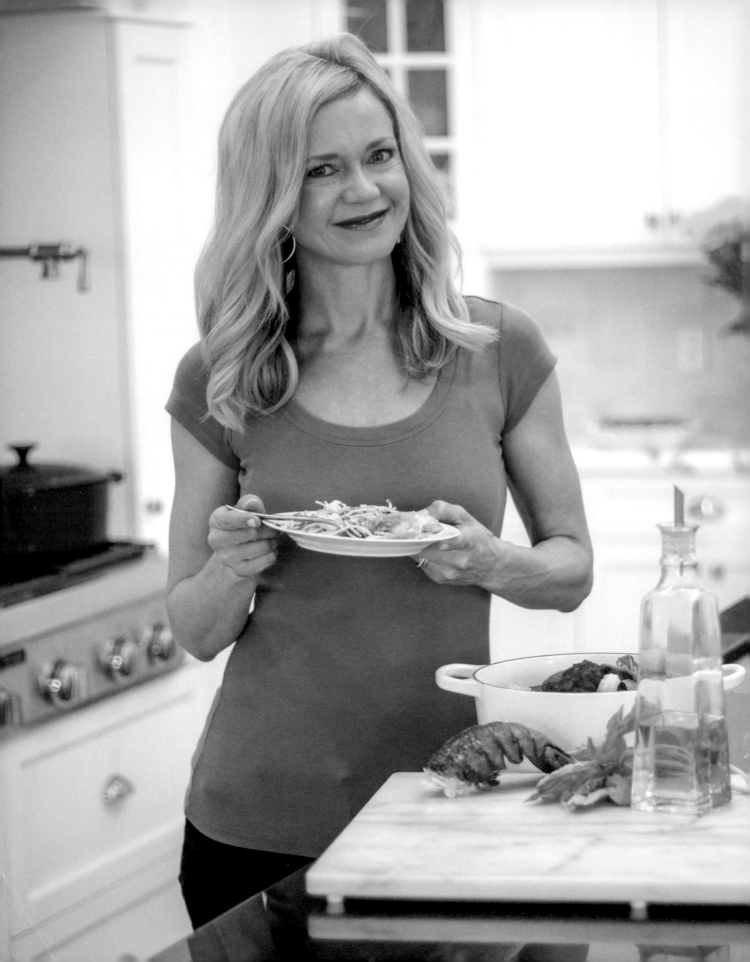

our story: in sickness and in health

If you are new to clean eating, we hope this book will inspire you but not overwhelm you. If you are already a devoted clean eater—perhaps more restrictive than we are—we hope this book will show you that healthy eating does not need to be complicated or restrictive. But before we get cooking, we want to tell you our story and how our clean-eating journey began.

We've been eating a clean diet for more than twenty years, and we've based our definition of "clean"—heavy on plants, light on animal foods, free of refined and processed foods, with some finer points we'll delve into later—on published medical research. Everything we recommend has been shown in scientific studies to improve health, and from our own experience, we know that it works to reduce inflammation, the cause of so many chronic ailments. So let's talk about how our clean-eating journey began and what we've learned along the way.

at the beginning

We were born exactly three years apart (Andy's birthday is April 4, 1973, and Ivy's is April 4, 1976), and we met in school in 1989. Ivy was in eighth grade, and Andy was the honor society student assigned to be her math tutor. Andy, who went on to be the class valedictorian, played on the high school football and soccer teams, and Ivy excelled in gymnastics, dance, and cheerleading. Those were the very good old days. We were both blessed with good health and happy lives.

Food didn't play too big a role in either of our lives at that point, although, like most kids, we both liked to eat! Dinner at our homes would have been something like meatloaf, green beans, mashed potatoes, and a salad of iceberg lettuce, with a glass of milk. Both of our families preferred

ice cream for dessert. At Ivy's house, fruit was also always on the table. Of course, the meat wasn't grass-fed, the potatoes were mashed with cream and butter, the green beans took up a teeny-tiny portion of our dinner plates, and the salad was smothered in some sort of creamy store-bought salad dressing made with refined vegetable oils. But back then, that would have been considered a very nutritious meal.

Fast-forward to the summer of 1998, when Ivy was twenty-two and had just started to experience a bizarre array of seemingly unrelated health issues. She was taking a full course of antibiotics once a month for recurring bladder infections and spent an entire summer battling debilitating fatigue while shuffling from one doctor to the next for an explanation of what could be causing the mysterious infections. Each visit was a dead end. Things got progressively worse. Soon bladder

5

urgency became a twenty-four-hour sensation, and Ivy was waking up six or seven times in the night to use the restroom. Her right leg became numb, and one day she woke up with a significant loss of strength in her right hip flexor muscle, making the simple act of lifting her knee to her chest nearly impossible. Then, one night, thinking she might be getting another bladder infection, Ivy followed her doctors' orders and downed nearly four cups of cranberry juice and water. Thirty minutes into the movie *The Horse Whisperer*, she thought her bladder might explode. Running to the ladies' room, panic set in when she was unable to void. She couldn't go a single drop. She called her parents, and they said they would meet her at the emergency room.

Leaving the hospital wearing a catheter, Ivy didn't need Google (which didn't even exist then!) to know that something was very, very wrong. Still wearing the catheter a few days later, she traveled several hours to the University of Miami. After extensive testing by a urologist there, Ivy was referred to a neurologist, who gave her a physical exam and then sent her to have an MRI scan of her head and spinal cord. She would soon know what was behind all her symptoms.

a life-changing diagnosis

The cause was not one that Ivy or her parents ever expected: multiple sclerosis (MS), an inflammatory autoimmune disease in which the immune system attacks the protective sheath that covers the nerves. She sat in the neurologist's pea-green office in a daze as he enumerated the symptoms of MS, many of which she already had: bladder problems, visual disturbances (including vision loss), depression, impaired memory, loss of mental clarity, debilitating fatigue, weakness, paralysis, inability to swallow, numbness, tingling in the extremities, difficulty walking, loss of coordination, and overwhelming dizziness. The disease sounded like

a living nightmare to Ivy. She worried she would wind up in a wheelchair or, even worse, never have children.

Ivy remained dazed as her doctor began to go over the treatment options: she could try one of the few approved medications that would treat the disease itself (this was 1998, and the medication options were very limited) or enter a trial study for a new medication. She was also given prescriptions for medications to help manage her symptoms, including amantadine, baclofen, and Valium. Most surprisingly, she was also advised to radically overhaul her diet and lifestyle. Again, keep in mind that this was 1998—before *The Dr. Oz Show*, before the term *clean eating*, before Whole Foods became a household name, and before the idea of using food as medicine was something the average person might be willing to accept. Things have changed radically in twenty years, but back then the idea of controlling a disease like MS with diet and lifestyle modifications seemed far-fetched—so far-fetched, in fact, that if her neurologist hadn't been a world-renowned expert in MS, Ivy might have dismissed his advice.

Ivy was told that it would be very important to reduce inflammation and keep stress to a minimum, and that diet would play a major role in reducing inflammation and preventing more attacks. She was also given the name of a book: *The Multiple Sclerosis Diet Book*, written decades earlier by Dr. Roy L. Swank.

As much as she wanted to, Ivy still had trouble believing that food could affect a disease like multiple sclerosis. Of course, she knew people dieted to lose weight or lower their cholesterol, but she had never heard of anyone changing his or her diet to manage the symptoms of an autoimmune disease. And besides, what on earth would be considered a "pro-inflammatory" or "anti-inflammatory" food? The whole idea of learning a completely new way to eat—and then implementing it, especially at twenty-two, when all her friends were still eating pizza and french fries—was overwhelming.

Where to start?

Dr. Roy L. Swank's research on MS dates back to 1948, long before modern disease-modifying MS drugs were available. Over the course of a nearly fifty-year career, Dr. Swank worked directly with thousands of MS patients, and his diet has been proven to reduce the frequency and severity of flare-ups in MS patients. After a period of five years, study patients who followed his diet functioned better than when they were first diagnosed with MS. After twenty years, most of the control-group patients were unable to walk, whereas the typical Swank patient was fully mobile and experiencing only mild symptoms.

The current edition of Dr. Swank's book, published in 1987, provides irrefutable evidence that diet can in fact improve symptoms of multiple sclerosis. Large-scale studies published in prestigious medical journals such as the *Journal of Neurology, Neurosurgery, and Psychiatry*, smaller-scale studies published in less widely known journals, basic science studies, and high-quality epidemiological studies have all linked the improvement of MS in real-life humans (not rats, not mice, not chimpanzees) with dietary changes.

call Andy

At the time of Ivy's diagnosis, Andy was studying at the University of Pennsylvania School of Medicine, one of the top medical schools in the country. Ivy trusted his opinion and asked him whether he thought the diet really could help slow the progression of her MS and manage her symptoms or whether it would be a big waste of time.

Despite his medical training, Andy's first reaction was skepticism. Of course, today it seems like common sense that anyone suffering from chronic illness should maintain a healthy lifestyle, but twenty years ago, many doctors remained highly suspicious of, or at least unimpressed with, nutritional therapies. But because of the respect Andy had for Ivy's neurologist, who was a full professor and had published more than sixty peer-reviewed papers, Andy decided to look seriously at the research. He spent one full day at the University of Pennsylvania's medical library reading all of the available literature. Only then, to his astonishment, was he able to confirm that the Swank MS Diet did have merit. Ultimately, it was with Andy's encouragement that Ivy made the commitment to radically overhaul the way she ate.

Although many relationships break apart when sickness strikes, it was actually Ivy's diagnosis that brought us together as more than friends. And it brought us together very quickly. We were married just two years later, in early 2000, and our son, Blake, was born almost exactly one year later. Through it all, Ivy stuck to her MS diet, but it wasn't easy. Although we were highly impressed with the results of the Swank program, Ivy had an increasingly difficult time following the prescribed diet to a T—it was so restrictive, and the food was incredibly bland and boring.

can an anti-inflammatory diet taste good?

Hoping that a more enjoyable but still healthful way to eat existed, we pored over countless medical and nutrition journals, reading everything we could about diet, lifestyle, and MS. After extensive research, we started to really understand what makes a food anti-inflammatory or pro-inflammatory. Ivy began making small changes to what she ate, creating an updated and revised Swank MS Diet that emphasized super anti-inflammatory foods like fruits, vegetables, and superfoods ultrarich in antioxidants and phytonutrients. Interestingly, the new diet was easier to follow and tasted better!

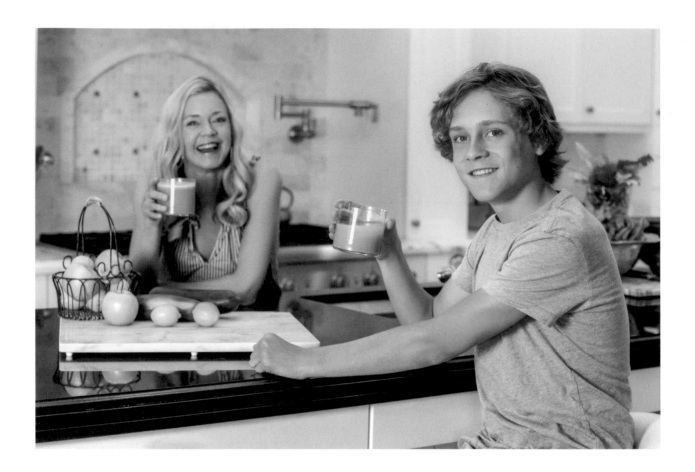

CLEAN EATING FROM BIRTH

When Blake was born, we decided to raise him on the same anti-inflammatory diet we were following. Now that he is almost eighteen years old, we feel strongly that our decision to raise him on a clean diet is one of the greatest gifts we have given him. Blake has enjoyed exceptionally good health over the years. He's never suffered from sore throats, asthma, allergies, ADD/ADHD, or eczema—he rarely even gets sick! He's taken antibiotics just once in his life, for an ear infection he got from swimming in a murky pond. A track runner who competed at the state level and a straight-A student who missed just two questions on the math portion of his SAT, Blake has excelled both physically and academically. And maybe the clean diet has absolutely nothing to do with how well Blake has done, but it certainly hasn't hurt!

One thing we do believe is the direct result of Blake's diet is that he has aged slower than his friends—he's been slower to reach his adult height and weight, and a bone-age study (done by X-ray) has shown his skeletal system to be younger than his real age. We are convinced that his slower growth is because the anti-inflammatory diet he follows is also antiaging, and it's low in exogenous hormones that can affect development. Aging slowly might not seem like a good thing when you are eighteen, but when you turn forty, it starts to seem like a major perk! Now that we are both middle-aged, we sure wish we had started our own clean-eating habits at birth.

One of the reasons the flavor improved so much was that we finally started to understand the big difference between pro-inflammatory animal fats and unrefined, phytonutrient-rich plant fats. You see, the main focus of the Swank MS Diet is to limit the intake of animal-based saturated fats to 20 grams a day. Although the focus there is on animal-based saturated fat, Ivy ended up eating much less fat overall, and consequently the food she was eating was not all that tasty. (From a culinary standpoint, fat is one of the most important conveyors of flavor; that's why fat-free foods are often so unappetizing.) Once Ivy finally started to realize the tremendous difference between fat from refined vegetable oils, fat from animals, and fats from plants such as avocados, nuts, and coconuts, and the benefits of whole fats over any type of oil, her culinary world changed tremendously. Her health also started improving even more. Learning how to get enough fat from the right sources and eliminate or reduce her intake of fat from pro-inflammatory sources—along with significantly ramping up her intake of nutrients in the form of antioxidants, phytonutrients, and fiber from unrefined plant foods (especially fruits and vegetables!)—made a major difference in Ivy's health. By the time our son was born in 2001, we were full-swing into the clean-eating thing. Ivy had stopped feeling as though her body was betraying her. The psychological burden of MS was finally gone, and we were both confident that the diet was helping tremendously.

The Science Behind Clean Cuisine

While this book is not the right forum for explaining the ins and outs of scientific research, we do want you to be confident that our recommendations are well-thought-out. When we decided that Ivy would hold off on multiple-sclerosis medications and instead follow an anti-inflammatory diet, we wanted to be as certain as possible that dietary therapy would be at least as effective as the available medications. In designing the Clean Cuisine program and creating these recipes for adults and children around the world,

we are careful to be just as certain, if not more certain, that we are truly offering an opportunity for better health.

We have never relied on any cellular or test tube studies, nor have we relied on any animal studies. Our favored approach has been to look for large studies called cohort studies, in which groups of people were followed for years and their diets monitored regularly. By looking at their medical records, it is easy to see which groups of people did better and which groups did worse. Dr. Swank's MS research amounted to a cohort study showing that those who followed his diet had far less disability as the years went on than those who didn't.

Unfortunately, though, there's not always a strong cohort study available on a particular dietary question. This is where the art of medicine comes into play. When Dr. Swank noted that MS was more common among Norwegians who lived in the mountains than among those who lived on the coast and surmised that the difference was due to the types of animal fat eaten by these two groups, he was relying on an observation, not a cohort study. This is perfectly acceptable, as observations allow researchers to come up with more powerful studies to prove the observation. Dr. Swank's observations in Norway motivated him to create a cohort study to prove his conjecture that reducing intake of animal-based saturated fats and increasing intake of omega-3-rich fatty fish would decrease the progression of disability in multiple sclerosis.

We have also looked at observational studies in coming up with our recommendations, even though we know these studies need more research to confirm their findings. We looked for cohort studies and randomized trials when forming our recommendations, but we also used good-quality observational studies, especially when multiple researchers have made the same observations. For example, if several researchers in different countries have noticed that regular coffee intake decreases the risk of type 2 diabetes, we start to wonder if it is a reasonable recommendation to include coffee in one's diet. When we dig into the research further and learn that coffee drinkers also have a reduced risk of Parkinson's, gallstones, hepatitis, and liver disease and that massive population studies find coffee innocent of contributing to heart disease, we start to wonder why coffee got such a bad reputation in the first place. And then when we learn that people who consume coffee regularly have a reduced risk of dying from all causes (that study was published in the *Journal of Epidemiology* in 2002, by the way), we start to think having one or two cups of coffee a day might actually be good for you!

The point is, sometimes arriving at a dietary recommendation requires looking at more than one source or study. This is how we can say that, for example, adding more turmeric makes the Mediterranean diet even more healthful than it already is. The Mediterranean diet has been proven to be more healthful overall than other diets in both randomized controlled trials and in cohort studies, and our advice with Clean Cuisine derives heavily from this. However, we also know from other studies that turmeric has potent anti-inflammatory benefits, so we recommend following Mediterranean diet principles but also using turmeric.

You can be confident that our recommendations are based only on proven or strongly suggested science. We never restrict food based solely on conjecture. We never rely on animal-only research. And we definitely do not follow fad diet trends. We would rather miss out on the latest unproven information than jump on the bandwagon and say that a food is bad when no evidence exists to support that statement. Remember, Clean Cuisine is about enjoying food, enjoying life, and enjoying good health—it's not about arbitrary restriction or deprivation.

it's not just for MS

The more we studied nutrition—and we studied it a lot—the more we realized that there is a common thread between MS and many other seemingly unrelated conditions, from arthritis to heart disease: inflammation. We slowly started getting our friends and family on board with our anti-inflammatory diet, and we started seeing impressive results, beginning with Ivy's mom, Gail, who was able to stop using the steroid inhaler she had been using for ages to treat her asthma. When she was finally able to throw away her rescue inhaler, too, we knew our program had real potential to help so many people with so many different conditions.

After sharing our nutrition recommendations with our friends and family, we brought our program to the public through a wellness class at the prestigious Atlantic Club in Red Bank, New Jersey (Bruce Springsteen and Jon Bon Jovi were among the members of the club). The class was advertised as a "5-Week Shape-Up" for club members who had health problems ranging from cardiovascular issues (such as unhealthy cholesterol ratios, high triglycerides, and high blood pressure) to inflammatory and autoimmune conditions like fibromyalgia and MS, as well as arthritis, asthma, obesity, and type 2 diabetes. Let's just say it was a broad spectrum of conditions!

While we were confident that we could improve the health of the people in our class, it took a leap of faith on Andy's part to believe that five weeks would be long enough. He had read in the *Journal of the American Medical Association* about a Canadian study in which four dietary changes reduced LDL ("bad") cholesterol as much as statin drugs in just four weeks. An abnormal cholesterol level is one marker of inflammation. Andy figured that if our anti-inflammatory diet really worked, then our class participants would see results just as quickly, but we decided to give ourselves one extra week to be safe.

For five weeks, the group met three times a week for nutrition classes and a thirty-minute "Full Fusion" workout taught by Ivy. ("Full Fusion" is the companion workout and DVD to our Clean Cuisine nutrition book.) Because we couldn't teach everything all at once, we had to teach the nutrition in baby steps. We surprised our participants up front when we said no to counting calories, fat grams, points, or anything else. Counting was popular back then, so it was a big deal just to recommend that people eat unrefined whole foods, with a heavy emphasis on plant foods, and add more super anti-inflammatory foods (especially those rich in omega-3s). It was really

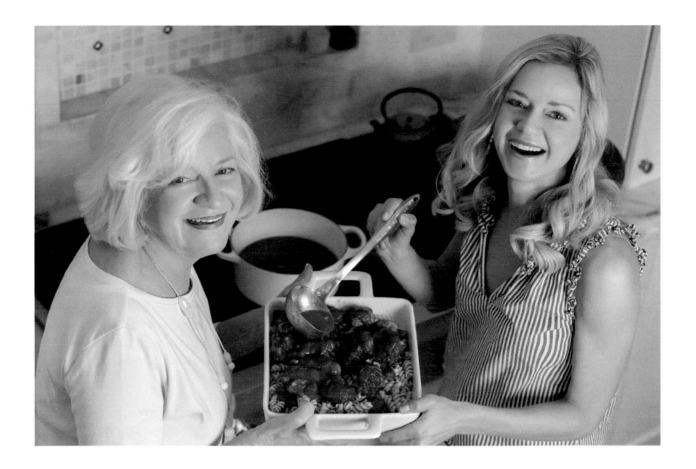

not at all complicated. In fact, it was very lenient, especially when you consider how strict so many diets—Paleo, raw, macrobiotic, vegan, and so on—are. Ivy had already begun cleaning up countless family recipes, so she was getting pretty good in the kitchen at that point. To supplement the class, she taught cooking on the side.

At the end of the five weeks, the results were nothing less than astonishing. Every single person lost weight, decreased their body fat percentage, and lost inches from their waist, their hips, or both. (We now appreciate that losing body fat is in and of itself anti-inflammatory because the less body fat you have, the lower your systemic inflammation.) Every person who had high triglycerides saw a decrease. Every person who suffered from an inflammatory disease such as asthma, allergies, arthritis, multiple sclerosis, or fibromyalgia enjoyed a significant improvement in their symptoms. Every person except one saw improvements in their overall cholesterol ratio.

write a book (and then a few more)

The results of that first class were impressive enough that we landed our first book deal. *The Gold Coast Cure* was published in 2005 and was a huge success; it was a number-one bestseller on Amazon, sold tens of thousands of copies, and was translated into seven different languages. That first book was based entirely on the principles we taught in the five-week class. Even though what we were promoting was actually a very lenient diet, it was still a drastic change from the way most people were eating. Cutting out things like processed foods, hydrogenated oils, refined vegetable oils, and high-fructose corn syrup was a big deal back then. The public still hadn't heard the term *clean eating*, and when we spoke to the media on our book tour, we had a hard time getting them to understand that our diet was an anti-inflammatory diet based on natural and unrefined foods. It was hard for producers and editors to understand that we were not promoting a low-fat or low-carb way of eating or advocating for the restriction of portions or calories. It was also hard for the public to believe that diet could have such a major impact on an autoimmune disease like MS, as well as so many other conditions. It all seemed too simple and too good to be true.

We followed up that first book with three more books. With each one, we emphasized plant foods more and more, but we have never strayed from the core principles presented in that first book. However, we have noticed that over the years, there's been a major shift in public opinion on food. Compared to when we started eating clean two decades ago, the average person today is much more open to the idea that food really is medicine. And yet, at the same time, diets have become increasingly more complicated and restrictive. Consequently, not nearly as many people are truly eating clean as you might think. Most people simply will not stick to a diet that is too restrictive. Yet the only way to get long-term results with dietary and lifestyle modification is to actually do it over the long term. For life.

we don't try to be "perfect" eaters

Our mornings start with coffee, not matcha tea, as you might expect. (We have that later in the day, though!) We have wine with dinner every single night, and we have done so for the entire eighteen years of our marriage (except when Andy is on ER call). We eat something sweet daily. True, our sweet treat is made with unrefined sugar, but it's still sweet! We haven't given up red meat, either, but we do make sure we buy the absolute highest-quality grass-fed meat, and we don't eat a lot of it. We aren't vegans, raw foodists, or even (gasp) gluten-free. In fact, we aren't even 100 percent dairy-free, because

we still eat a bit of high-quality cheese here and there. (We do, however, recognize that dairy is not a health food, so we have eliminated it from this book for the sake of simplicity.) The point is, we don't try to be "perfect" clean eaters. Instead, we aim for balance. Our anti-inflammatory Clean Cuisine way of eating does not fit into any of the popular diet categories: we are not vegan, vegetarian, macrobiotic, grain-free, Paleo, raw, low-carb, keto, Atkins, or anything else. We feel strongly that a diet or lifestyle program cannot be overly strict or people just won't stick to it, which means it won't work.

With Clean Cuisine, we have taken all the available research on nutrition and put together the most effective way of eating that will still allow you to enjoy the widest possible range of delicious foods. Could you adopt a more extreme way of eating? Absolutely! Will doing so substantially improve your health, energy level, or appearance? Based on all the available science, that's highly doubtful. Our primary goal is life enhancement; we want to enjoy life—and food!—as much as possible. So our way of eating is strict where it counts most and lenient where it doesn't matter so much. And it's worked for us! After two decades, we are still doing it.

life isn't always perfect

Changing our plates most definitely did change our fates! But eating clean hasn't been the answer for all of our health woes. By far, the most difficult challenge of the past twenty years was a health crisis related to Ivy's femoral retroversion, a congenital hip disorder that started causing Ivy pain shortly after the birth of our son. The pain intensified over the course of ten years to the point that she was unable to find a single comfortable position to sit or lie down, much less walk or even stand. It took two lengthy operations to fix her hip, one of which required breaking her thigh bone in half. In addition to having a terrible complication from that surgery, Ivy wasn't prepared mentally for the horrible postoperative pain or for being unable to walk for six months.

In many ways, the hip ordeal was far worse than the MS health hurdle years prior. One of the main reasons is that nothing Ivy tried seemed to help. Sure, she probably did better than she might have had she been eating donuts and Ding Dongs, but this was a major health hurdle that was not much helped by clean eating. However, it taught her a lot about the importance of stress management for pain, mood, and overall well-being. In the past, exercise had been Ivy's "drug" of choice because it relieved stress like nothing else, but the hip ordeal prevented her from exercising for months on end and forced her to learn new ways to manage stress. She also finally understood what her neurologist had meant years ago when he'd emphasized the importance of managing stress in MS patients. This advice applies to almost any inflammatory or autoimmune disease. You can have the cleanest diet in the world, but if you are not managing stress properly—or if an overly strict eating or lifestyle regimen is actually contributing to the stress—you won't reap the full benefits of the dietary changes.

No matter how clean we make our diets, life won't always be picture-perfect. What we have learned over the last twenty years is that food can totally change your life, but it doesn't need to dominate your life, and clean eating alone will not solve all your health woes. Controlling stress through meditation, mindfulness, and exercise is important, too.

From our family to yours, we hope you and your loved ones enjoy the recipes in this book as much as we have enjoyed making and eating them over the years.

Wishing you good health and happiness always,

Ivy & Andy
(Blake too!)

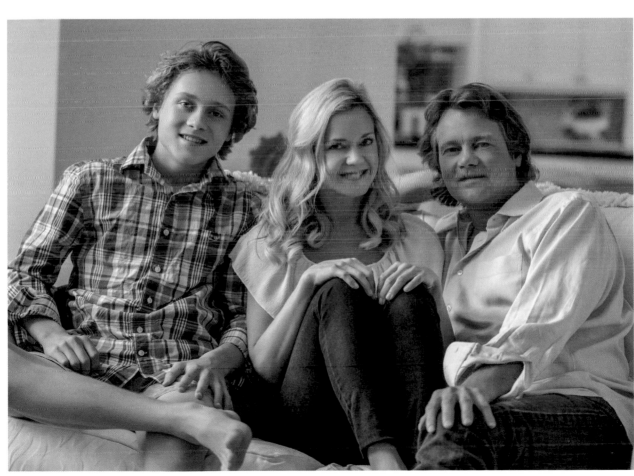

"It's fun to get together and have something good to eat at least once a day. That's what human life is all about— enjoying things."

—JULIA CHILD

Part 1

EATING
clean cuisine

clean cuisine defined

Clean means many things to many people—perhaps tidy or fresh, safe or simple. *Cuisine*, of course, refers to food, but more than just the food sold at the local takeaway. The word *cuisine* implies that the food is special and that the experience of eating it is special and enjoyable. So what, then, is *clean cuisine*, and why do we call this *The Clean Cuisine Cookbook*? Let's dig in!

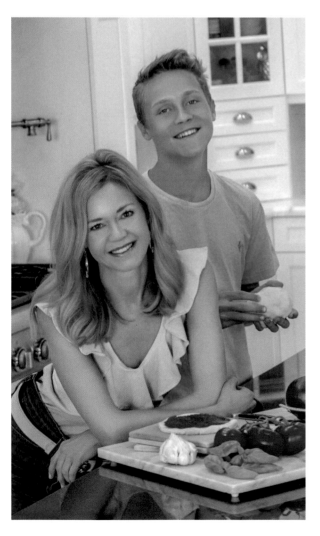

what is clean cuisine?

Let's start with the first word, *clean.* To us, clean food is unprocessed, unadulterated, and natural, without dirty chemicals or additives that are not found in food in the wild. Clean food provides the nourishment people grew accustomed to eating over hundreds of thousands of years. It is food that is in harmony with nature and with our bodies' needs. Clean food can be prepared elaborately, but it can also be as simple as an apple plucked from a tree.

Cuisine, on the other hand, is always imaginative, delicious, and inspired. Cuisine is food you would be proud to serve your family and friends. Cuisine tastes good.

In our recipes, we combine clean food with cuisine to create meals that taste good and are good for you—not just *sort of* good for you, like the food in many diet books and cookbooks. Clean Cuisine recipes are incredibly nutritious. They are recipes you can feel good about feeding to your entire family. And they are recipes that even the kids will like!

While Clean Cuisine blends clean food and delicious preparations, it does not fit into any of the popular diet categories. It's not plant-based, vegetarian, Paleo, low-fat, raw, keto, grain-free, macrobiotic, or any of the rest. Instead of basing Clean Cuisine on which foods are eliminated (there aren't very many, by the way!), we designed Clean Cuisine to do two things: reduce inflammation and optimize nutrition.

If we had to define Clean Cuisine in one sentence, it would be this: **"It's a plant-rich diet based on a wide variety of anti-inflammatory whole foods in their most natural and nutrient-rich state."**

Two Important Clean Cuisine Principles

Clean Cuisine is good for you. Our recipes fight inflammation. They are also nutrient dense and satisfying. Let's discuss these two points more.

Inflammation is the cornerstone of the body's healing response, bringing more nourishment and more immune activity to a site of injury or infection. But when inflammation persists or serves no purpose, it damages the body and causes illness. Stress, lack of exercise, genetic predisposition, and exposure to toxins (like cigarette smoke) can all contribute to chronic inflammation, but dietary choices also play a critical role. Learning how specific foods influence the inflammatory process is the best strategy for containing it and reducing long-term disease risks. Many modern illnesses are made much more symptomatic by inflammation. Autoimmune diseases such as rheumatoid arthritis and multiple sclerosis, in which the immune system attacks part of the body, become more symptomatic when there is more inflammation in the body. Inflammation also affects any disease related to the quality of blood flow, including atherosclerosis, which causes heart attacks and strokes and is largely responsible for senility.

Nutrient density—the amount of nutrients a food contains per calorie—is also very important. Your body craves nutrients. It does not necessarily crave a certain number of calories. If you are eating empty-calorie foods that have few nutrients (like most processed foods, such as potato chips), your body will crave more food (and thus more calories) because it has not received the nutrients it needs to keep you alive and healthy. That's one reason regularly eating foods without nutrients leads to obesity, which significantly increases your risk of

diabetes and cancer. What's more, because fat cells themselves create more inflammation, regularly overeating foods without nutrients (which is very easy to do) also increases your risk for any disease related to inflammation. Nutrient-dense foods make you feel fuller and offer hunger-free weight loss as a side benefit.

While many lifestyle choices affect health, diet is among the most important. The way you eat reinforces good health on a daily basis. When your way of eating reduces inflammation and helps you lose excess weight, you will be amazed at how much less stress you feel and how much easier and more enjoyable it is to exercise. We believe that it's easier to start an anti-inflammatory lifestyle by focusing on eating delicious food than by trying to control all the stress around you or to commit to an overly strict exercise regimen. So let's start with our plates!

We want you to be healthy, so we want you to choose foods that fight inflammation and that are as nutrient dense as possible. We will show you what those foods are and help you understand how to prepare them so that they taste great.

It's Not About Restriction— There Are Many Good Foods

We are lucky to live in a time when nutritionists and chefs fully agree on the value of eating and enjoying real, whole foods, from ancient grains to healthful fats and even the occasional glass of wine. Today, clean eating and eating delicious (even gourmet!) food are one and the same. We take great pride in making clean foods taste delicious and allowing as many great tasting foods as possible. No whole food is eliminated unless there is a very good reason for eliminating it. Our rules are simple. We won't ask you to weigh your food, fret about the glycemic index, rank oranges against bananas, or count calories.

The science is complicated, but it is now known that all calories are not equal in terms of overall health, the actual amount of energy absorbed by your body, or your tendency to gain weight. The calories from processed food are metabolized much differently than the calories from whole foods. Our motto, dating back to our first book, has always been, "Don't count your food; make your food count!" As you eat more of the good foods, you will then naturally eat less of the bad foods. And there are so, so many good foods to choose from.

We also don't try to micromanage macronutrient ratios. By that, we mean we are not going to tell you that your diet must be precisely X percent fat, Y percent carbohydrate, and Z percent protein. In ancient times, thousands of cultures flourished on a wide range of diets, with a wide range of macronutrient ratios. And when you look at places around the globe where the healthiest and longest-lived people are today, called Blue Zones, diets are varied. That said, they do have definite similarities. For one thing, the diets are very rich in unrefined plant foods and low in meat, sugar, animal fat, and the toxic processed foods of modern civilization.

We have looked closely at how the world's healthiest and longest-lived people eat and at the nutrition science literature, and we've based our Clean Cuisine way of eating on studies that look at real people, not animal studies or cellular or test tube studies. Once we started piecing the pieces of the diet puzzle together, we discovered a way of eating that is incredibly rich in variety. Most importantly, it's also easy and enjoyable. And isn't that what life is all about—feeling good and enjoying yourself?

That's especially important because the only way you will reap the benefits of clean eating is if you actually do it consistently. Both of us are very motivated when it comes to healthy eating, but even we would be unable to follow an unnecessarily austere diet program. We feel firmly that a diet cannot be overly strict or people just won't do it, and therefore it won't work. That's why we designed Clean Cuisine to be both enjoyable and effective. Could you adopt a more extreme way of eating? Sure! Would doing so substantially improve your health? Based on all the available science, that's highly doubtful. Clean Cuisine is strict where it counts most and lenient where it doesn't matter so much. We even incorporate

coffee and wine, and we will show you how to prepare and enjoy delicious unprocessed sweets for dessert.

Clean Cuisine is all about choice and variety. Unless there is scientific proof that you are harming yourself by eating a particular food or by preparing your food a certain way, we're going to let you make the call. The one exception is if you have a definite food allergy or sensitivity. Strawberries, for example, might be brimming with nutrients, but if you are allergic to them, then they are going to create an inflammatory response in your body. Everyone is different, and not everyone can tolerate the exact same foods.

But for the most part, clean eating does not need to be nearly as complicated as people have made it. If you simply focus on consistently eating a wide variety of nutrient-rich whole foods (mostly plants!) and get rid of the processed stuff, you will be amazed at how much better you will feel. The key is *consistency*.

It's About More Plants, Less Animal Foods

In general, Clean Cuisine favors plant foods over animal foods. Animal foods contain pro-inflammatory saturated fat and inflammatory peptides like carnitine, lecithin, and choline. These foods alter the trillions of microbes living in the gut and promote bacteria that has been linked to inflammation and intestinal disease. These bacteria produce inflammatory substances that increase your risk of heart disease, stroke, cancer, dementia, and many inflammatory conditions. Plus, the more animal foods you eat, the less room you have for plant foods.

That being said, most animal foods can be enjoyed in reasonable portions. But while almost all unprocessed plant foods are great for your health, many animal foods have been shown to be less than perfectly healthful, especially when they are

MAKE IT SIMPLE _____

The closer a food is to its natural state, the healthier it will be. This means you want to choose whole foods that are unadulterated, just the way nature intended. You want to go for corn instead of cornflakes, steel-cut oats instead of a granola bar that is made with oats (but also with a bunch of junk, like high-fructose corn syrup and processed corn oil). If push came to shove, you would even want to choose whole olives over olive oil.

consumed in excess. And it's important to remember that for every step you climb up the food-chain ladder, toxins found in the environment accumulate in the animal, and toxic overload can tip the body's balance toward inflammation, illness, weight gain, and accelerated aging. While it would be ideal to eat 100 percent organic foods, if this is not possible (and it usually isn't), you will normally consume fewer toxins by choosing nonorganic whole plant foods over even the cleanest organic animal foods.

Unrefined whole plant foods are also the best source of anti-inflammatory phytonutrients and gut-healthy fiber. Both phytonutrients and fiber play key roles in the many overlapping health benefits obtained from eating Clean Cuisine.

Phytonutrients are substances that protect the plant and fortify it against illness, but for you, the plant eater, they also offer invaluable disease protection and anti-inflammatory benefits. Phytonutrients act in a myriad of health-promoting ways. Many are sources of natural antiaging antioxidants, and others act as powerful inflammation extinguishers. Some phytonutrients enhance immune function and promote healing. Others stimulate enzymes that detoxify carcinogens. In a nutshell, the more phytonutrients you get into your diet, the better!

Fiber is the indigestible part of plant cells, so it's found in fruits, vegetables, whole grains, nuts, seeds, and beans. Fiber acts in a myriad of ways to promote good health and decrease inflammation. Fiber is nature's detoxifier, working to safely and effectively flush toxins—including potential carcinogens—from the body. It also helps slow digestion so that nutrients can be absorbed more evenly and blood sugar stays stable. And it plays a critical role in keeping the colon healthy and promoting gut health. Fiber is also very filling and can cut down on overall calorie consumption, which comes particularly in handy for preventing obesity and diabetes. Fiber prevents constipation, which can be uncomfortable and medically dangerous. Simply adding more fiber-rich foods to your diet appears to be associated with decreased inflammation. Not surprisingly, people who eat the most fiber from whole plants have trimmer waistlines, lower insulin levels, and a reduced risk of type 2 diabetes and many other diseases. And finally, fiber helps lower cholesterol and improve your cholesterol profile.

OPTIMIZING GOOD GUT BACTERIA

It's well known that the composition of your gut bacteria influences your risk for many health problems, from obesity and type 2 diabetes to certain autoimmune diseases. There is now growing evidence that fiber from plant foods is critical for nourishing good gut bacteria.

The two most common kinds of bacteria in the gut are Firmicutes and Bacteroidetes; together, these two make up more than 90 percent of the gut's population of bacteria. The ratio of these two groups controls levels of inflammation and correlates directly to conditions such as obesity, type 2 diabetes, and coronary artery disease. Scientists do not yet know the ideal ratio, but they do know that having more Firmicutes than Bacteroidetes is strongly associated with more inflammatory conditions and higher rates of obesity. A higher level of Firmicutes also has the ability to change our genetic expression, paving the way for more inflammation, more risk of obesity, more risk of type 2 diabetes, and more risk of coronary heart disease. Studies show that simply increasing your intake of fiber-rich carbohydrate foods can improve the Firmicutes-to-Bacteroidetes ratio. We also know that gut microbes feed on fiber and produce short-chain fatty acids that help regulate the immune system and tamp down inflammation. So if you are not eating enough dietary fiber to support these microbes, your immune system may be in a constant pro-inflammatory state.

But you can't just load up on fiber-fortified processed foods and call it a day. Studies done on inulin and other fibers added in isolation to processed foods show that they don't have the same beneficial effects as the fibers that occur naturally in whole foods. Your gut loves diversity, and eating a wide variety of plant-based whole foods is the best way to give your gut the fiber diversity it needs to promote more good bacteria and less bad bacteria. (We'll talk more about the gut microbiome on page 42.)

As long as it is from whole foods (and not supplements!), there is no upper limit on fiber consumption. Ancient humans ate far more fiber than we do today, as processing and refining foods to remove the fiber was not technologically possible. Humans evolved to thrive on a high-fiber diet, and many modern diseases, including obesity, diabetes, and cancer, have increased in prevalence over the years largely as the result of our fiber-deficient diets.

The only possible way to get more phytonutrients and fiber in your diet is to eat more plants and less animal foods. There's just no way around it. Thus, Clean Cuisine places a heavy emphasis on plant-based nutrition.

It's Not Vegan

Having given such praise to phytonutrient- and fiber-rich plant foods, now would be a good time to once again state that Clean Cuisine is neither vegan nor vegetarian. It does, however, take advantage of the fact that plant-strong diets are more nutrient dense than animal-rich diets.

We should also emphasize we don't eat animal foods for the protein they provide, because we know we can get the protein we need from plant foods. Instead, we eat animal foods because we like the taste and because they contain certain nutrients (such as iron, vitamin B_{12}, vitamin D, zinc, and DHA) that are difficult to get in adequate amounts from plant foods. Nutritional supplements are an option for strict vegans, but it is best to use supplements as just that, supplements, not as the sole source of a nutrient. It is far better to get the nutrients your body needs from whole foods.

Furthermore, even though studies do show that whole-food vegetarians have fewer heart attacks, less incidence of cancer, lower weight, lower blood pressure, and longer life spans, if you dig deep into the research you'll see that even people who do not completely avoid animal foods enjoy equally impressive health benefits—as long as the bulk of their calories come from unrefined, whole plant foods, with plenty of fruits and vegetables. Also, when we look closely at the research, we cannot find scientific evidence to support health reasons for eliminating fish from your diet.

The take-home message here is that science supports the idea that you can reap the health and weight-loss benefits of a vegan diet without being vegan. Even Colin Campbell, one of the biggest champions of vegan diets in the medical community, acknowledges that it has not been proven that a zero-animal-food diet is best. We would go further: we believe that a plant-heavy diet that includes wild-caught, low-mercury, omega-3-rich seafood is the most healthful.

Our goal with Clean Cuisine is not to set the bar for dietary purity so high that it guarantees failure; instead, we want to help you learn to eat and cook in a way that is doable and enjoyable for the long haul. Less than 0.5 percent of the population is vegan, meaning that they eat no animal foods whatsoever; you don't need to go to those extremes to improve your health.

the clean cuisine food pyramid

The Clean Cuisine food pyramid, just like the old USDA food pyramid, will help you visualize which foods to eat more of and which foods to eat less of.

Treats like cheese are positioned at the top of the pyramid—they are allowed, but since they are less nutrient dense and less able to fight inflammation than foods lower down on the pyramid, they should be consumed in smaller quantities. (Note: All the recipes in this book are dairy-free, but at home we do still eat a teeny bit of high-quality cheese now and then.) If you are a chocolate lover, you will probably spot chocolate at the top of the pyramid right away. Because, yes, you can still have chocolate and other treats on Clean Cuisine! Research even shows that compounds found in tea, coffee, wine, and chocolate cause beneficial changes in gut bacteria that may help prevent diabetes. What you won't find among the allowed treats are foods that contain partially hydrogenated oils and trans fats (found in many processed foods). And you won't find refined sugar in any food we eat. Again, we are strict where it counts most and lenient where it doesn't matter as much.

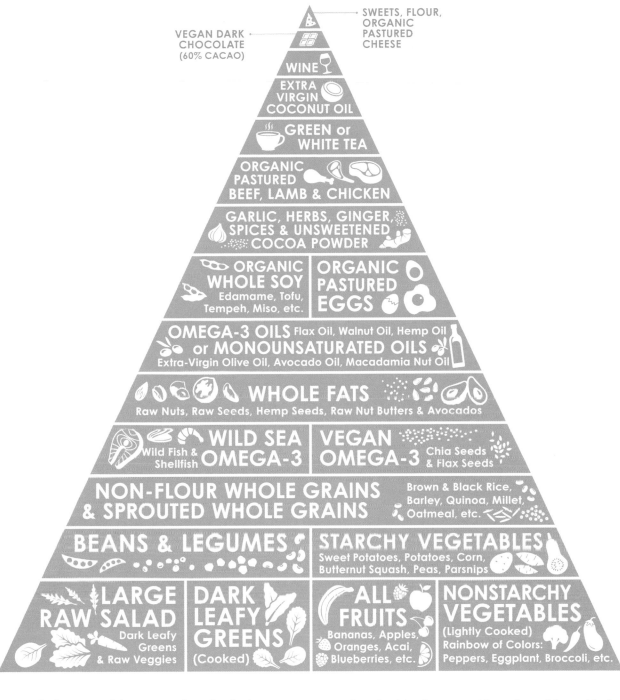

The Clean Cuisine food pyramid:

SWEETS, FLOUR, ORGANIC PASTURED CHEESE (top)

VEGAN DARK CHOCOLATE (60% CACAO)

WINE

EXTRA VIRGIN COCONUT OIL

GREEN or WHITE TEA

ORGANIC PASTURED BEEF, LAMB & CHICKEN

GARLIC, HERBS, GINGER, SPICES & UNSWEETENED COCOA POWDER

ORGANIC WHOLE SOY Edamame, Tofu, Tempeh, Miso, etc. | **ORGANIC PASTURED EGGS**

OMEGA-3 OILS Flax Oil, Walnut Oil, Hemp Oil **or MONOUNSATURATED OILS** Extra-Virgin Olive Oil, Avocado Oil, Macadamia Nut Oil

WHOLE FATS Raw Nuts, Raw Seeds, Hemp Seeds, Raw Nut Butters & Avocados

WILD SEA OMEGA-3 Wild Fish & Shellfish | **VEGAN OMEGA-3** Chia Seeds & Flax Seeds

NON-FLOUR WHOLE GRAINS & SPROUTED WHOLE GRAINS Brown & Black Rice, Barley, Quinoa, Millet, Oatmeal, etc.

BEANS & LEGUMES | **STARCHY VEGETABLES** Sweet Potatoes, Potatoes, Corn, Butternut Squash, Peas, Parsnips

LARGE RAW SALAD Dark Leafy Greens & Raw Veggies | **DARK LEAFY GREENS** (Cooked) | **ALL FRUITS** Bananas, Apples, Oranges, Acai, Blueberries, etc. | **NONSTARCHY VEGETABLES** (Lightly Cooked) Rainbow of Colors: Peppers, Eggplant, Broccoli, etc.

At the bottom of the pyramid are foods that can be eaten in nearly unlimited quantities. These foods are extremely nutrient dense and contain phytonutrients that offer additional health benefits, especially when it comes to fighting cancer. Dark leafy greens, vegetables, and whole fruits are great examples. In the middle of the pyramid are foods that you should eat, but not necessarily every day.

Any food in the pyramid can be safely avoided if you don't enjoy it or are allergic to it. Examples include shellfish, tofu, nuts, and eggs. There are no foods on the Clean Cuisine program that are absolutely essential for optimal health. Regardless of whether you have food sensitivities, allergies, or simply very specific taste preferences, you can make Clean Cuisine work for you!

ten clean cuisine dos and don'ts

The original idea was to call this chapter "Ten Clean Cuisine Anti-inflammatory Rules," but we decided the word *rules* was a bit too rigid for our approach. Clean Cuisine has a lot of leniency. As already mentioned, it doesn't require perfection or counting, measuring, or in any way restricting yourself. It just requires consistently choosing more of certain foods over others. The most important thing is to choose more of the good anti-inflammatory and nutrient-rich foods and less of the pro-inflammatory and nutrient-poor foods. But you don't need to be perfect. For example, we recognize that cheese is not an anti-inflammatory superfood, and we do not include it in any of the recipes in this cookbook, but as we mentioned in chapter 1, we do still eat a wee bit of real cheese now and then in real life. Why? Because we love cheese and we know that having a little bit is not going to destroy our health, especially since the rest of our diet is brimming with nutrient-rich and anti-inflammatory foods. Don't strive to be a perfectionist with your food. It's much healthier to seek balance, enjoyment, and nutrition.

Having said all that, here are the ten nutrition dos and don'ts that we choose to live by.

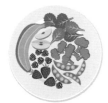
1. eat vegetables and/or fruits with every meal

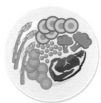
2. think plant strong

3. consume both land and sea omega-3s

4. slash refined empty carbs

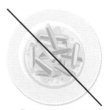
5. never eat trans fats

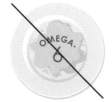
6. avoid omega-6-rich oils

7. eat more beans and legumes

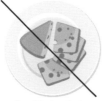
8. ditch dairy

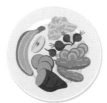
9. increase your intake of prebiotic and fermented probiotic foods

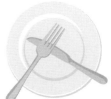
10. don't eat when you aren't hungry

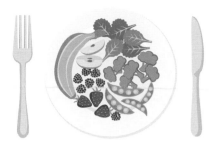

1. eat vegetables and/ or fruits with every meal

The biggest diet mistake people make is not eating anywhere near the amount of fruits and vegetables they should. When people decide to clean up their diets, they automatically start by nixing processed foods, sugar, and fried goodies from the menu, which is a great start, but just as important is eating enough fruits and vegetables. One of the most consistent findings in the scientific literature is that as fruit and vegetable consumption increases, chronic disease decreases across the board. Did you know that, other than quitting smoking, no lifestyle change will extend your life more than eating more fruits and vegetables? The second benefit of eating more fruits and vegetables is weight loss. It is almost impossible to be overweight if your diet is rich in fruits and vegetables.

One of the reasons it's so important to eat fruits and vegetables in abundance is that they offer such incredible nutrient bang for such a teeny-tiny calorie buck. Vegetables in particular pack a major nutrient punch in hardly any calories. For example, eating 1 cup of raw spinach delivers hefty amounts of fiber, minerals, and phytonutrients for a paltry 10 calories.

All of our recipes are designed to make this nutrition basic easy to accomplish because they all contain fruits and vegetables (or a superfood), and many contain several. There is no limit on the amount of fruits and vegetables you can eat on Clean Cuisine, as long as no extreme liberties are taken with their preparation. In other words, we're not recommending fried vegetable tempura. Raw is always okay; cooked is also okay as long as you avoid "dirty" oils (we'll talk more about these on page 34) and unhealthful coatings or cooking techniques. Juice is the only exception: we don't recommend it, and we'll explain why on page 32.

Should You Limit Your Consumption of Mother Nature's Candy (Fruit)?

One of the foods Andy's patients are consistently most confused about is fruit. They repeatedly ask whether the sugar in fruit is unhealthy. It is absolutely true that fruits contain sugar—certainly more sugar than ultra-low-calorie dark leafy vegetables and nonstarchy vegetables. But we don't want you to get hung up on the sugar in fruit, because as long as you're eating the whole fruit, with all its water and fiber, it will cause blood sugar and insulin levels to rise very slowly. In other words, the sugar in whole fruit doesn't disrupt your blood sugar like the sugar from a lollipop or a can of soda. If you avoid fruit juice and instead eat the whole fruit, which is what we recommend, you'll be getting plenty of blood sugar–blunting fiber, not to mention tons of antioxidants, phytonutrients, and vitamins, too! (We talk more about fruit juice on page 32.)

Many people worry that fruit could somehow be fattening, but this is just not the case. Fruit consumption has actually been shown to be inversely associated with body weight—in other

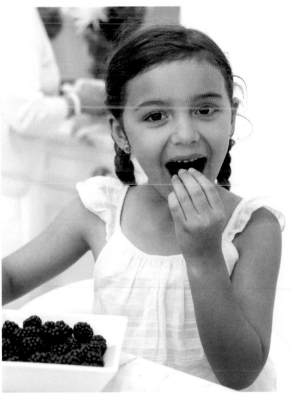

words, people who eat more fruit weigh less. In a study published in the journal *Nutrition,* seventy-seven overweight and obese dieters enrolled in a six-month randomized controlled trial testing the effects of a computer-assisted dieting intervention program. The goal was to decrease energy intake, increase fruit and vegetable consumption, and maintain a balanced diet. Although vegetable consumption increased as a result of the intervention, fruit consumption did not. However, after controlling for other factors, higher fruit consumption was associated with a lower body mass index at both the beginning and end of the study, and those participants who did increase their fruit consumption lost more weight. The results suggest that eating more fruit by no means reduces the likelihood of weight loss.

Besides, the vast majority of people don't eat anywhere close to the amount of fruit they should, so worrying about eating too much fruit is probably not where you should focus your energy. And in Clean Cuisine, there are no off-limits fruits. Even high-sugar fruits like bananas (a great source of prebiotics, by the way!), mangoes, and dates are nutrient-rich choices.

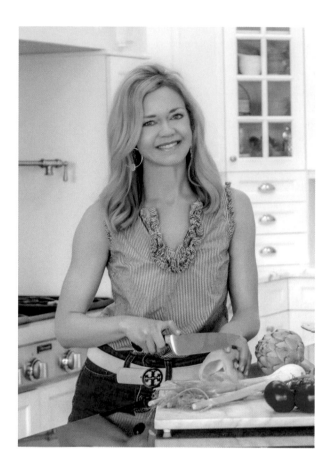

Are Raw Vegetables Best?

"Not necessarily" is the short answer. We are well aware of the growing popularity of the raw-foods diet, and we borrow a number of our preparation techniques from the raw-food culinary world. However, we still eat plenty of cooked foods, including cooked vegetables. In fact, some of the nutrients in vegetables, including certain phytonutrients, are better absorbed after the vegetables have been cooked. For example, the carotenoids in carrots, the lycopene in tomatoes, the zeaxanthin in red peppers, and the lutein in dark green leafy vegetables, red peppers, and corn are all significantly more bioavailable after these foods have been exposed to heat. (All vegetables with these phytonutrients are even more readily absorbed when eaten with a little fat, too. That is one of the reasons you never want to use fat-free salad dressing—not to mention that fat-free salad dressing tastes downright terrible!)

Although they're not technically vegetables, mushrooms contain toxic compounds that are broken down and eliminated by cooking. And heat actually increases the variety of health-promoting, sulfur-containing substances found in members of the allium family, such as onions and garlic. Since sulfur is required for the synthesis of glutathione, your body's master antioxidant and super detoxifier, your body can manufacture much more glutathione from cooked onions and garlic. This does not mean you should only eat your onions and garlic cooked, however. There are benefits to eating both cooked and raw onions and garlic. The idea is not to be too extreme with your food in general.

The point here is that putting some heat to your vegetables is not always a bad thing! Having said that, heat does destroy certain nutrients, such as vitamin C, and overcooking can damage the pigments that give vegetables color, such as the chlorophyll in green vegetables. While you certainly do not have to eat all of your vegetables raw, don't overcook them, either.

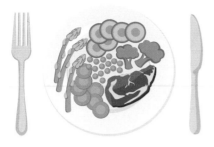

2. think plant strong

Every meal and snack should have more plant food on the plate than animal food. Plant foods can be bad for you if they are processed and refined or prepared using the wrong oils and cooking techniques, but the whole plants, as they're found in nature, are almost universally healthful. Plant food is the only source of phytonutrients and fiber, and it is more nutrient dense than animal food. Studies also clearly show that when your diet leans more toward plant foods, you carry around less weight and body fat—and the less body fat you carry, the less systemic inflammation you're burdened with. Furthermore, having a plant-based diet lets you avoid a large amount of the disease-promoting inflammation that occurs when you consume too many animal foods. (We'll talk more about the downside of eating too many animal foods on page 26.)

Ditch the thinking that animal protein is somehow superior for your health. Assuming that you, like us, eat a little animal food here and there throughout the day—or even just for dinner—you will be getting plenty of protein. In fact, unless you are eating a diet with too few calories or one with almost no variety,

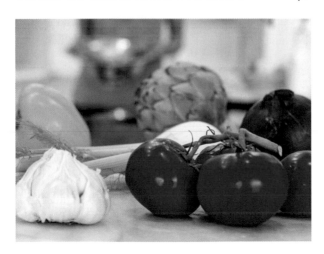

you will get all the protein and essential amino acids you need even if you eat no animal food. If you choose to be vegetarian or vegan, you can still follow Clean Cuisine! (We explain why we are not vegans or vegetarians ourselves on page 20.)

Fiber Is Found Only in Whole Plant Foods

Fiber is a critical nutrient naturally present in all plant-based whole foods. (We've talked about the health effects of fiber on page 19.) As a general and bariatric surgeon, Andy frequently sees the negative complications associated with a low-fiber diet, including obesity, colon cancer, and intestinal diseases.

Fiber that is eaten the way nature packages it, in whole foods, has been proven to provide tremendous health benefits. However, the scientific literature does not support fiber supplements for promoting health or weight loss. This means you cannot spike your Lucky Charms with a sprinkling of Metamucil and expect to reap the same benefits you would get from eating a breakfast of unrefined whole carbs, such as steel-cut oats. The benefits of fiber from whole and unprocessed foods are many, as discussed on page 19. In addition, fiber-rich whole plant foods:

- **offer significant protection against cancer.** In fact, eating a diet high in fiber from whole foods could reduce colon and rectal cancer by as much as 50 percent. Almost every week, Andy treats a patient with colon cancer, and he would love to have half of those weeks off! Researchers have concluded that if Americans simply ate an additional 13 grams of fiber a day from whole carbs, then about one-third of colorectal cancers in the US could be avoided.

- **prevent diverticulitis and diverticulosis,** potentially lethal diseases of the colon that Andy deals with in his surgical practice on a weekly basis. In countries with high-fiber diets, these diseases are very rare. Studies suggest that about half of all symptomatic cases of these diseases could be prevented by eating a fiber-rich diet.

- **create a sense of fullness, satisfy hunger, and minimize the overconsumption of calories.**

The Downsides of Animal Foods

The first thing people worry about when we tell them not to overdo it with animal foods is protein deficiency. We'll talk about that in depth in chapter 4, but for now, just know that the vast majority of people are not in the state of protein emergency that the manufacturers of protein bars and protein shakes would like us to believe. In fact, most people eat far more protein than their bodies need.

That excess protein pushes plant foods that are rich in antioxidants, fiber, and phytonutrients right off your plate! Your stomach can hold only so much food in a day, so the more animal foods you eat, the less room you have for plant foods. This is a problem because your body needs the nutrients in plant foods more than those in animal foods. We are not saying you should eliminate animal foods altogether, because certain key nutrients (such as heme iron, DHA, and vitamin B_{12}) are available only in animal foods, but we are saying that you shouldn't overdo it. (We talk more about why we are not vegan or vegetarian on page 20.)

A diet rich in animal foods, especially meat, can also interfere with healthy hormone levels. Meat consumption is known to raise estrogen, and a high-meat diet can contribute to estrogen dominance, a problem that has become more and more prevalent in the Western world. In addition, a diet rich in animal foods, especially meat, is associated with less fiber consumption, which raises "bad" estrogens and grows the wrong bacteria in your gut.

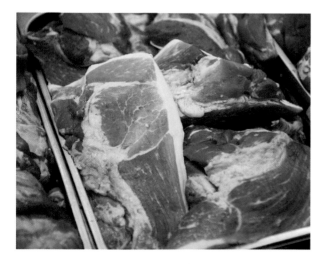

On top of all this, three components of animal food are particularly problematic: saturated fat, inflammatory peptides, and arachidonic acid.

Animal-Based Saturated Fat

One of the most inflammation-provoking substances in animal food is saturated fat. The saturated fat in animal food is not the same as the saturated fat in plant food. For example, coconut oil is a rich in saturated fat, but most of it is in the form of medium-chain triglycerides (MCTs). Your body handles the MCTs from coconut oil in a completely different manner than it does the saturated fat from animal foods like dairy and beef. The same goes for plant-based saturated fat in foods like olives and nuts. So it's important to note that we are not saying all saturated fat is bad—just that in animal foods.

One of the main concerns about the saturated fat from animal foods is that it disrupts your gut microbiome and can contribute to many of the problems that prebiotics and probiotics are trying to correct. A 2016 review article in the *World Journal of Gastroenterology* summarizes findings that saturated fats and a high-fat diet in general can disrupt the microbiome in a way that contributes significantly to the severity of many gastrointestinal illnesses. Intestinal conditions made worse by saturated fat from animal foods include inflammatory bowel diseases such as Crohn's disease and ulcerative colitis as well as mechanical conditions such as diverticulitis. Even if none of these conditions apply to you, the disruption to your microbiome can lead to irritable bowel syndrome and chronic nuisance diarrhea. There is also growing evidence that dietary fat–induced changes in how microbes in the gut signal the brain can affect the nervous system both functionally and structurally. If you have a neurological condition such as multiple sclerosis, depression, ADD, vascular dementia, or peripheral neuropathy, it is especially important to limit your consumption of animal-based fats.

In addition to disrupting the gut microbiome, the saturated fat from animal foods interferes with your body's ability to utilize the super-important omega-3 fats, which most people are already seriously deficient in. It is also well researched that saturated fats from meats increase your risk of developing colon cancer. And finally, that *World*

Journal of Gastroenterology article also showed that a diet high in animal-based saturated fat (and trans fat) is closely linked to obesity and metabolic syndrome as well as gastrointestinal disease.

Inflammatory and Cancer-Causing Peptides

Red meat (grass-fed or otherwise), egg yolks, and cheese contain inflammatory peptides such as carnitine, lecithin, and choline. These peptides change the bacteria in your gut, making them produce inflammatory substances that are absorbed into the bloodstream, increasing the risk of heart disease, stroke, cancer, and dementia, not to mention wrinkles and impotence. Meat-consumption also raises insulin-like growth factor 1 (IGF-1), a hormone that stimulates cell growth. Elevated IGF-1 levels have been linked to hormone-sensitive cancers such as prostate cancer and breast cancer.

Arachidonic Acid

Found only in animal foods, this is a type of pro-inflammatory omega-6 fat that can be very harmful to health when eaten in excessive quantities. In addition to contributing to inflammation, high blood levels of AA are associated with platelet aggregation (or "stickiness"), which is a major contributing factor to heart disease.

As bad as that sounds, we do need some AA in order to maintain optimal health and a well-functioning immune system. It is no accident that AA is present in breast milk—again, our bodies do need some of it. We just need to make sure we don't overdo it. The key is to balance it with anti-inflammatory omega-3s. You can dramatically reduce your AA consumption simply by choosing foods from animals whose diet is as nature intended. For example, grass-fed beef has less AA than conventional grain-fed beef. Pastured hens and their eggs have less AA than factory-farmed chicken and eggs. When it comes to fish, the difference is rather astounding. For example, 4 ounces of farmed Atlantic salmon contains 1,306 milligrams of AA, while the same amount of wild-caught Atlantic salmon contains just 303 milligrams of AA. We can't emphasize enough the importance of eating only the highest-quality animal foods, as we'll discuss in a moment. There are a wide variety of reasons why, but limiting AA consumption is a big one!

Choose Animal Foods Wisely

Clean Cuisine is plant-strong nutrition, but we do recognize that meats contain valuable nutrients and were enjoyed by our ancestors for millennia. Meats that are properly chosen and prepared can be part of a healthy diet.

Our advice for animal-food consumption can be summed up as follows:

 Always choose the highest-quality animal foods. Look at the animal's diet; choose only animals that were fed the diet nature intended the animal to eat. (See page 65 for more.)

 Choose organic when possible. (We'll talk more about this in chapter 5.)

 Find a dairy-free substitute for milk and cream. There is no nutritional reason to drink milk, and there are plenty of tasty milk and cream substitutes. For what it is worth, Andy drinks his coffee black and Ivy uses coconut cream for her dairy-free coffee creamer. (See page 74 for more.)

 Eat real cheese in very small quantities. Cheese is not a health food, but eating a small amount is not the end of the world.

 Recognize that fatty fish will give you the most nutritional bang for your animal-food buck owing to its omega-3 fats (EPA and DHA) and nutrients (vitamins B_{12} and D, iron, and zinc).

 Eat animal foods in moderation. Consider being an ovo-vegetarian (eating only plant foods and eggs) until dinner and then eating animal foods only as a modest part of your dinner, not the main attraction.

 Consider having Meatless Monday. (We have a whole collection of recipes in this book and on the blog to help you with this one!)

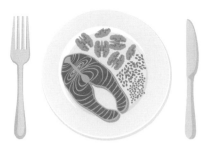

3. consume both land and sea omega-3s

Omega-3 fats support the health of your immune system, reproductive system, cardiovascular system, and central nervous system. These are the most powerful anti-inflammatory substances available without a prescription and are therefore beneficial for any condition that's related to inflammation, such as asthma, allergies, multiple sclerosis, chronic pain, coronary artery disease, and many others. Omega-3 fats also play a vitally important role in supporting healthy skin, hair, and nails, as well as in improving cognitive function, attention span, and the ability to retain and process information. They even improve your mood and make you happier! And when it comes to weight loss, omega-3 fats are incredibly important. One particular type of omega-3, EPA, improves your body's ability to burn fat while also making your cells more sensitive to insulin. The more sensitive your body is to insulin, the easier it is to lose weight and maintain a healthy body weight.

Unfortunately, modern diets are more deficient in omega-3s than just about any other nutrient. We make it a point to eat at least one serving of omega-3-rich foods every single day. The omega-3 found in fish and shellfish is more bioavailable than that found in plant foods, so this is one very good reason to consider including fish in your diet even if you are otherwise vegetarian or vegan. (Be sure to read pages 86 and 87 for how to choose the cleanest and healthiest seafood.) But whether you're vegan or not, we recommend supplementing with a high-quality fish oil (we suggest 2,000 to 3,000 mg daily).

We also encourage the consumption of vegan land-based foods rich in omega-3s and consider these to be superfoods. They include flax seeds, hemp seeds, chia seeds, and certain nuts, like walnuts and almonds. Vegan omega-3 fat is complementary to sea-based omega-3 fat, and ideally both should be eaten in large quantities. Unless you make a conscious effort to eat more omega-3s on a daily basis, chances are you will fall short on this critical nutrient.

Kinds of Omega-3s

There are three kinds of omega-3 fats that are most important for health: alpha-linolenic acid (ALA), eicosapentaenoic acid (EPA), and docosahexaenoic acid (DHA).

ALA (also known as LNA) is found in walnuts and hemp seeds, but it's most concentrated in flax seeds and chia seeds. Although eating the whole food in the form of nuts and seeds is the superior choice, you can also get ALA from unheated, cold-pressed flax oil, hemp oil, or walnut oil—just drizzle it on vegetables, salads, grains, or beans. The benefits of this type of omega-3 fat are many, including reduced inflammation, lower blood pressure, and improved insulin sensitivity (which means less risk of obesity, heart disease, and type 2 diabetes).

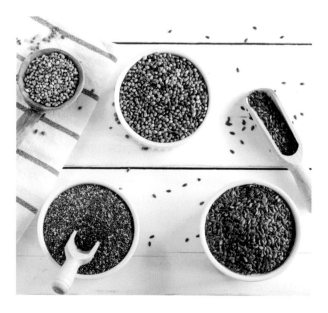

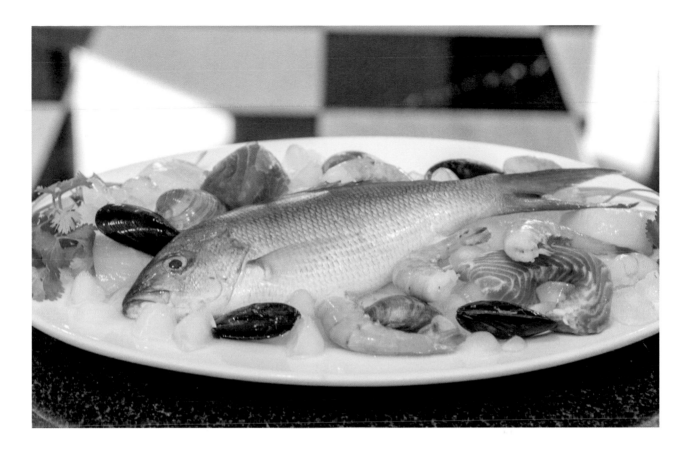

EPA and DHA are only found in nonvegan sources. EPA and DHA are really the key omega-3s, and because they each do different things, you need them both. The richest sources of EPA and DHA are fatty fish and fish oil supplements. Egg yolks also contain DHA. When it comes to reducing inflammation in the body and brain, EPA plays a critical role because it inhibits multiple steps in the inflammatory process. But don't think DHA is useless! Quite the opposite. DHA plays an essential role in optimizing brain function, vision, and whole-body health. Among many other benefits, your body uses DHA to manufacture a critical protein called brain-derived neurotrophic factor (BDNF). BDNF is essential for learning, thinking, and higher levels of brain function. DHA is the reason omega-3s have been publicized as "smart nutrients." There are some areas in which EPA and DHA appear to be equally beneficial. For example, both are equally effective in reducing triglyceride levels. Also, both EPA and DHA contribute to the maintenance of normal blood pressure and healthy heart function.

Your body can convert ALA to EPA and then EPA to DHA, but the conversion process does not happen optimally or reliably. For example, eating too much omega-6 fats, animal-based saturated fat, or trans fats can interfere with the conversion process and create an omega-3 deficiency even if you are eating plenty of ALA. So even though a well-planned plant-rich, whole-foods vegan diet can contain plenty of ALA, we still recommend a pharmaceutical-grade fish oil supplement for EPA and DHA because individuals differ in how well their body converts ALA to EPA and DHA. In addition, inflammatory autoimmune conditions, metabolic issues, and numerous lifestyle factors can create a DHA deficiency even if your diet is rich in ALA. The greatest weakness of many otherwise healthful, plant-strong vegan or nearly vegan diets is their lack of optimal amounts of EPA and DHA. The Okinawans are among the longest-lived people in the world, and they traditionally consume approximately three servings of fish per week in addition to eating a clean, plant-strong diet.

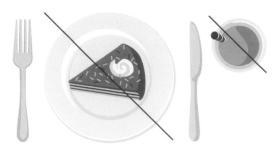

4. slash refined empty carbs

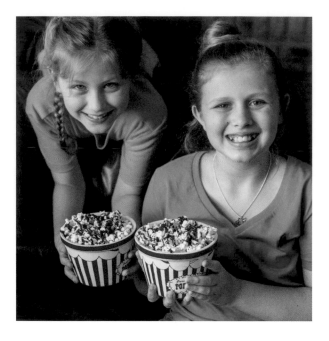

Unlike the carbs found in whole, unrefined plant foods (such as potatoes, apples, and steel-cut oats), refined carbs are a nutritional nightmare. These foods are no longer nutritionally intact, the way nature designed them. The fiber and most of the naturally occurring nutrients have been removed during processing, and you are left with a calorie-rich, nutrient-poor, empty-calorie food. And because refined carbs are not bulky, they don't take up a lot of space in your stomach, and you therefore need to eat massive amounts of them to feel full. They contribute to malnutrition, excess hunger (what we call the "malnourished munchies"), out-of-control food cravings, weight gain, and inflammatory disease. Empty carbs are rapidly absorbed, so they create a sharp glucose surge into your bloodstream, which forces your pancreas to pump out the hormone insulin, which moves glucose from the bloodstream into cells. The problem is, insulin is also your body's primary fat-storing hormone; it forces your liver to convert the excess sugar in your blood into fat.

The more frequently you assault your body with quickly absorbed, blood sugar–spiking refined carbs, the greater the demand you place on your pancreas, the more fat you gain, and the more you increase your chance of developing type 2 diabetes. A diet rich in empty carbs is also linked to heart disease and even increased cancer risk.

But that's not all! If you are not particularly active and the empty carbs you eat are not burned for energy, your body can convert them into pro-inflammatory saturated fat, specifically palmitic acid, a very dangerous type of saturated fat associated with an increased risk of heart disease.

The saturated fat your body manufactures will also increase inflammation in your body, exacerbating symptoms of inflammatory conditions such as MS, asthma, fibromyalgia, psoriasis, and arthritis.

If that's not bad enough, insulin also activates the main enzyme responsible for making cholesterol in your liver. This means that even if you eat a 100 percent cholesterol-free, animal-free diet, your LDL ("bad") cholesterol can still increase if you eat too many processed, empty-calorie carbohydrates.

Luckily, there really are only a few refined carbohydrates you want to avoid. Unfortunately, they're all ubiquitous in modern society and found in numerous processed food products. Keep your eyes open and avoid consuming the following processed empty-calorie carbs in the recipes you make and in the packaged foods you buy.

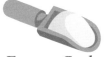

Empty Carb #1: Refined Flour

The vast majority of baked goods sold in the United States are made from refined flour derived from wheat. In refining whole wheat berries into flour, the nutrient-rich wheat germ, which contains antioxidant vitamin E along with a vast array of trace minerals and phytonutrients, and the fiber-rich wheat bran are removed. This leaves behind nutrient-poor, fiber-free starch. No nutrients equals empty calories. Refined flour is found in hundreds of processed food products, and eating it is basically just like eating sugar. And along with sugar, refined flour is the ultimate empty carb.

Refined flour is "enriched flour," "wheat flour," "all-purpose flour," or any other flour that does not have the word *whole* in front of it on the list of ingredients. "Enriched flour" and "all-purpose flour" certainly sound healthier than "refined white flour," but they are all the same thing. "Enriched" refers to the government-mandated addition of small amounts of synthetic vitamins and minerals to refined flour after it has been processed. The only reason flour is "enriched" is that all the good stuff was removed during processing! Whole foods are not enriched; only processed foods are enriched. But even enriched flour does not contain fiber, and the synthetic vitamins and minerals that are added to it represent only a small portion of the nutrients that were removed during processing. Furthermore, your body does not recognize or utilize synthetic nutrients as it does naturally occurring nutrients. In addition, the disease-fighting phytonutrients are lost forever during the refinement process and are not added back.

FOODS LIKELY TO CONTAIN REFINED FLOUR

(But read the ingredients list on all foods you purchase!)

Bagels	Crackers
Baked goods	Muffins
Breadcrumbs	Pancakes
Breaded meats and vegetables	Pasta
	Pizza
Breads	Pretzels
Breakfast bars	Rolls
Cakes	Waffles
Cookies	

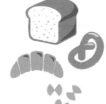

SUGAR BY ANY OTHER NAME IS STILL SUGAR!

Don't be fooled by common sugar pseudonyms

Cane juice	Glucose
Corn sweetener	High-fructose corn syrup
Corn syrup	Maltose
Dextrose	Modified food starch
Evaporated cane juice	Raw sugar
Fructose	Sucrose
Fruit juice sweetener	Syrup

Empty Carb #2: Refined Sugar

Even a first grader can tell you that eating too much sugar is not good for you! The problem is that sugar is everywhere. Start reading labels and you'll find sugar hidden in everything from spaghetti sauce to breakfast cereals to frozen entrees. According to the United States Department of Agriculture, the average American adult consumes more than sixty-four pounds of sugar every year. Yikes! To put that in perspective, sixty-four pounds of sugar translates to a whopping 116,120 empty calories. Ugh.

Not only is sugar the perfect example of the ultimate empty calorie, it can also be a toxic age accelerator. Eating excess amounts of sugar can wreak havoc with your cells on the inside and also damage your skin on the outside. In healthy youthful skin, collagen fibers twist together in linear strands, but according to findings in the *British Journal of Dermatology*, sugar binds to the collagen, so the fibers can't pack together as tightly ... and the skin begins to look wrinkled and old. The older you get, after about age thirty-five, the less resilient your skin becomes and the less capable it is of repair after repeated sugar attacks. So while that cookie might look good today, it might not look so good ten or twenty years from now.

But if you love sweets (like us!), don't worry; we'll show you how to enjoy unrefined sweeteners and whole-food sweeteners in moderation on page 72.

Empty Carb #3: Fruit Juice

Juice fasting, juice detox programs, and drinking cold-pressed raw juice at a juice bar might seem like incredibly healthy ideas, but the truth is that nothing about juicing is as healthy as it sounds. Okay, so maybe fresh-pressed, raw, 100 percent fruit juice (which is different in every way from the heated and pasteurized stuff found at the supermarket) is not all empty calories, but it's not optimal, either.

Juice is a much more concentrated source of calories than whole fruit, with fewer nutritional benefits. It's also very easy to overconsume juice because it's fiber-free and therefore substantially less filling than whole fruit.

Juicing advocates claim that removing the fiber from whole fruits and vegetables is a good thing, making the nutrients more readily available to the body. The problem is that removing the indigestible fiber allows your body to very quickly absorb a massive amount of fructose (the sugar found in fruits and vegetables), something that is particularly undesirable if you are overweight, have type 2 diabetes, or suffer from any inflammatory condition. Drinking pure juice is like injecting pure fructose right into your body. That might be desirable if you just ran a marathon and your body's glycogen reserves have been depleted, but for the average person who is only moderately active, ingesting a large amount of fructose is not a good idea.

Fiber is also an essential component of detoxification and is crucial for helping rid your body of toxins, so drinking fiber-free juice as a means of detoxifying your body just doesn't make a lot of sense. Fiber-rich whole fruits and vegetables also keep you feeling full longer. Fiber-free juices do an awful job of filling you up, which is another reason juicing is not a good idea if you are trying to lose weight or maintain your weight.

Fans of juice fasting and juice detox programs claim that drinking pure juice gives your digestive system a rest so that your body can heal itself. This is completely untrue and not based on any science. Start poking around in medical journals for research on juice fasting and you won't find any. What you will find are studies that link drinking juice to obesity and type 2 diabetes.

The only juice that is really healthful to drink is juice made from the entire fruit, pulp and all. When we make orange juice, we peel an orange, quarter it, then put the whole orange segments in our Vitamix and blend it; we do not squeeze the juice from the orange and throw out the pulp. In fact, most of the phytonutrients in oranges are concentrated in the inner white pulp. Why on earth would you want to throw out the fiber- and phytonutrient-rich pulp and drink just the sugary liquid? (Our watermelon juice recipe on page 288 is unstrained and made from the pulp of whole watermelon.)

Although cold-pressed, fresh, and raw juices are by far nutritionally superior to the pasteurized packaged juices that can sit in perpetuity on grocery store shelves, any way you pour it, juice is never as healthy a choice as the whole fruit or vegetable or a smoothie made from whole fruits and vegetables.

Empty Carb #4: White Rice

Just use brown rice—or better yet, black rice—instead. White rice is brown rice that has had the bran and germ removed. As a result, white rice lacks the nutrients present in brown rice: antioxidants, B vitamins, minerals, fats, fiber, and a small amount of protein. Short-grain brown rice tastes basically the same as white rice, and black rice is just delicious. We really have no idea why on earth the white stuff is ever eaten in the first place.

SWEET ENDINGS:
HOW TO HAVE A SMALL SWEET TREAT EACH DAY

Considering how much we both love sweets (Ivy in particular), we wish we could tell you that candy is dandy and that dessert should be a guiltless pleasure. But that would not be truthful (sigh). By definition, desserts are sweet and therefore contain sugar. So while we can't advise you to leave your dietary conscience at the door once the dessert tray arrives (even if one of your favorite European chocolate tortes happens to be among the display!), we can share some sensible strategies for incorporating sweet treats into your diet without causing too much harm.

The strategy we find most helpful is to sneak in nutrition wherever possible, mostly by adding fruits, nuts, seeds, and superfoods, and keep your dessert portions small. If you have totally eliminated sugar elsewhere in your diet and you otherwise eat nutrient-dense Clean Cuisine, then eating one small sweet treat each day is really not the end of the world. And besides, all of our dessert recipes in this book include healthy ingredients such as nuts and fruits. None of the dessert recipes are empty-calorie foods. (Note: Desserts are one thing we pretty much have to make ourselves if we want to eat them because there are not many truly clean ready-made desserts on the market.)

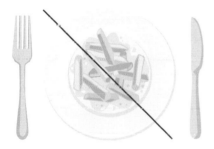

5. never eat trans fats

Trans fats are found in processed foods, though fortunately not as often as in the past. They are the absolute worst fats and should not be eaten in any quantity. The US National Academy of Science's Institute of Medicine, the organization responsible for determining the recommended dietary allowance for nutrients and their maximum safe amounts, concluded that there is absolutely no safe level of intake for trans fats. Any food whose list of ingredients includes partially hydrogenated oil or hydrogenated oil of any type, margarine, or vegetable shortening always contains at least some deadly trans fat. Also assume that all fried foods at restaurants (including fast-food places) contain trans fats.

Trans fats increase inflammation and contain no essential nutrients. They are worse than empty calories because they not only cause weight gain and leave you feeling hungry but also increase inflammation in your body and therefore make you more predisposed to modern chronic diseases, including multiple sclerosis, arthritis, Crohn's disease, and asthma. Plus, trans fats block healthy fats from being converted into helpful inflammation fighters.

Trans fats are also directly linked to heart disease. Alarmingly, these terrible fats are capable of altering your cholesterol profile toward the most dangerous ratio. They also raise your triglyceride level and impair artery dilation, a one-two punch that further increases your risk for coronary artery disease. In a 1993 study published in the prestigious medical journal *The Lancet*, almost ninety thousand healthy women were followed for eight years. Women who ate, on average, 5.7 grams of trans fat daily had 50 percent more heart attacks and deaths than women who ate only 2.4 grams per day of trans fat. Statistically, this difference is highly significant. The difference between 2.4 and 5.7 grams is less than one medium order of McDonald's french fries or one standard-sized glazed donut.

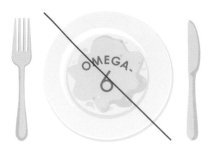

6. avoid omega-6-rich oils

Avoid omega-6-rich oils when purchasing packaged foods and preparing recipes at home. You will see that on our Clean Cuisine plan, we typically use extra-virgin olive oil, unrefined nut-based oils such as macadamia nut oil, or extra-virgin coconut oil. We do not use vegetable oils such as corn oil, soybean oil, sunflower oil, canola oil, and grapeseed oil. It probably goes without saying that we also avoid regular vegetable oil. These oils all contain a lot of omega-6 fats, which counteract much of the anti-inflammation work that omega-3 fats do. Most people are already struggling to eat enough omega-3 fat, so the last thing you want to do is to eat a bunch of omega-6 fat that interferes with the little bit of omega-3 fat you're eating.

As you already know, we are not big fans of counting or measuring our food, nor do we favor plotting out the perfect ratio of macronutrients for each and every meal. However, we do recognize the importance of the ratio of omega-6 to omega-3 in the diet. Although antiaging experts suggest the optimal ratio of omega-6 to omega-3 is 2:1, for most people, a ratio of 4:1 is a good one to shoot for. The ratio in the typical American diet is a very unhealthy and pro-inflammatory 12:1 to 25:1. That is way too much omega-6 and hardly any omega-3.

Having a good ratio of omega-6 to omega-3 in your diet is one of the most important factors for lasting good health, especially if you are already fighting an inflammatory disease. Eating an unbalanced ratio of omega-6 to omega-3 increases inflammation, which exacerbates inflammatory conditions and makes your body less sensitive to insulin, which in turn contributes to obesity, type 2 diabetes, and heart disease. Ominously,

studies have even linked diets rich in omega-6 fat to cancer. Inflammation also damages our ability to produce and balance important hormones. Very high amounts of omega-6 might interfere with your ability to produce sex hormones and mood-stabilizing hormones, and can interfere with thyroid activity.

But don't worry! It's easy to optimize your omega ratio if you follow our suggestions for getting more omega-3 on page 28 and reduce your omega-6 by eliminating all vegetable oils. That includes regular vegetable oil, corn oil, soybean oil, sunflower oil, canola oil, and grapeseed oil. (Note: This can be tricky when buying packaged foods. You really need to read the ingredients list carefully.)

The reliance on highly processed convenience foods is one reason so many people consume an unhealthy ratio of omega-6 to omega-3 fats. Processed foods like crackers, frozen foods, baked goods, cereals, and snack bars often contain highly refined omega-6 fats from vegetable oils and are almost always completely devoid of omega-3 fats. Even if you buy packaged foods labeled "organic," "all-natural," "gluten-free," and so on, you are likely consuming too many vegetable oils and therefore too much omega-6 fat, not to mention empty calories. Remember, these vegetable oils are super cheap and therefore highly profitable for food manufacturers.

The only widely available vegetable oils that naturally contain a better-than-average, healing omega ratio are canola oil, flax oil, walnut oil, and hemp oil. Flax oil, walnut oil, and hemp oil are very fragile and cannot be used for cooking. Canola oil does contain some omega-3 fat, but not nearly as much as the other three. And the mass-market processing of canola oil destroys most of the good fats anyway.

Unlike vegetable oils, extra-virgin olive oil and most nut-based oils contain a large percentage of a type of fat called monounsaturated fat. This fat does not interfere with the good effects of omega-3 fat and does not increase inflammation. In fact, monounsaturated fats have the unique ability to boost your body's utilization of omega-3s. Hence, these types of oils are the ones we use most. When appropriate, we also use extra-virgin coconut oil, which offers special nutritional benefits and is great for high-heat cooking.

More Problems with Vegetable Oils

Despite their healthy-enough-sounding names, vegetable oils—whether they are organic or "all-natural" or not—are anything but healthy. Their high amount of omega-6, which we've already discussed, is just one reason why. Here are two more.

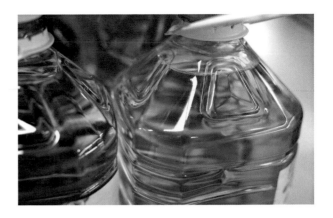

1. **Standard vegetable oils are processed improperly.** For the most part, vegetable oils are made from omega-6-rich grains and seeds like corn kernels, sunflower seeds, and soybeans. While these foods are healthy in their whole and unadulterated state, they become harmful when processed and handled improperly. Omega-6 fats, like all essential fats, are unable to withstand high temperatures without becoming damaged and rancid, yet high temperatures are exactly what these fats are exposed to when they're processed into oil: vegetable oils are refined at very high temperatures, processed, and then deodorized to make their taste "acceptable." The vast majority of vegetable oils are not processed properly because cold-pressing and expeller-pressing, both of which do not harm omega-6 fats, cost more money.

2. **Vegetable oil is an empty-calorie food.** The typical innocent-looking bottle of vegetable oil squatting on the supermarket shelf is an empty-calorie food. Since we are already eating too much omega-6 fat as it is, we do not need to eat more of it in our cooking oil. At least if you are eating a whole omega-6-rich seed, you're getting fiber and other phytonutrients. If you only eat the oil, you get nothing at all except for more empty calories … which is the last thing most of us need.

The easiest way to avoid eating too much empty-calorie omega-6 fat is to ban processed vegetable oils from your diet and to avoid eating processed foods, convenience foods, and salad dressings that contain these oils. Read the ingredients on all of the foods you buy, and when you prepare food at home, use healthier oils that contain either more omega-3 fats or more monounsaturated fats. And always, always look for unrefined oils of any type.

"HEART-HEALTHY" VEGETABLE OILS LINKED TO
HEART ATTACK AND OBESITY _____

Although vegetable oils have become popular for their ability to lower cholesterol, we can assure you eating a vegetable-oil-rich diet will do nothing to improve your heart health or slim your waistline. The Israeli paradox illustrates this point perfectly. Israeli cooking techniques relied heavily on omega-6-rich vegetable oils and margarine. At the time of the discovery of this paradox, even though the people living in Israel were noted for having one of the lowest cholesterol levels in Western countries, and even though Israelis ate much more polyunsaturated fat than saturated fat, they also had exceedingly high rates of heart attack and vascular disease. The simple takeaway is that, while both omega-3 and omega-6 have the power to reduce your cholesterol level, only by eating more omega-3s can you reduce your risk of cancer, heart disease, and obesity. Just remember that more omega-3 fats and fewer omega-6 fats equals less inflammation and better health.

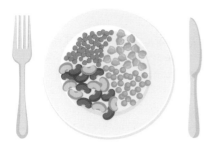

7. eat more beans and legumes

Beans and legumes are filling and contain a lot of fiber, a nutrient we all could use more of. All beans are healthful, and all types can be and should be included if you are eating Clean Cuisine. Beans have been eaten since antiquity and are a staple food in many cultures. They contain unique micronutrients not available in other plant-based foods. The fiber in beans and legumes, such as lentils and peas, protects against colon infections, intestinal cancers, and diabetes.

Beans and legumes are just about the best source of fiber and resistant starch on the planet. In fact, nearly half of the starch in beans comes from resistant starch, meaning the starch is not digested, making beans an incredibly powerful weight-loss ally (more on this on page 38). Although you will certainly be getting plenty of fiber by eating fruits and vegetables, adding just ½ cup of beans or legumes to your diet daily will boost your fiber profile by approximately 8 grams. The National Cancer Institute recommends at least 25 grams of fiber a day—we believe you should eat a lot more fiber than that, but 25 grams is a good start.

But that's not all! Beans and legumes are truly a fountain-of-youth food, bursting with antiaging antioxidants and phytonutrients, as well as a nutritional storehouse of vitamins and minerals, including folate, iron, potassium, and ultraclean plant protein. Like all plant foods, each kind of bean and legume has its own unique nutritional, antioxidant, and phytonutrient profile. So don't play favorites! All you need to know is that all beans and legumes are healthy. Many public health organizations, including the American Diabetes Association, the American Heart Association,

and the American Cancer Society, recommend legumes as a key food group for preventing disease and optimizing health. The *Dietary Guidelines for Americans*, developed by the US Department of Health and Human Services and the US Department of Agriculture, recommends 3 cups of beans or legumes per week.

That old catchy rhyme "Beans, beans, they're good for your heart … " also rings true. The resistant starch in beans can bind to cholesterol and other fats in your colon for removal. Regular bean consumption has been linked with reduced levels of homocysteine (an amino acid that, in high concentrations, has been linked to an increased risk of heart attack and stroke), lowered blood pressure, and reduced risk of heart disease. In a large study of almost ten thousand men and women in the United States, those who ate beans and legumes four or more times a week had a 22 percent lower risk of coronary heart disease and an 11 percent lower risk of cardiovascular events than those who ate them less than once a week.

Bean eaters not only have healthier hearts, they also have trimmer waistlines. A Canadian study of 1,475 men and women found that those who consumed beans regularly tended to weigh less and have a smaller waist circumference than those who did not eat them. The regular bean

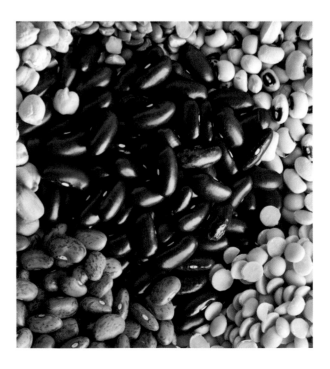

eaters were also 23 percent less likely to become overweight over time. Bean eaters weighed, on average, 7 pounds less and had slimmer waists than their bean-avoiding counterparts, yet adults consumed 199 calories more per day and teenagers consumed an incredible 335 calories more per day. It is important to note here that, as we discussed in chapter 1, all calories are not equal. Calories from fiber and resistant starch do not contribute to weight gain. Also, some foods increase cellular metabolism and encourage increased energy burn to a greater extent than others. It is very possible to eat more calories yet still lose weight—as long as you choose the right foods.

A number of factors contribute to the weight-loss benefits of beans, including their fiber and resistant starch and their high nutrient-to-calorie ratio. Beans and legumes are also one of the best foods you can eat for weight loss because they absorb water and expand in your stomach, keeping you feeling full and satisfied for hours. And since they are slowly digested, they slow the utilization of glycogen (stored glucose), thus improving insulin sensitivity and increasing your body's fat-burning potential.

Lentils, black beans, adzuki beans, cannellini beans, navy beans, white beans, red kidney beans, garbanzo beans, pinto beans, and black-eyed peas are all very healthful. Every single bean and legume has something special to offer, so try to mix it up and eat a wide variety every week.

Spilling the Beans on the "Dangers" of Phytates

Phytates, found in all edible plant foods, like whole grains, nuts, beans, and seeds, perform an essential role in plants: they are an energy source for the sprouting seed. So anyone who eats plant foods consumes phytates, but some plant foods have more than others. Unfortunately, beans and legumes have gotten a very undeserved bad rap the last few years, especially within the Paleo community, because of phytates.

The chief concern about phytates is that they could impair the absorption of certain dietary minerals, including iron, zinc, manganese, and, to a lesser extent, calcium. But science doesn't back this up. There is actually no solid evidence that eating a balanced diet that includes some animal foods along with phytate-containing beans, nuts, whole grains, seeds, and whole soy is detrimental in any way. In fact, just the opposite!

Science shows the healthiest people in the world eat unrefined phytate-containing plant foods as part of a healthy and well-balanced diet. Places with the highest concentrations of centenarians (people who live to be one hundred years old) are called Blue Zones, and Blue Zone residents are considered to be the world's healthiest people. No matter where in the world they live, residents of Blue Zones eat plant-rich diets (in particular, lots of beans), which means that they eat phytates. In fact, phytic acid has health perks! Phytates have been shown to decrease inflammation and have been found to protect against bone, prostate, ovarian, breast, liver, colorectal, blood, and skin cancers. And because phytates slow the absorption of sugars, they help lower blood sugar levels, thus indirectly helping prevent obesity and type 2 diabetes. Phytates are also known to reduce triglycerides and increase HDL ("good") cholesterol, helping prevent heart disease. Phytates have even been shown to protect against conditions such as Parkinson's and Alzheimer's. The point is, phytates are certainly not all bad. Far from it!

There might be cause for concern if your diet consisted only of foods rich in phytates. It is true that raw vegans and even some vegetarians are at slightly increased risk of nutrient deficiency, not only because they eat diets rich in phytates but also because they don't eat animal foods that contain important nutrients.

However, simply cooking your food dramatically reduces its phytic acid content. If you want to be doubly safe, you can also soak or sprout your beans, grains, nuts, seeds, and soy. Sprouting and soaking releases all the vital nutrients stored within the plant and maximizes nutrition. Also, simply making the switch from regular whole-grain bread to sprouted whole-grain bread can enhance nutrition and reduce overall phytic acid in your diet. Traditional fermentation methods (such as making tempeh or miso from soy) are also extremely effective at reducing phytic acid.

And if you are still concerned about foods that contain phytates, there is a simple solution: eat a diverse diet that is plant-rich but not vegan. That's what Clean Cuisine is. At the end of the day, you have to use common sense; when you investigate dietary patterns from epidemiological studies, you discover that the people whose diets are rich in phytate-containing whole plant foods are among the healthiest people in the world, and to us, that counts for a lot.

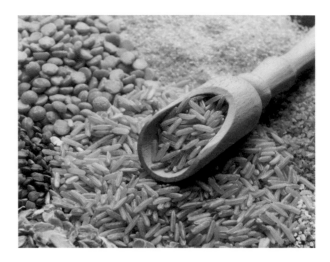

The Weight-Loss & Health-Promoting Starch

One reason beans are excellent for weight loss is that nearly half of their starch is resistant starch. Most people know that starch is found only in carbohydrate-containing foods, and most people think starch is unhealthy. But not all starch is bad. In fact, resistant starch is as close to a miracle starch as it gets.

Resistant starch actually resists digestion, meaning the calories in resistant starch are much less likely than the calories in other foods to be stored as fat. And because resistant starches are only partially digested yet even more satiating than simple starches like sugar and flour (which are completely digested), you end up with lower blood sugar levels, fewer insulin spikes, and a better ability to burn fat after resistant starch–rich meals. In other words, you feel like you've eaten more due to the taste and volume satisfaction that resistant starch brings, but your body treats these foods as if you've eaten less because only a small portion of the food is metabolized. If your body needs more energy than can be absorbed from the resistant starch, it has no choice but to burn fat!

The fact that plant-based whole carbs rich in resistant starch make up the bulk of the rural Chinese diet might help explain the findings, outlined in Colin Campbell's *The China Study*, that per kilogram of body weight, the rural Chinese eat a generous 30 percent more calories than the average American, yet they weigh 20 percent less, despite having comparable activity levels. This is a perfect example of how not all calories are created equal. It is time to retire calorie counting from the weight-loss vernacular for good.

Not only will resistant starch help you shed pounds, but it can also improve your health in many other ways. Resistant starch helps heart health by removing dietary cholesterol from the body, thus lowering blood cholesterol levels. Diets rich in resistant starch also help remove toxins from the body and can lower the risk for colon cancer. Finally, because resistant starch is a prebiotic fiber that promotes good bacteria and suppresses bad bacteria, it can help normalize bowel function and support a healthy digestive system and gut microbiome. Having more good-for-you bacteria in your digestive system will also improve your immune function and make it easier for your body to fight disease.

CLEAN CUISINE–APPROVED PLANT-BASED WHOLE CARBS RICH IN RESISTANT STARCH

Bananas	Millet
Barley*	Oatmeal
Beans	Peas
Brown rice	Polenta
Corn	Potatoes
Lentils	Yams

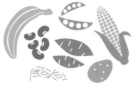

* Barley contains gluten and should be avoided by those with celiac disease or gluten sensitivity.

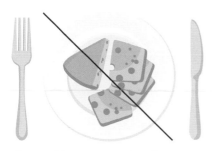

8. ditch dairy

None of the recipes in this book include any dairy products. There is, in fact, no dairy food group now, and we feel strongly that there never should have been one. Dairy foods are primarily a source of protein, and they are in no way superior to any other proteins. Since we already eat plenty of protein, why eat even more when we are not also obtaining any unique essential nutrients? There are many other foods that provide everything dairy provides but in a much more nutrient-dense and anti-inflammatory package.

Animal milk is not necessary in any way for either human adults or children and is basically an added-calorie food containing protein, pro inflammatory animal-based saturated fat, and sugar, all of which most of us already get plenty of. We do not need to drink milk for calcium, as calcium is more prevalent per calorie—and more bioavailable—in many plant foods. The few other nutrients in milk are added artificially and can be obtained without the empty calories by taking supplements or, ideally, by eating other whole foods.

Admittedly, we do eat a bit of cheese here and there, but this is a true treat. We don't eat cheese for any reason other than we love the taste—we aren't fooled into thinking cheese is a health food! Having said that, properly prepared fermented dairy products without added sugar or artificial ingredients, such as plain, unsweetened goat's milk yogurt or kefir, can be enjoyed in moderation, as they provide unique health benefits. We'll talk more about fermented foods on page 42.

Dairy Q & A

Dairy consumption is often controversial, and there are a lot of misunderstandings and confusion about its health effects. Let's look at some of the most common questions about dairy.

1. **Is the protein in milk good for you?** Dairy milk contains two proteins, casein and whey, and neither one do a body good. Whey increases insulin levels, which can hinder the ability to control blood sugar and reduce inflammation. Casein promotes the release of a hormone called insulin-like growth factor 1 (IGF-1), which helps cells reproduce and regenerate—but in excess, it can fuel the growth of cancer. Casein has also been shown to trigger an immune response in some people, which of course increases inflammation. Skim milk in particular has more casein and whey than full-fat milk. However, yogurt's fermentation process reduces IGF-1 levels, so if you had to choose between milk and plain, unsweetened yogurt, the yogurt would definitely be your best bet, and not just because it has probiotics.

2. **Does drinking milk prevent osteoporosis?** No. While dairy foods have some components that promote calcium retention, such as magnesium, vitamin D, and potassium, they also have other components, primarily animal protein, that promote calcium excretion through the urine. Studies show that people who live in parts of the world where cow's milk is not a dietary staple are less likely to develop osteoporosis than people who live in places where it is, such as the United States. Countries that have the highest consumption of dairy also have the highest incidence of hip fractures, and a major finding from the Nurses' Health Study, which followed 121,701 women ages thirty to fifty-five, was that milk consumption does not protect against hip or forearm fractures. Epidemiological studies actually link osteoporosis not to low calcium intake but to a diet high in animal protein, which causes excess calcium loss.

3. **Are there any good nondairy sources of calcium?** Yes! Dark leafy greens are one of the most outstanding sources of calcium because they result in far greater net calcium retention than you'd get from dairy, since the animal protein in dairy promotes calcium excretion. Plus, they come jam-packed with all sorts of nutritional perks in the form of fiber, phytonutrients, antioxidants, and vitamins, all for a fraction of the calories found in dairy! A cup of milk contains 291 milligrams of calcium, but did you know that a cup of cooked collards has 358 milligrams of calcium? Or that a cup of cooked spinach has 244 milligrams of calcium? A cup of cooked kale has 94 milligrams, a cup of cooked mustard greens has 150 milligrams, and a cup of cooked Swiss chard has 102 milligrams. The point is, plant foods are incredibly nutrient-dense and provide plenty of calcium.

4. **Does milk naturally contain vitamin D?** No, vitamin D is added to milk—it's not naturally occurring, like the vitamin D found in fatty fish, egg yolks, or mushrooms exposed to ultraviolet light, and the amount added to milk is not nearly as much as your body can manufacture from sunlight.

5. **Is it true that 75 to 80 percent of the world's adults are lactose intolerant?** Yes. Lactose is a sugar found in milk. Babies have an enzyme called lactase that breaks lactose apart for digestion, but after the age of weaning, the vast majority of people in the world lose that enzyme and are therefore lactose intolerant.

6. **Is it true that dairy is the most common food allergy?** Yes! In fact, cow's milk protein, not nuts, is the leading food allergen in children. Cow's milk consumption has been linked to food allergies in general, too.

7. **Has milk consumption been linked to autoimmune diseases and cancer?** Yes. The consumption of animal foods, especially cow's milk, is associated with increased risk of autoimmune disease. The link between milk consumption and type 1 diabetes is well documented in prestigious medical journals such as the *New England Journal of Medicine*.

Milk consumption is also linked with various cancers, including prostate cancer. Nine separate studies have linked prostate cancer with high consumption of milk, including a 2010 study in the journal *Prostate* showing more than a doubling of risk. Cow's milk consumption has also been linked to multiple sclerosis.

8. **Is it true that one glass of milk can contain 180 million white blood cells and still be considered safe to drink?** This is downright gross, but true. White blood cells—the cells that make up pus—are found naturally in milk because they are important for the immune-system development of the calves that are supposed to drink the milk. Humans aren't really meant to drink cow's milk, and the white blood cells don't do anything to support human health or the human immune system.

9. **Is it true that many nonorganic dairy cows are given a hormone called bovine somatotropin (BST), also known as rBGH, in order to increase milk production?** Yes, and this hormone often leads to udder infections (mastitis). The sick cows are then given antibiotics, which make it even more difficult to treat infections in the future, both in livestock and in humans.

10. **Is it true that the vast majority of dairy cows are fed a diet of grain and are not free to graze on pasture the way nature intended?** Yes, and the health of the cow and the nutrients in her milk are directly affected by the foods she eats. Cows evolved to eat grass, not grain, and when they don't eat the foods nature intended, they produce poor-quality milk that does not have the same nutrient profile as milk from grass-fed cows.

So while there are beneficial nutrients in milk, including calcium, vitamin D, magnesium, vitamin A, vitamin B_{12}, potassium, and protein, milk is not exactly the cleanest source of these nutrients, and you definitely don't need to drink milk to get them! There are far better sources for all of these nutrients than dairy, particularly dark leafy greens. Dairy foods are not a nutritional requirement.

GOT GREENS?

If you are concerned about preventing osteoporosis, maintaining a healthy weight, and boosting your intake of bone-building nutrients, one of the most important things you should do is swap milk for greens. Instead of making an effort to consume three servings of dairy a day, try getting one or two large servings of dark leafy greens. You will do your body—and your bones—a big favor!

Calcium alone is not enough for strong bones—you also need magnesium and vitamin K to help your body absorb and make use of the calcium you consume. Dark leafy greens such as spinach, collards, turnip greens, and parsley are a fabulous source of these nutrients (as well as calcium!). The magnesium in dark leafy greens helps your body absorb and retain calcium and works like calcium's teammate to build and strengthen bones and prevent osteoporosis. Since your body is not good at storing magnesium, it is vital to get enough of it in your diet on a daily basis. The vitamin K in dark leafy greens helps activate certain proteins that promote bone health. Epidemiological studies and clinical trials consistently indicate that vitamin K has a positive effect on bone mineral density and decreases fracture risk. In fact, in the Nurses' Health Study, women who got more than 109 micrograms of vitamin K a day were 30 percent less likely to break a hip than women who got less than that amount.

One bone-building nutrient that dark leafy greens do not contain, however, is vitamin D. (As mentioned earlier, dairy products don't naturally contain vitamin D, either; they are artificially enriched with vitamin D.) To get a natural vitamin D fix, eat fatty fish like salmon and egg yolks from pastured hens, and make it a point to get a bit of sun exposure.

Instead of asking "Got Milk?" ask "Got Greens?" Greens are the true superfood; they just don't have a multibillion-dollar industry like the Dairy Council behind them for marketing!

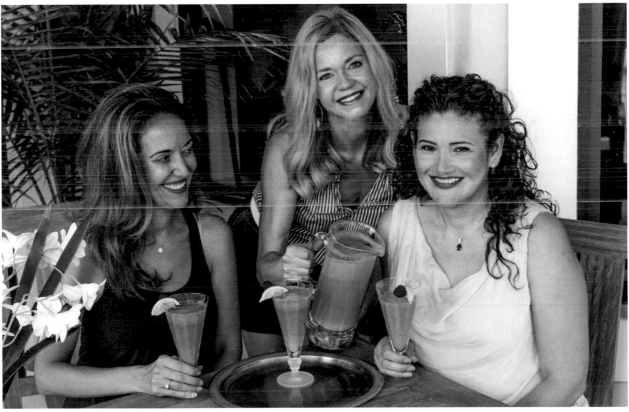

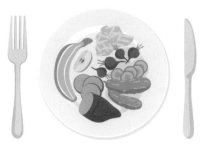

9. increase your intake of prebiotic and fermented probiotic foods

When we started researching clean eating back in 1998, we didn't come across a lot of information regarding the importance of gut health. But as the years have gone by, we've come to realize the bacteria in our gut play an essential role in fostering a strong immune system, removing toxins from our systems, and optimizing our overall health. Our gut microbiome even determines how well we absorb the nutrients from our food! Other beneficial actions of certain strains of gut bacteria include:

- boosting energy production and supporting a healthy metabolism
- assisting with the absorption of vitamins and minerals
- improving digestion
- enhancing cognitive function
- reducing stress and promoting a positive mood
- supporting a normal inflammatory balance

Things like poor diet, stress, medication, illness, aging, and even travel can throw our microbiome totally out of balance, but eating a diet containing a wide variety of naturally fermented probiotic- and prebiotic-rich foods can help—in fact, it's crucial for having a healthy and strong gut microbiome. The "wide variety" part of that statement is important, because when it comes to optimizing gut health, microbial diversity is critical.

There are many nutrient-rich prebiotic- and probiotic-rich foods to choose from. With the exception of raw cheese and yogurt, they are all plant based.

PREBIOTIC FOODS

Apples
Avocados
Bananas
Barley
Beans
Cabbage
Cacao
Chickpeas
Flax seeds
Jicama
Lentils
Oats

Onions (both cooked and raw)
Potato skins
Raw asparagus
Raw dandelion greens
Raw garlic
Raw leeks
Seaweed
Soybeans
Sweet potatoes
Unrefined apple cider vinegar
Wheat germ
Whole-grain and sprouted whole-grain breads

PROBIOTIC FOODS

Coconut kefir
Cured olives
Fermented vegetables (such as sauerkraut and kimchi)
Kefir (including plant-based kefir)
Kombucha
Kvass
Miso

Namu shoyu (an unpasteurized soy sauce)
Natto
Organic natural wines (see page 44)
Raw cheese
Tempeh (fermented soy)
Traditional pickles (as well as pickled carrots and beets)
Yogurt (including plant-based yogurt)

Note: Any food that is naturally fermented contains probiotics.

Many health-conscious people these days know about the importance of probiotics, but prebiotics are every bit as important for gut and whole-body health. Probiotics contain live beneficial bacteria that flourish in your bowels, and prebiotics contain fibers that support their growth. Prebiotics are high-fiber, nondigestible carbohydrates, but while your body can't naturally digest them, they're the preferred food of the bacteria in your gut.

You can absolutely get your probiotics from a high-quality supplement (we take a broad-spectrum probiotic supplement daily), but we prefer to get them from naturally fermented foods. Fermentation creates many of the same strains of good bacteria naturally found in your gut, making live-culture fermented foods one of the best sources of probiotics. Plus, we don't just eat them for their health benefits; we love how they taste! Keep in

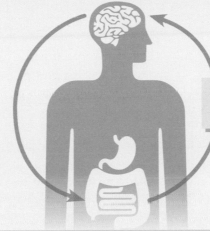

HEALTHY GUT = HEALTHY MIND

HEALTHY GUT
A healthy diet affects how you feel not only physically but also mentally.

A good diet can lead to...
A healthy gut starts with the right nutrients and a healthy balance of probiotics, prebiotics, and phytobiotics in your diet. Good nutrition can increase both your physical and mental wellness.

HEALTHY MIND
A healthy gut microbiome provides optimal mental wellness benefits.

Science shows...
the gut affects the brain and the brain affects the gut

Probiotics, Prebiotics, Phytobiotics
oh my!

PROBIOTICS	PREBIOTICS	PHYTOBIOTICS
Probiotics are good bacteria that live in the gut. Probiotic foods contain live good bacteria that support a range of benefits, from mental wellness to digestion aid.	Prebiotic foods contain fibers and carbohydrates that can be fermented and digested by gut bacteria and encourage growth of beneficial bacteria.	Phytobiotic foods are rich in flavonoids, which protect good bacteria and establish a hospitable environment for the growth of good bacteria.
EXAMPLES: yogurt, kefir, kimchi, kombucha, sauerkraut, miso, tempeh, probiotic supplements	EXAMPLES: asparagus, bananas, green leafy vegetables, garlic, leeks, onions, chicory, artichokes, ginger, prebiotic supplements	EXAMPLES: apples, grapes, dark chocolate, berries

Think probiotics don't work? Maybe you don't have the right strain...
There are two main things to consider when choosing a probiotic supplement:

The Strength: Your body needs a certain strength of probiotics to be effective. Consuming too many or too few CFUs (colony-forming units) can cause problems. Ten billion CFUs is right in the sweet spot of what science has shown to be effective.

The Strains: Probiotic benefits are very strain-dependent, just like vitamins. If you need vitamin A, you're not going to take vitamin E and expect the same results. Similarly, a probiotic strain that supports the immune system may not support mood at all. A strain that benefits digestion may do nothing to help inflammation. You need the right strain to get your desired benefit.

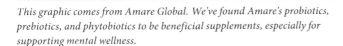

This graphic comes from Amare Global. We've found Amare's probiotics, prebiotics, and phytobiotics to be beneficial supplements, especially for supporting mental wellness.

mind, it is always best to get your probiotics from food rather than supplements. If you rely only on supplements, then you miss out on the other health benefits offered by the food itself. For example, the cabbage in sauerkraut is an excellent source of vitamins C and K and a great source of fiber and various B vitamins. Different strains of probiotics offer different health benefits, which is why it is very important to obtain a broad spectrum of probiotic strains from a wide variety of foods.

Prebiotic- and probiotic-rich foods also help prevent numerous digestive diseases, such as colitis, diverticulitis, and infectious diarrhea. They are especially important if you are taking antibiotics or have recently been treated with antibiotics. As a surgeon, Andy recommends that all his patients who are taking antibiotics consume a probiotic- and prebiotic-rich diet along with a broad-spectrum, high-quality probiotic and prebiotic supplement.

CHEERS! ORGANIC NATURAL WINES CONTAIN PROBIOTICS & PREBIOTICS

Wine is alive. Like all fermented beverages, it plays host to beneficial bacteria while it ferments. It's full of probiotics and prebiotics that not only help optimize gut health but can also improve your overall health. For example, the anthocyanins in red wine are prebiotics that support a balanced gut microbiome by helping the good bacteria take over the bad bacteria. And one bacterium found in wine, *Pediococcus pentosaceus,* attaches to your intestinal wall and protects it from pathogens like *E. coli.* Wine also contains lactic acid bacteria that have similar health benefits as fermented foods, like kimchi and miso.

However, commercial processing techniques like extreme filtration can damage or remove many of the good compounds in wine. Manufacturers often replace them with artificial coloring and lab-created yeast strains. That's why we recommend natural wine. There are two criteria for a wine to be considered "natural": First, the grapes must be sustainably farmed, which usually means they are organic and/or biodynamic. Second, there should be nothing added or taken away from the wine—so the beneficial probiotics and prebiotics remain. Some wines can be given a low dose of sulfur dioxide and still be considered natural enough to be sold in natural wine establishments, but be aware that sulfites are used to kill bacteria, so the lower the sulfites, the more "alive" a wine remains. You can see the difference under a microscope—low-sulfite wine is vibrant with a diverse spectrum of wild bacteria and yeast. And that's what you want for the best gut and health benefits.

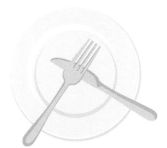

10. don't eat when you aren't hungry

Ivy here. For me, fasting does not sound appealing, but I recently realized that twelve-hour intermittent fasting—basically, not consuming food for a twelve-hour period—has been part of my lifestyle for years now, entirely unintentionally. And the health benefits are definitely worth taking note of.

Although the idea of eating five or six small meals throughout the day has been popular among dieters, it's never made sense to me to eat when I'm not hungry, and science is now starting to agree that keeping your stomach filled with food all day long might not be the healthiest thing to do. Fasting to improve health dates back thousands of years; Hippocrates and Plato were among its earliest proponents. The research supporting the health benefits of fasting are impressive. Here are just a few reasons why you might want to consider fasting:

 Improved brain health. Fasting has been shown to support the health of mitochondria—the famous "powerhouses of the cell" that generate energy—and anything that supports mitochondrial health also improves brain health. There is even some evidence that intermittent fasting may reverse progressive brain disorders.

 Enhanced detoxification. The body uses a great deal of energy on detoxification, but it also uses a great deal of energy to digest food. When your body is not busy digesting food, it can focus its energy on eliminating toxins and repairing cells.

 Reduced inflammation. Fasting triggers a set of cellular changes that produce a dramatic increase in antioxidants and decrease inflammation.

 Weight loss / weight management. In general, it takes between six and eight hours for the body to burn through its supply of glycogen, the glucose stored in the liver and muscles. Only when glycogen is depleted will the body turn to fat cells for energy, so eating throughout the day makes it much harder for the body to burn fat. Fasting forces your body to tap into stored fat reserves.

There are many different ways to fast. You can skip dinner. Avoid food for a twenty-four-hour period once a week. Consume nothing but water for an extended period of time. But none of these fasting options sound all that desirable to me.

Twelve-hour intermittent fasting is a different story. In my opinion, it's the easiest, least painful, and most natural way to fast. In fact, if you are following a nutrient-dense, clean diet, it should actually be easy. As mentioned, I have been doing it more or less by accident for years. That's partly because for more than half the duration of the fast I am asleep!

The easiest way to fast is to leave at least twelve hours between your evening meal and your morning meal. In other words, if you typically eat dinner at 8 p.m., wait until at least 8 a.m. before eating again. The great thing about this is that if you sleep for eight hours, that leaves just four hours when you're awake and fasting.

We have always believed it's not a good idea to eat if you are not hungry. Andy is never hungry for breakfast, so he skips it altogether. I find I typically can go about fourteen hours between dinner and breakfast. Because of Andy's demanding work schedule, we typically don't eat dinner until around 8 p.m., and I find I am not hungry for breakfast until at least 10:30 a.m.—sometimes as late as 11!

I should point out, though, that if you are new to clean eating, you may find it difficult to go for long periods between meals. Before I changed my diet, I vividly remember always needing an after-dinner snack and still waking up in the morning ravenous. I think you need to be eating a nutrient-dense diet and have stable blood sugar before you can go for long stretches without eating and still feel comfortable.

And speaking of feeling comfortable: while it's not a good idea to eat when you are not hungry, it's also not a good idea to let yourself be miserable and hungry for hours on end. Having said that, if you are eating a nutrient-dense diet and a solid and healthy dinner, you should find it rather easy to go twelve hours without eating. You could potentially be doing your body a big favor, too!

CHAPTER 3

the diet rx

Andy here. As a doctor, I've seen firsthand that mainstream medicine is excellent at saving and improving lives: we're good at treating formerly deadly infections, replacing joints and restoring mobility, and handling mass trauma situations. But when it comes to treating systemic inflammatory conditions and autoimmune diseases, we often fall short. In some cases, the side effects of the prescription medications used to treat inflammatory conditions and autoimmune diseases can be as bad as—or worse than—the disease itself.

The immune-modifying medications used to treat multiple sclerosis can have some serious side effects, and when Ivy was diagnosed with MS at twenty-two years old, she was nervous about starting on the prescription-medication route. She was especially concerned about the potential effects of disease-modifying medications on a future pregnancy. For these reasons and others, Ivy felt it was appropriate to at least try a natural approach to manage her disease first.

This was back in 1998, when the idea of food as medicine was not exactly mainstream. (It is still a far cry from mainstream, but today the idea is much more accepted than it was twenty years ago!) Ivy's neurologist at the University of Miami introduced her to the Swank MS Diet for multiple sclerosis, and both of us read up on it extensively, spending time at the medical library (the internet was not the best place for research in 1998) and reading the medical literature on which this diet is based in order to understand it better. Swank's *The Multiple Sclerosis Diet Book* is decades old, but its general advice still holds true today. Animal-based saturated fat and trans fats should be avoided and unrefined plant-based oils (such as extra-virgin olive oil) used instead. Fish is favored over the meat of land animals, based on Dr. Swank's observation that Norwegians who lived in the interior of the country and ate mostly beef and dairy foods had a seven-times-higher rate of multiple sclerosis than genetically identical Norwegians who lived on the coast and ate mostly fish. Finally, added sugars should be avoided, as excess sugar is converted to saturated fats in our body for storage. (This body fat is now known to be a constant source of inflammation and part of the reason chronic diseases are more common in overweight persons.)

Dr. Swank's book motivated Ivy to change her diet, and her health rapidly improved. She was able to avoid taking immune-modifying medicines completely and eventually stopped taking medications for her symptoms as the symptoms went away. To this day, our family has enjoyed complete freedom from inflammatory conditions and autoimmune diseases such as multiple sclerosis. In studying nutrition as it relates to multiple sclerosis, we learned why nutrition works, and we learned how nutrition can help in the fight against many chronic diseases, some of which seem unrelated at first.

the first step to health: reducing inflammation

The common thread between multiple sclerosis and many other seemingly unrelated conditions (such as coronary artery disease, asthma, arthritis, obesity, type 2 diabetes, and vascular dementia) is inflammation. If you can reduce systemic inflammation, you can potentially slow the progression or greatly reduce the symptoms of these conditions.

The symptoms of multiple sclerosis occur because your own body is attacking the sheath that covers the nerve fibers. This process is called autoimmunity because your immune system is being tricked into attacking part of your body. Researchers speculate that a virus might be the root cause, but people with the condition are mostly concerned with minimizing symptoms, not finding the exact source of the problem. This is where anti-inflammation diets come into play.

If your body is inflamed, many processes work in overdrive, including immune processes. If the foods you eat increase inflammation, then the processes that make autoimmune diseases symptomatic will be more active. The reverse occurs if you choose foods that decrease inflammation—autoimmune symptoms abate. Following all of the advice in this book will decrease inflammation in your body. Clean Cuisine is a more modern and more effective version of the Swank MS Diet that synthesizes decades of additional research to help you enjoy a more vibrant, healthful life while still enjoying a wide variety of delicious foods.

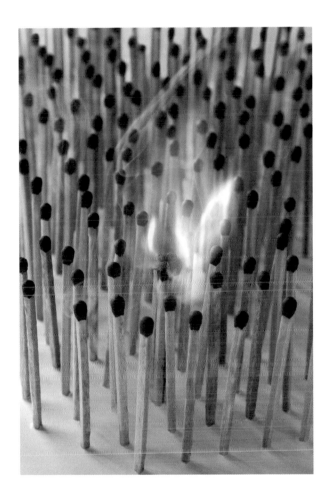

Other autoimmune conditions made worse by inflammation include rheumatoid arthritis, asthma, seasonal allergies, Crohn's disease, ulcerative colitis, lupus, and fibromyalgia. These are all conditions in which the body inappropriately attacks its own tissue. Basically, any disease for which your doctor might prescribe a steroid will get better if you follow the Clean Cuisine nutrition plan.

healing specific diseases

Inflammatory bowel diseases such as Crohn's disease and ulcerative colitis respond well to an anti-inflammation diet, with occasional modifications when there are active intestinal issues, such as reducing intake of normally healthful fats (such as olive oil) and substituting them with easily digested fats (such as coconut oil). For those suffering from antibiotic-related diarrhea and irritable bowel syndrome, we emphasize an increased intake of probiotics and prebiotic foods. Once the intestine is healthy enough for all of the clean foods we recommend, an abundance of new health benefits can be enjoyed, even by those who have been told that they will never be able to eat normally again.

Another huge group of diseases caused by inflammation are the diseases caused by atherosclerosis (hardening of the arteries). Inflammation is carried by the bloodstream throughout the body, so it makes sense that the blood vessels bear the brunt of the damage. Hard arteries dramatically increase the risk of heart attack, stroke, and dementia or senility. A large portion of senile dementia is in reality vascular dementia caused by years of poor blood flow to the brain, not genetic disease such as Alzheimer's. The Clean Cuisine diet can dramatically reduce your risk of artery-based chronic disease and, when followed regularly, is more effective than aspirin, cholesterol medication, and blood thinners, and it has no side effects.

Diet also has a substantial effect on preventing osteoporosis and osteoarthritis. Even though osteoarthritis is sometimes caused by injury and factors unrelated to diet, some of its symptoms are indeed inflammation-mediated. Joint pain that is helped by medicines like Advil or Aleve will respond to an anti-inflammatory diet as well. Pay special attention to eating substantial amounts of omega-3 fat and avoiding processed vegetable oils and saturated fats from animal foods (see pages 26 and 34 for more on these). Osteoporosis can be prevented by eating more omega-3 fat and more fruits and vegetables. Calcium helps, but remember that the calcium in dark leafy vegetables is better absorbed than the calcium in dairy, and dark leafy vegetables contain far more nutrients per calorie. (We talk more about osteoporosis on page 39.)

There are also conditions that are not directly related to inflammation that are improved or prevented by following the Clean Cuisine way of eating. In chapter 1, we defined Clean Cuisine as a plant-rich diet based on a wide variety of anti-inflammatory whole foods in their most natural and nutrient-rich state. Although they are not directly related to inflammation, type 2 diabetes and obesity can both be beaten by following this way of eating. If you are filling up on nutrient-dense foods like fruits and vegetables, you will have far fewer cravings for empty calories. If you avoid rapidly absorbed processed sugars and starches, your body will naturally produce less insulin, preventing you from ever becoming insulin resistant and prediabetic in the first place. If you already have type 2 diabetes, you cannot cure it by making more insulin or by injecting artificial insulin; you must attack it at its root by losing weight and eating foods that naturally keep sugar levels in your blood low and therefore eliminate the need for insulin to be secreted in high levels to begin with.

Diabetes and obesity are terrible conditions because they feed off of each other and end up causing inflammation in your body. Here is how: the high blood sugar levels caused by eating the wrong foods force your body to make more insulin; this insulin forces your body to store the excess blood sugar as saturated fat; the saturated fat itself releases the mediators of inflammation into your bloodstream; and these mediators then exacerbate all the problems we just talked about, including heart artery disease and autoimmune conditions. No medicine can break this cycle; only a long-term commitment to healthy eating will ultimately be effective. It is also very important that people with an inflammatory condition (such as multiple sclerosis or fibromyalgia) keep their body fat percentage low because excess body fat indirectly increases whole-body inflammation.

Clean Cuisine's increased attention to fruits, vegetables, nuts, and legumes offers other benefits as well. Cancer is less prevalent among persons who eat this way, partly due to decreased inflammation and partly due to the anticancer phytochemicals, fiber, and micronutrients found only in plant-based foods. Cancer is also less prevalent when our bodies are not carrying excess saturated fat, which, as we just explained, increases inflammation on a constant basis.

High blood pressure is less common in persons who eat more fruits and vegetables and less processed food. Those of you who have read about the DASH diet, which has been proven to reduce blood pressure and improve health, will recognize the overlap between DASH and Clean Cuisine. Our diet also decreases cholesterol levels, in particular "bad" LDL cholesterol. If it is followed regularly, our way of eating is as powerful as the popular statin drugs, with no risk of side effects. Studies in medical journals such as the *Journal of the American Medical Association* have shown just how powerful a few dietary changes can be for heart health.

of popular diets that exist today (such as Paleo, vegan, low-carb, and macrobiotic). Having looked at the medical research on nutrition and disease, it is our firm belief that you do not need to go to extremes to enjoy optimal health and maintain a healthy body weight. And you definitely don't have to give up great-tasting foods! The nutrition and diet world can be a very confusing space to navigate these days, but we hope we have given you hope that you can eat a wide variety of great-tasting food while looking and feeling your best.

Finally, keep in mind that no diet will work if you are not able to stick to it for life—and the more restrictive your diet is, the higher the risk of noncompliance. The idea of eating a plant-rich diet based on a wide variety of anti-inflammatory whole foods in their most natural and nutrient-rich state might initially be a little more difficult to grasp than the idea of eliminating one thing (such as grains, fat, or carbs), but once you get the concept, eating Clean Cuisine is much more doable in the real world. The more doable something is, the more likely you are to stick to it. And if you stick to it, you will see (and feel!) results.

eating well for life

It would be rare to find a person over the age of fifty who does not have one of the health concerns discussed above; thus, it would be rare to find a person who would not benefit from improved nutrition. Food is part of our daily life and has greater effect on our long-term health and length of life than any other factor, with the exception of smoking. But food and nutrition do not need to be as complicated as some people have made them.

When we started our research into nutrition two decades ago, people thought the idea of eliminating processed foods was extreme. Now that so many people have embraced the idea that food can in fact be medicine, diet recommendations that actually *are* extreme have become the norm. People aren't just eliminating processed foods, refined sugars, and refined oils; they are slashing carrots and bananas from their diets, too! We do not endorse fad diets, and we don't believe in extremism. Clean Cuisine is far less restrictive than the vast majority

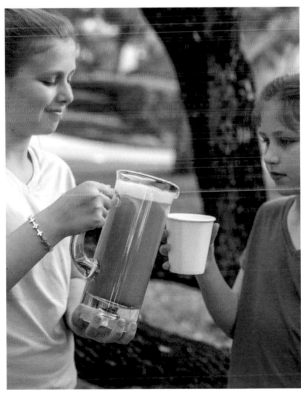

examining the autoimmune protocol diet

Clean Cuisine is designed to be the least restrictive healthful diet possible. We like to limit rules and maximize flavor. We are very skeptical of diet protocols that eliminate natural, unprocessed foods. Modern chronic and autoimmune diseases have much more to do with eating processed and empty-calorie foods that did not exist in the past and much less to do with eating the wrong natural foods. Eliminating "high-sugar" natural foods like carrots and bananas from your diet is not the best place to focus your energy.

The autoimmune protocol is a way of eating that is intended to reduce inflammation and heal those suffering from autoimmune diseases. It's a very restrictive diet that eliminates nuts, seeds, grains, beans and legumes, dairy, eggs, nightshades (tomatoes, potatoes, peppers, and more), and other foods. We know a lot of people suffering from autoimmune diseases are trying it, so we wanted to weigh in here and compare it against what we recommend in this book.

But first, it is important to understand a few concepts before analyzing a dietary protocol. Very few specific diets have been proven to be better than others. Probably the best diet study ever done showed very strong evidence that the Mediterranean diet is better for good health than the traditional low-fat diet previously recommended by the American Heart Association, but studies of this quality are rare. In developing Clean Cuisine, we considered if there might be any way to improve upon the Mediterranean diet or to identify which parts of it are most beneficial. Among our many conclusions was that using extra-virgin olive oil for dressings and for cooking is indeed very healthful and likely a key component of the Mediterranean diet's success. We also concluded the Mediterranean diet might be even better with less bread and pasta, but certainly eating whole-grain pasta is better than eating a bag of chips. In other words, no diet is perfect, and no diet has been proven perfect. But with over twenty years of experience in clean eating, we believe Clean Cuisine is very close to optimal and will help prevent chronic diseases and reduce the symptoms of autoimmune diseases in the vast majority of people.

Unlike the Mediterranean diet, the autoimmune protocol is not backed by any adequately strong studies proving it is better than any other diet. That does not mean it is a bad diet, but it does mean we need to analyze it using our experience and our understanding of nutrition as it relates to disease, and we will not have the benefit of proven research. Let's give it a try.

How the Autoimmune Protocol Affects Inflammation

First, we need to look at the different types of inflammation. The most common type of inflammation, and the type that kills the most people and shortens lives the most, is inflammation of the blood vessels. This causes heart attacks, strokes, dementia, complications of diabetes that result in wounds and limb loss, kidney disease, high blood pressure, and many other conditions. The severity of these conditions depends significantly on the types of fats you eat (animal-based saturated fat is bad and omega-3 fat is good, for example) and on how much processed carbohydrates you eat (these foods are stored in your body as inflammatory saturated fat if you eat them in excess). The autoimmune protocol diet does not really address this type of inflammation because it eliminates very beneficial foods like nuts and seeds and encourages you, to some extent, to eat foods that can make this type of inflammation worse, such as red meat. Remember, this is the most common type of inflammation, and it is the type of inflammation we are almost all going to have to deal with as we get older. This type of inflammation needs to be priority one.

Another way we experience the ill effects of inflammation is through suffering the symptoms of autoimmune disease. In people predisposed to these conditions, increased whole-body inflammation levels trigger the body to attack itself, causing symptoms of an autoimmune disease. Ivy knows this inflammation well since she has multiple sclerosis. As we've talked about already, other autoimmune conditions include rheumatoid arthritis, lupus, asthma, fibromyalgia, and Crohn's disease. Some autoimmune conditions are directly related to intestinal health and some are not, but they are all improved by eating a plant-rich diet of anti-inflammatory whole foods, primarily because fat and carbohydrate intakes are modified in a highly beneficial way to decrease inflammation. It is possible that a gut-friendly program such as the autoimmune protocol diet could also benefit specifically intestinal autoimmune conditions, but this is not proven. Eating more meat, no nuts, and less variety of fruits and vegetables may help some people with some conditions involving the intestine (again, there's no proof), but again, for the deadliest, most problematic modern chronic diseases, including heart attacks, strokes, and vascular senility, this diet is going to be counterproductive.

Other types of inflammation have to do with pain responses and your ability to fight cancer. Fruits and vegetables collectively have been proven to decrease cancer risk, and many plant-based spices and substances have been shown to help with the type of inflammation that causes pain—turmeric and the capsaicin in peppers come to mind. There is no evidence that eating one type of fruit or vegetable is always better for all conditions. And unless you have a food allergy (more on this in a bit), there is no evidence that avoiding some types of fruits or vegetables is always better for all conditions. Each and every fruit and vegetable has its own unique nutrient, antioxidant, and phytonutrient profiles; it is far better to include as much variety as possible. In fact, it is believed that intolerances to foods can actually be brought about by eating the same foods over and over—and the more foods you eliminate from your diet, the more likely you are to be eating the same foods day after day.

Some of the recommendations in the autoimmune protocol diet just don't make sense to us. For example, we cannot find any credible research showing a benefit from avoiding nightshade vegetables, which include tomatoes,

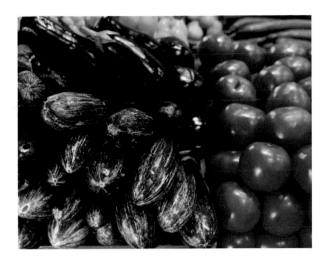

potatoes, peppers, and eggplants—whereas there is extensive research showing a wide variety of overlapping health benefits from eating these foods and the micronutrients and phytonutrients found within them. Take tomatoes, for example. If you search PubMed, a database of millions of articles from medical and science journals published internationally, you can find more than one hundred studies over the last twenty-five years discussing the incredible benefits of lycopene, a phytonutrient found in tomatoes. However, on the autoimmune protocol diet, tomatoes are eliminated. Unless you have an allergy or a legitimate sensitivity to one or more nightshades, we cannot find a logical reason for excluding them from your diet. All fruits and all vegetables are healthful, anti-inflammatory, and good for us, and we should consciously make an effort to eat more of them. And the more variety, the better!

Food Sensitivities

Now we get to another concept that comes up in the autoimmune protocol diet. This has to do with sensitivity, allergy, and tolerance. Among other foods, dairy, nuts, and grains (wheat in particular) are eliminated in the autoimmune protocol diet, presumably because many people have gut-related issues with these foods. Let's look at these one by one.

As you'll recall from the previous chapter, we discourage consuming dairy products. We feel that dairy products do not offer any necessary nutrition that you cannot get from more nutrient-rich foods and are basically empty calories. It is also true many people do not tolerate dairy foods very well. Typically, but not always, this is an intolerance and not an allergy; that is why it's called a "lactose intolerance" and not a "lactose allergy."

Intolerance basically means that you get annoying side effects like bloating and diarrhea from eating these foods, but you do not release antibodies against them—there is no systemic allergic response. Since the vast majority of people are not truly allergic to dairy, it is highly unlikely that avoiding it will improve your autoimmune disease symptoms. On the other hand, filling up on dairy foods that contain minimal nutrition per calorie will, in the long run, hurt your health. Dairy is also a significant source of pro-inflammatory animal-based saturated fat, which, as we have already discussed, is not healthy. Bottom line, dairy is not encouraged on either Clean Cuisine or the autoimmune protocol diet.

Nuts and legumes are very healthy and have been eaten by humans and primates since the dawn of time. They are potent anti-inflammatory foods. Studies show they help with weight control and protect against heart disease. The main problem with nuts and legumes is that some people have true allergies to them. A peanut allergy can be severe, even fatal, and introducing peanuts into a child's diet should be done cautiously and with the guidance of your pediatrician. (Interestingly, mothers who breastfeed and also eat peanuts can reduce their child's likelihood of developing a peanut allergy.)

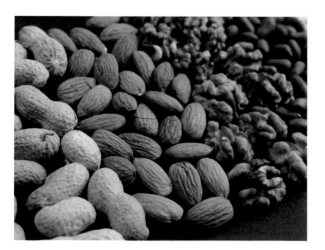

Tree nut allergies, on the other hand, are rarely life-threatening. We recommend having food allergy testing for tree nuts only if you believe you have had an allergic reaction. Be aware, however, that false positives are common, and it is worth noting that some people grow out of allergies over time. We recommend going to a physician who's an allergy specialist for testing so that you'll have professional clinical expertise guiding the interpretation of the results; food allergy test kits sold at drugstores and online are not reliable and are likely to result in false positives. For the vast majority of people, nuts, legumes, and seeds are healthful and highly beneficial.

Finally, we get to the most controversial issue of all: grains and gluten. Whole grains in general are healthful and are part of Clean Cuisine. We recommend eating a variety of grains, not just wheat, for the same reason we recommend eating a variety of fruits and vegetables: different kinds of grains offer different nutrients.

About 94 percent of people can eat modest amounts of wheat with no negative effects on their health. Perhaps 1 percent of people have celiac disease, an autoimmune disease that damages the small intestine and requires the complete elimination of gluten. Celiac disease can be suggested by a blood test and proven by a small-bowel biopsy. The only cure for celiac is to avoid gluten. Perhaps one-tenth of 1 percent of people are allergic to wheat but don't have celiac disease. These people may get hives or have throat swelling if they eat wheat, but they have no long-term health problems associated with it. These folks should avoid wheat, just as a person allergic to peanuts should avoid peanuts.

Another 5 percent of the population may have a condition called non-celiac gluten sensitivity (NCGS). It causes symptoms such as fatigue, diarrhea, bloating, and perhaps an increased risk of infections or worsened symptoms of preexisting autoimmune conditions. While researchers acknowledge this is a real phenomenon, they know little about what long-term effects it might have on the body and how much people with NCGS would benefit from avoiding gluten. Also, there is no reliable medical test for NCGS, so the diagnosis must be made by carefully obtaining a medical

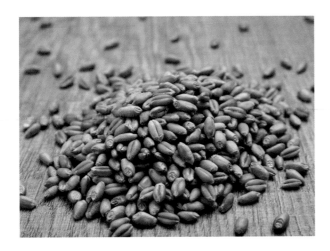

and dietary history. Given that 5 percent of the population is a significant number of people, we have no problem with those who in the interest of good health choose not to eat gluten, even if they are just playing it safe.

We do, however, believe that once they strengthen and balance their gut health by following a plant-rich whole-foods diet that includes plenty of probiotics and prebiotics, fiber, fruits, and vegetables, many people will be able to work gluten back into their diets in moderation. (Again, the exception would be if you have celiac disease, in which case you need to completely eliminate gluten from your diet permanently.) For what it's worth, taking a teaspoon or two of apple cider vinegar before every meal is an effective way to help stimulate your body's digestion process, which will enable you to break down gluten (and all proteins) better. And finally, taking a high quality multistrain probiotic (see page 404 for recommendations) will help restore balance in your gut microbiome and improve digestion, which will also make it easier for your body to break down gluten. We are not trying to convince anyone to eat gluten if they are dead set against it; we are just trying to provide options and be honest about what has worked for our family.

We chose not to include gluten in the recipes in this book in order to be as inclusive as possible. Eliminating gluten from your diet can be rather restrictive, but thanks to the widespread popularity of gluten-free diets in the last decade or so, it is far easier to healthfully go gluten-free today than it was twenty years ago. However, we do eat gluten-containing grains ourselves; neither of us is in the 6 percent who are in any way sensitive to gluten, so we don't want to deprive ourselves unnecessarily. Having said that, we do not eat large quantities of gluten-containing foods, nor do we eat large quantities of any one particular grain.

A Final Word on the Autoimmune Protocol

Even if you choose to avoid gluten, there is no evidence that following any of the other recommendations of the autoimmune protocol diet will improve an autoimmune condition. Any small studies showing benefits from the autoimmune protocol diet are likely comparing its results to simply eating a standard unhealthy modern diet, and certainly eliminating processed foods, processed grains, added sugars, and vegetable oils is good for you. But the other restrictions of the autoimmune protocol are not necessary and will not improve your health unless you truly have an allergy. In fact, following all the autoimmune protocol recommendations will likely hurt your health by depriving you of many potentially healthful nutrients (including anti-inflammatory antioxidants and phytonutrients) and may cause some people to eat too much meat. There are very strong studies showing that excess meat consumption increases the risk of heart disease and cancer and contributes to weight gain. Red meat consumption also contributes to hormonal imbalances (specifically estrogen dominance).

We encourage you to eat a wide variety of healthful and nutrient-dense whole foods and to explore new tastes and gastronomy in general. We are very much against eliminating natural foods without proof that doing so is necessary. Please don't be misled by the latest fad.

understanding carbohydrates, fats, and proteins

There are three calorie-containing macronutrients that make up all of the food we eat: carbohydrates, fats, and proteins. Some diets recommend eating a certain percentage of each macronutrient. Some recommend nearly eliminating one or another. Neither of these approaches is necessary for optimal health, and we discourage counting your food like this. Some carbohydrates are good, and some are less good. The same applies to fats. Assuming your are eating enough calories and are also eating a whole-foods diet, It is almost impossible to not eat enough protein, so instead of adding up your protein intake, focus on eating healthy foods that happen to contain protein. Overall, focus on eating more nutrients (especially antioxidants, phytonutrients, and fiber!) and not on counting or measuring macronutrients.

Having said that, it's good to have a general understanding of carbohydrates, fats, and proteins and the roles they play in good health. We'll spend the rest of this chapter discussing the macronutrients and the foods they're found in.

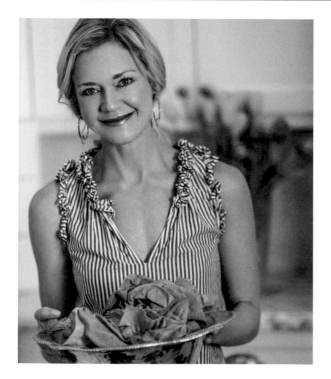

carbohydrates

Many common foods consist primarily of carbohydrates. These foods are nearly universally healthful in their natural, whole, unprocessed form. On the other hand, simple sugars and refined starches are empty calories and contribute to a host of undesirable conditions, including obesity, type 2 diabetes, and the many inflammation-mediated diseases discussed in chapter 3.

Let's start with the healthful carbohydrates. All fruits and all vegetables are encouraged on the Clean Cuisine program. These should be eaten in their whole form and can be eaten as often as you like. Fruits and vegetables can be purchased either fresh or frozen; both forms are about equally healthful. Organic produce is great, but if money or availability is a concern, conventional is fine, too. We are stricter about organic when it comes to animal foods because organically raised animals actually have a far better nutrient profile than factory-farmed animals, whereas with fruits and vegetables, the difference is less stark.

Fruits and vegetables contain fiber, which slows digestion, fights diabetes, decreases cancer risk, and helps with digestive health. More fiber is better, so try to eat the skins of fruits whenever possible. Fruits and vegetables also contain phytonutrients, which fight inflammation and decrease cancer risk. *Eating more fruits and vegetables has a greater effect on your lifespan than any other dietary change.* We do recommend avoiding fruits canned or packaged in sugar-based liquid or sauce. Canned produce is okay, but it should be packed in water without added sugar. Dried fruit is okay as well, as long as there is no added sugar. Avoid fruit juices, as these lack fiber (unless the skin and pulp are included), their sugars are absorbed quickly by the body, raising blood glucose, and they do not offer the lasting satisfaction that whole fruit offers. (For more on juice, see page 32.)

Other carbohydrate-rich foods include starchy vegetables like potatoes and beets. These foods are great and contain unique nutrients, so the more variety you eat, the better. Where people go wrong with potatoes is in the processing and preparation. A simple baked potato is much more healthful than creamy, milky mashed potatoes and certainly more healthful than fried potatoes. Beans and legumes are also encouraged on Clean Cuisine; they are a healthful source of clean protein and are high in fiber.

Perhaps the most controversial good carbohydrate is whole grains and the flours made from these grains. If you refer to the Clean Cuisine pyramid on page 21, you'll see that whole grains do not form the base of our pyramid, meaning we don't think you should be eating large amounts of these foods every single day. You can eliminate these foods from your diet if you want, but doing so will make following Clean Cuisine far more restrictive than necessary. Keep in mind, if you eliminate one major source of calories from your diet, you are likely going to replace it with something else—and if you replace whole grains with protein or fat, you won't be getting the health-promoting fiber, antioxidants, and phytonutrients found in whole grains. Whole grains, which, unlike refined grains, contain the outer fiber in addition to the starchy core, are filling, nutritious, and healthful and are featured in many of our recipes. Whole-grain pasta can also be enjoyed, but you do have to be careful about portion size, as it contains more sugar and starch than fruits and vegetables and is less filling per calorie. Whole-grain flour should be used instead of refined flour. In this cookbook, we use a variety of whole-grain flours.

We have chosen not to use gluten-containing grains in our recipes because we know a lot of clean eaters appreciate, or require, gluten-free recipes. Understand, though, that we are not gluten-free ourselves, and we believe that once you optimize the health of your gut and reduce whole-body inflammation, gluten sensitivity can often be overcome. (We talk about gluten in more depth on page 52.) It is our opinion that the overwhelming majority of people who have a sensitivity to gluten developed that sensitivity because they consume it at every meal in the form of bread, pasta, crackers, cereal, and so on. Even worse, most people are consuming gluten in the form of empty-calorie *refined* grains! In general, our advice is to enjoy as wide a variety of whole grains as your own body can tolerate and to always eat more fruits and vegetables rather than more grains.

Bad carbohydrates tend to be processed foods. Cookies, crackers, chips, white flour, and standard baked goods are poor choices because they not only are nutrient-poor but also are quickly absorbed, thus spiking blood sugar levels and elevating the fat-storing hormone insulin. When purchasing packaged foods, look for whole grains and a substantial amount of fiber. (Note: We are not big fans of reading the nutrition facts on food labels because they can often be deceiving. However, if you are buying packaged foods, a good rule of thumb is to look for whole grains that have at least 2 or 3 grams of fiber per 25 grams of carbohydrate.) Never choose products that contain added sugars (see the list of pseudonyms for sugar on page 31—you'll see them on a lot of lists of ingredients). Never choose products containing enriched flour of any kind. *Enriched* is a code word meaning that the flour has been processed and is not whole grain anymore. It refers to the fact some of the vitamins that were removed during processing have been added back, but many of the grain's phytonutrients that were removed are not added back. None of our recipes make use of processed carbohydrate products, and all of them contain fruits, vegetables, or a superfood among their ingredients.

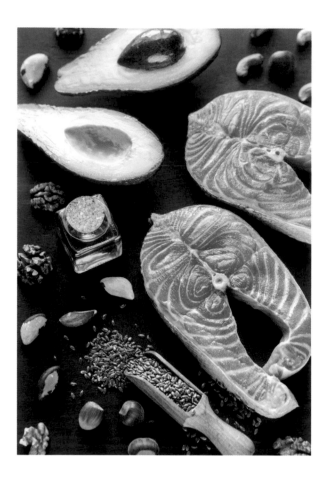

fats

Fat is a powerful macronutrient that significantly affects the inflammation response in our bodies. Just as with carbohydrates, there are good fats and bad fats. In general, whole, unprocessed fat-containing foods and oils are more healthful than refined, packaged products. Furthermore, most of us eat more of some types of fats and oils than we should, while there are some types that most of us can benefit from eating more of. We categorize fats as omega-3 fats, omega-6 fats, saturated fats, monounsaturated fats, and trans fats. Saturated fats are further categorized as animal-based or plant-based.

We talked in depth about omega-3 fats in chapter 2. These anti-inflammatory fats, which reduce your risk of chronic disease, are found in fish, shellfish, almonds, walnuts, flax seeds, and chia seeds. The only thing to be wary of here is cooking with omega-3-rich oils like flaxseed oil, as the heat will destroy the good fat. Cooking doesn't harm the omega-3 in whole foods like fish and seeds, however, as the foodstuff surrounding the omega-3 fat protects it from destruction.

We also talked about omega-6 fats—and the importance of eating only a little bit more omega-6 than omega-3—in chapter 2. Omega-6 fats are found in nuts and seeds and to a lesser extent in many whole grains, and as long as you are consuming these fats as part of a whole food, you really don't have to worry about getting too much. However, omega-6-rich oils should not be eaten or used in cooking. The reason is that we already get too much omega-6 in our food, and high heat damages these oils. It's especially important to avoid omega-6-rich vegetable oils like regular vegetable oil, soybean oil, canola oil, corn oil, grapeseed oil, and sunflower oil, which are damaging for health in many different ways (see page 34 for details). We make a strong point in our recipes to include only the most healthful unrefined oils that are low in omega-6 fat.

Monounsaturated fats are found in high quantities in olive oil, avocados, and many nuts. These are healthful fats, and they are great for cooking because they're not damaged by heat. In general, though, you want to eat these fats in whole foods rather than in large amounts of oil, as the whole foods contain most of the nutrition. Save the oil for cooking, and use minimal amounts as dressings for flavor.

Saturated fats are generally pro-inflammatory and have been known to contribute to many inflammatory conditions, including coronary artery disease and multiple sclerosis. However, plant-based saturated fats, found in foods like nuts and coconut oil, tend to have an anti-inflammatory effect, and many studies show benefits to eating these foods. We often cook with extra-virgin coconut oil, which isn't damaged by high-heat cooking and adds nutrition (and flavor!) to our recipes. We avoid cooking with butter and other animal-based saturated fats, however. In the past, we've recommended limiting total saturated fat intake to 15 to 20 grams per day. This remains good advice as far as animal-based saturated fat is concerned.

Finally, the most dangerous fats of all are trans fats. These are found in very small quantities in dairy products from cows, sheep, and goats. But industrial trans fats are found in processed foods, including baked goods and many restaurant and fast-food fried items. Look for partially hydrogenated oil or hydrogenated oil on the label, and avoid those foods! Trans fats interfere substantially with the good work that the healthy fats do and increase inflammation in the body while adding no necessary nutrition.

Although Clean Cuisine is definitely not a low-fat diet, in general we strongly encourage eating whole-food sources of plant-based fat, consuming animal fat no more than once a day, eating fatty fish for its omega-3 fat, and limiting the use of oil to what is necessary for cooking. Plant-based fats tend to contain more nutrients than animal-based fats and are gentler on the gut as well. There is substantial research showing that animal-based saturated fats increase the risk of colon cancer and disrupt the optimal bacterial balance in your intestines.

It's also important to point out that when it comes to fats and oils, the whole fat is always nutritionally superior to the oil. Avocados are healthier than avocado oil. Raw walnuts are a better choice than walnut oil, and flax seeds trump flaxseed oil. Oil is a processed food: nutrients, fiber, and important phytonutrients are removed when plant foods are pressed into oil. Although a fairly high-fat diet rich in good fats is acceptable, nobody should be eating an oil-rich diet. It is not good for your heart or any other part of your body to eat any type of oil in excess. Oil is a condiment, a flavoring, and an element of cooking. You do not need to eat any oil at all to be healthy because you can get all the fat you need from whole foods. For the most part, the less oil you eat, the better. Having said that, we definitely do not encourage an oil-free diet by any means—that's because the taste of our food is extremely important to us, and oils have tremendous culinary benefits. But we want to make sure that you are not misled into thinking that you will be doing your heart or waistline any favors by pouring extra-virgin olive oil onto your food by the cupful. If you swap oils for whole plant foods high in healthy fats, such as nuts, seeds, olives, coconuts, and avocados, you'll be getting a lot more fiber, phytonutrients, disease-preventing plant sterols, and a number of other nutrients that are much more useful for protecting your heart and your health than oils.

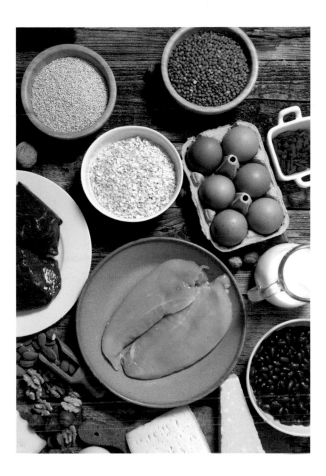

proteins

It is interesting that of the three macronutrients—carbohydrates, fats, and proteins—the only one that seems to get off scot-free when it comes to its potential role in disease and weight gain is protein. Nobody ever seems to want to blame protein for anything harmful. Carbs and fats get blamed for obesity, heart disease, type 2 diabetes, and so on, yet somehow protein has remained unscathed in the eyes of the general public. In fact, everyone seems to be scrambling to get *more* protein! We've never heard of someone saying, "Oh no, I can't have more chicken; I'm trying to limit my protein intake." You don't see many manufacturers advertising the fact that their products contain "extra fat" or "extra carbs." But processed protein bars, protein powders, protein shakes, and protein supplements are ubiquitous. It's as if we're all in some sort of enormous protein emergency. But there is absolutely no reason to eat above and beyond the protein your body needs for maintenance and repair.

Protein is not a free food. If you eat more protein than your body needs, the extra can be stored as body fat. That means the calories in that extra piece of chicken don't just vanish. Eat too many skinless chicken breasts or too much whey protein powder or too many egg whites, and you can absolutely put on unwanted pounds. And that extra body fat ends up causing more inflammation. Eating more protein (or any other macronutrient, for that matter!) than your body needs will also accelerate the aging process and create oxidative stress, which damages cells and DNA and is linked to diseases such as cancer and Alzheimer's.

To us, protein is a bit of an afterthought, as most people already eat more than adequate amounts of good-quality protein. We care more about whether that protein is consumed with good carbohydrates and good fats.

Plants for Protein

If you polled random people on the street, they would most likely tell you that protein and animal foods such as beef and chicken go hand in hand. This means if you are eating a diet high in protein, you are likely eating a diet rich in animal foods. One of the problems there is that your stomach can hold only so much food in one day; if you are filling up on animal foods, you are basically pushing antiaging, anti-inflammatory, disease-fighting, and gut health–optimizing plant foods right off your plate. Most people aren't eating nearly enough unrefined whole plant foods as it is, so the last thing we need is to displace plant foods with large portions of protein-packed beef, chicken, milk, and protein shakes.

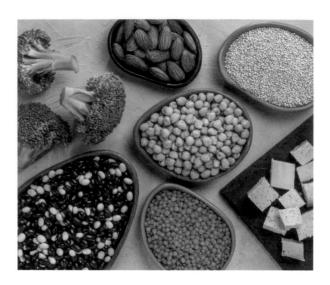

What we really need to be eating is more unrefined plant-based foods, which contain fiber and disease-fighting phytonutrients that are essential for reducing inflammation, preventing DNA damage, helping us stay youthful, and protecting against disease—and which animal foods lack. And here's the surprising news: you do not need to eat animal foods just to get enough protein. You can get plenty of protein from a plant-based diet!

We can see the meat lovers shutting this book right now. But don't get nervous! Just because we tell you that you can get plenty of protein from plants doesn't mean we are trying to convert you to a vegan diet. (Andy, in particular, isn't about to give up his salmon, and our son would be very disappointed if we were to tell him that the Blake Burger on page 188 is not healthy.) But there are far too many nutrients that we need from plant foods, and if we overconsume animal foods because we are under the misguided impression that we will be protein deficient if we don't, then we end up shortchanging ourselves in overall total nutrition.

DITCH THE PROTEIN SHAKES

The vast majority of protein shakes have been processed so heavily that they have had pretty much all other nutrients removed, leaving behind pure protein and usually some filler fats and carbs. These are not, of course, natural, whole foods, and we don't recommend consuming them. It is particularly important to avoid protein shakes made with whey, a milk protein.

The vast majority of our protein should come from unrefined whole plant foods. Animal foods should be consumed in much smaller quantities than are standard in the modern-day diet. So yes, you can still have some steak, but in moderate portions, and not at every meal.

How Much Protein Is Enough?

How much protein do you need to eat? A lot less than you think. Some experts estimate that you need 1 to 2 grams of protein per kilogram of lean body mass. The Institute of Medicine recommends that we consume 0.8 gram of protein for every kilogram that we weigh. For example, a 120-pound woman would need to eat only about 44 grams of protein a day. This isn't a whole lot! It's not that you have to tally up precisely how much protein you eat each and every day, a tiresome bore of a chore if there ever was one, but it is good to have a general idea of how much protein you need.

We like to say that you should consume roughly 0.5 gram of protein per pound of body weight. If you are overweight, you should calculate your protein needs based on your *ideal* body weight, not your current weight. Any excess amount of protein over this amount is likely to be empty calories. (The exception to this is if you are recovering from major surgery or you exercise *intensely* for more than six hours a week.) Based on this guideline, a healthy-weight 120-pound woman should eat about 60 grams of protein per day. When you start to look at the protein content in your food, you soon realize that it is *extremely* easy to get 0.5 gram of protein per pound of body weight. In fact, because of our animal food–rich diets, the average American consumes 100 to 120 grams of protein per day. That amount should really be eaten only by people whose *ideal* body weight is between around 200 and 300 pounds.

Trust us, the prevailing nutrition problem with modern society is not that we are not getting enough protein; instead, we aren't getting enough unrefined whole plant foods! If anything, people eat way more protein than they should.

Protein on Your Plate

So how do we put our protein beliefs into practice? Typically, we put protein on the side of the plate. If we're having chicken or fish, the meat is a small portion on the side and the vegetable takes up the majority of the plate. Consider eating more plant-based proteins as well. Tofu, beans, and lentils contain good-quality protein and are more nutrient dense than any animal protein (except cold-water fish, which contains the good omega-3 fat we need so much more of). Many other plant foods also contain surprisingly high amounts of protein per calorie; wild rice and spinach are both protein rich on a per-calorie basis even when compared to meats such as steak or pork.

It is possible to get all the protein you need following a vegan diet, but we choose not to be vegans (for reasons discussed on page 20). Certain animal superfoods, like whole eggs from properly raised birds and wild cold-water fish like salmon and sardines, contain nutrients that are essential for optimal health and are not readily available in plant foods. In particular, animal protein contains vitamin B_{12}, an absolutely essential nutrient that's very hard to find in plant foods unless it is added artificially.

However, if you do choose to eat only plant-based foods, Clean Cuisine can still work for you. Just make an effort to get enough omega-3 fat and vitamin B_{12} (supplement if you have to), but do not waste time trying to make sure you're getting all nine essential amino acids every day. As long as you get enough calories, your body can mix and match the essential amino acids over a period of days. Also, certain vegan foods, such as whole soy products, contain all the essential amino acids in adequate quantities even if they are not eaten in combination with other foods.

We believe strongly that eating organic animal protein increases the nutrient profile of the meat and minimizes the buildup of harmful compounds, like excess saturated fat. If you're on a budget, we suggest you prioritize organic, grass-fed, cage-free, ethically raised animal food over organic produce. There is much more to be gained nutritionally from organic animal food than organic produce, though both are a great improvement over conventional.

" No one is
born a great cook.
One learns
by doing. "

—JULIA CHILD

Part 2

COOKING
clean cuisine

CHAPTER 5

stocking your
clean cuisine kitchen

Ivy here. When I was growing up, my parents did not know the terms *clean eating* and *whole-foods diet*, but they knew eating processed junk food was not healthy. Consequently, at our house, you would never find Doritos, Ding Dongs, or Cheez-Its, but you would find jars of all shapes and sizes filled to the brim with dried beans, pasta, rice, grains, and nuts and seeds. We also had lots of canned items, especially beans, all sorts of tomato products, and numerous exotic condiments, along with spices galore. There were also things like canned olives, baby corn, roasted red peppers, hearts of palm, and marinated mushrooms and artichokes. We had nut butters, teas, coffee, chocolates, vinegars, and oils from all around the world. And you could always find a wide range of canned seafood, from caviar to tuna and anchovies to oysters.

One of the things I remember most about our incredibly well-stocked pantry was that every time I had a friend over, they would comment on how there was nothing to eat! All we had were "ingredients," not "food." It was the same thing in the refrigerator and freezer: we had butter, milk, cheese, fruits, vegetables, and meats, but no tater tots or frozen pizza. I remember thinking that when I got old enough to have my own house, I was going to have everything from chips to cookies to a wide assortment of sugary breakfast cereals and lots of packaged snack foods.

Of course, by the time I grew up and finally had my own pantry, I had already started to learn that having a pantry full of "ingredients" was not only the healthiest way to eat but also could be the tastiest. In many ways, the items I stock in our pantry, refrigerator, and freezer are very similar to the foods I grew up with in my parents' house. The main difference is that I've substituted gluten-free, whole-grain, or bean pasta for pasta made with refined wheat flour. I use almond or hemp milk rather than cow's milk. I use only raw nuts and seeds rather than those roasted in oil. I have a much wider selection of whole grains and unrefined flours than my mom ever cooked with. I purchase sprouted whole-grain bread and only unrefined oils. The sugar jar contains unrefined coconut sugar rather than highly processed white sugar. And so on. I also buy superfoods that most people in my parents' generation didn't even know about, such as chia seeds, hemp seeds, flax seeds, and goji berries.

If you are inspired to give clean eating a try, or even if you just want to slowly replace processed foods with healthier options, this chapter can help you get started. The more you can stock your cupboards and refrigerator with good stuff, the easier clean eating will be. You can shape up your pantry gradually, or you can have fun going through your kitchen and tossing or giving away all the unhealthy packaged and refined foods that you don't want to eat anymore. And once you have a well-stocked pantry, refrigerator, and freezer, clean eating will soon become second nature. Really.

on choosing organic

One of the decade's biggest culinary buzzwords is *organic*. The concept is nothing new: before the introduction of chemicals into agriculture, all farming could have been considered organic.

But just because a food is labeled "organic" does not mean that it is automatically nutritious. One of the world's junkiest junk foods, Oreo cookies, is now made organic, but if you have a choice between an organic Oreo or a conventionally grown apple, choose the apple!

So does buying organic really matter? And are some foods more important to buy organic than others? The answers vary, so let's look first at plant foods and then at animal foods.

Organic Plant Foods

The difference between conventional and organic farming lies in how the farmers grow the crops. For a food to be labeled USDA-certified organic, it must be grown and processed according to federal guidelines that prohibit the use of synthetic pesticides, fertilizers, herbicides, irradiation, sewage sludge, and genetic engineering. Conventionally grown, nonorganic foods don't follow these restrictions, which means they are often loaded with toxic chemicals that can harm health. For example, pesticides and herbicides have been linked in study after study to ailments from allergies and ADD to autism and even cancer.

The fact that organic food is not genetically modified is also very important. Genetic modification combines DNA from different species, messes with natural selection, and introduces novel proteins that have the potential to increase food allergies and stimulate autoimmune response. In theory, this could be particularly harmful to people with autoimmune conditions such as multiple sclerosis or rheumatoid arthritis. If you knew nothing else about genetic modification, this would be enough to justify concern. And indeed, more than sixty countries around the world—including all of the countries in the European Union, Australia, Japan, the United Kingdom, Russia, China, and India—currently require labels that indicate whether a food has GMOs or not.

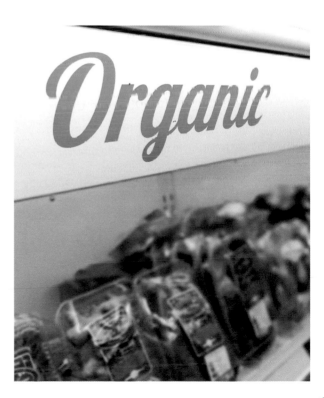

Unfortunately, the United States is not on board (yet) with labeling GMO foods. In addition to produce and plant foods, livestock, agriculture, and aquaculture foods can also be sources of GMOs since genetically engineered ingredients are common in animal feed; this impacts animal foods such as eggs, milk, meat, and seafood. Although those in favor of not labeling GMO foods are quick to point out that no large-scale human research on GMOs and their health impact has ever been conducted, I still believe it is safest to avoid GMO foods whenever possible. Buying USDA-certified organic food ensures that what you are buying is GMO-free.

But the benefits of organic produce go beyond not having bad things—they also have more good things. Dozens of studies have shown that organic fruits and vegetables have more nutrients than conventional produce. For example, a ten-year study at the University of California, Davis, found that organic tomatoes have almost double the quantity of antioxidants called flavonoids, which can reduce blood pressure and help prevent heart disease and strokes. In another study, from Newcastle University in England, researchers discovered organic produce has up to 40 percent higher levels of vitamin C, zinc, iron, and other key nutrients. And scientists from the University of Florida found that organically grown produce has up to 25 percent more cancer-fighting phytonutrients.

Part of the problem is that conventional produce is almost always picked when still unripe and hard so that it won't get bruised or damaged when it's shipped hundreds (and often thousands) of miles. But plants have to fully ripen on the vine to reach their peak nutrient levels. Immature produce that gets transported long distances is often chemically ripened in warehouses before it heads to the supermarket, a process that makes fruits and veggies look ripe, beautiful, and colorful but doesn't let them develop their full nutrient potential. Picking produce before it is ripe also negatively affects its flavor. You simply can't get the same flavor from a tomato that was not allowed to ripen naturally on the vine.

I try to buy organic fruits and vegetables whenever possible. However, there is no way I could stick to a clean-food diet if I had to commit to eating 100 percent organic foods. For one thing, if I were only to eat organic, I would almost never be able to eat at a restaurant! When grocery

THE DIRTY DOZEN AND THE CLEAN 15

The Environmental Working Group has a very useful "Dirty Dozen" guide that lists the fruits and vegetables most impacted by chemicals (often, the skin is consumed or is particularly permeable). On the flip side, the fruits and veggies in the "Clean 15" list absorb a minimal amount of pesticides and fertilizers, so there's little difference between organic and conventionally grown.

CLEAN 15

	Corn
	Eggplants
	Honeydew melons
Asparagus	Kiwis
Avocados	Mangoes
Broccoli	Onions
Cabbages	Papayas
Cantaloupes	Peas
Cauliflower	Pineapples

DIRTY DOZEN

	Hot peppers
	Nectarines
	Peaches
Apples	Pears
Bell peppers	Potatoes
Celery	Spinach
Cherries	Strawberries
Grapes	Tomatoes

shopping, though, I try to avoid the "Dirty Dozen" (see sidebar on previous page). Simply avoiding the produce on the Dirty Dozen list will go a long way toward reducing your exposure to toxic chemicals. You can also reduce your exposure by washing your produce well. Use a vegetable wash solution with 1 tablespoon apple cider vinegar in 1 gallon of water, and be sure to rinse well.

Organic Animal Foods

You might assume that organic animal foods are the cleanest sources of animal protein. And it is absolutely true that by choosing organic animal foods, you are taking one giant step toward healthier animals and better food quality. To be USDA-certified organic, animals must be raised free of genetic engineering, have year-round access to certified organic land, receive 100 percent organic feed, and never receive antibiotics or growth hormones. So eating organic instead of conventionally raised meat will lessen your exposure to pesticide residues, synthetic hormones, antibiotics, and toxins in general.

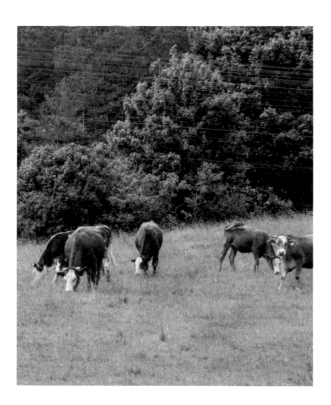

But when it comes to buying the highest-quality animal foods, it's essential to think about going beyond organic and consider the diet of the animal. This is because the animal's diet affects the health of the animal, which ultimately affects the health of the person who eats it.

Modern conventional farming is designed to grow and fatten animals at an unnaturally rapid rate; the animals eat a calorie-rich grain-based diet rather than the nutrient-rich grass-based diet they would naturally consume in the wild. That diet of dry grain directly contributes to the development of pathogens such as *E. coli* (in cattle) and salmonella (in poultry). Did you know that mad cow disease is unknown among cattle fed entirely on pasture and hay? When cows eat the foods nature intended them to eat, they are healthier. So even if ranchers feed cows organic grain, that doesn't mean grain is optimal for cow health. And ultimately, grain-fed beef is not desirable for you, either.

Grain-fed animals (and the milk from those animals) are less nutritious than grass-fed, pastured animals. For example, compared with grass-fed beef, grain-fed beef has only one-quarter as much vitamin E and one-eighth as much beta carotene. Chickens that are raised on fresh pasture and free to roam and forage for a naturally healthy chicken diet of insects, worms, grass, and wild plants are nutritionally superior to caged chickens fed an unnatural diet of grain alone.

Grain-fed animals also have far more pro-inflammatory omega-6 fat and much less anti-inflammatory omega-3 fat. As we discussed on page 34, most people today consume far too much omega-6 and far too little omega-3, and the consumption of conventionally raised meat is a major reason why. The fat in grass-fed animals is much closer to a healthy balance.

So while organic grain-fed meat may be free of unwanted toxins, it is still nutritionally inferior to grass-fed meat.

The bottom line is that there is more to choosing a healthful animal food than simply picking organic. And as we talked about in chapter 2, limiting animal food overall is good for your health.

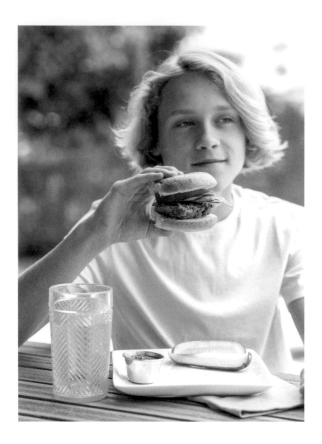

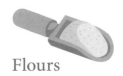

Flours

The recipes in this book use only gluten-free flours. It is very important to note that not all gluten-free flours are nutrient-rich. In fact, many all-purpose gluten-free flour blends contain refined, nutrient-poor flours, and many of the single-ingredient gluten-free flours are also refined. The four most popular gluten-free flours, and the ones we try to avoid, are tapioca flour, potato starch, white rice flour, and sweet rice flour.

All of the flours I buy are unrefined, and whenever possible, I look for sprouted flours, which are ground from grains that are sprouted and then dehydrated. Sprouting activates enzymes in the grains, which greatly enhances your body's ability to digest and utilize all of their important nutrients. It is worth noting that some people with gluten sensitivity find they can eat sprouted flours, as sprouting can reduce the gluten content. As for the taste, most people do not notice much of a difference between sprouted flours and conventional flours. However, if you have extremely sensitive taste buds, chances are you will like sprouted flours better because they are ever-so-slightly more flavorful.

It is definitely cheaper to buy flour in bulk. If you don't have a natural foods store near you, online is your best bet. One last tip: If you don't plan to use your flours within a month or so, then you will want to store them in the freezer to optimize freshness.

in the pantry

When you're ready to stock your pantry with clean foods, start by throwing out the processed stuff! Then it's time to add the healthful clean ingredients. Here's what you can find in our pantry at any given time.

CASSAVA FLOUR SWAP: SPROUTED SPELT FLOUR

If you are not gluten-free/grain-free, you can substitute sprouted spelt flour for cassava flour in any recipe in this book. Sprouted spelt flour is also the perfect flour swap in any recipe that calls for all-purpose or whole-wheat flour. Like whole-wheat flour, it has a nutty and slightly sweet flavor, but sprouted spelt flour has more copper, iron, zinc, magnesium, and phosphorous. Although it does contain gluten, spelt is an ancient grain that is easier for most people to digest than wheat. *Sprouted* spelt flour is even easier to digest than conventional spelt flour, and since sprouting reduces the gluten content, some people with gluten sensitivity find they can tolerate sprouted spelt. Although conventional spelt flour can also be used as a substitute for cassava flour, sprouted spelt flour is the nutritionally superior option. If you are on a budget, it is also worth noting that sprouted spelt flour is less expensive than cassava flour. Assuming you are not gluten-free/grain-free, sprouted spelt flour is a very good all-purpose flour.

Although I buy a wider variety of unrefined flours than what I have listed below, the following flours are the ones used in this book:

- **Blanched almond flour**
- **Brown rice flour**
- **Coconut flour**
- **Corn grits or polenta**
- **Masa harina.** Spanish for "dough flour," this finely ground corn flour is made from dried hominy, or hulled corn kernels, and is traditionally used to make tortillas and tamales. Masa harina corn flour is available from any natural foods store.
- **Medium-grind cornmeal**
- **Oat flour.** Oats are naturally gluten-free but are usually processed in facilities that also process wheat and other grains with gluten, so if you absolutely need to avoid gluten, look for certified gluten-free oats.
- **Cassava flour.** This is one of our all-time favorite flours, though we only recently discovered it. It has a neutral taste and, unlike other gluten-free or grain-free flours, it doesn't give foods a dry or odd texture. In fact, in many instances we prefer the cassava flour version of baked goods to the conventional wheat versions. (Note: If you're neither gluten-free nor grain-free, you may swap sprouted spelt flour for cassava flour in any recipe in this book; see the sidebar on page 66.)

Just like tapioca starch, cassava flour is made from cassava root (also known as yuca root). However, unlike tapioca starch, cassava flour is unrefined, making it a "whole food" root vegetable flour that also contains fiber. Cassava flour is a much more nutritious option than tapioca starch, and it is exceptionally high in vitamin C. It is also a naturally good source of manganese, potassium, and folate.

Because it is totally grain-free, cassava flour is an excellent choice for those with gluten-intolerance symptoms, sensitive digestive systems, celiac disease, or disorders such as irritable bowel disease.

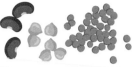

Beans and Legumes

All beans and legumes are superfoods. There are so many varieties that it is impossible to list them all here, so I have only included the ones that I use most frequently:

- **Black beans**
- **Black-eyed peas**
- **Cannellini beans**
- **Chickpeas (aka garbanzo beans)**
- **Great Northern beans**
- **Kidney beans**
- **Lentils (both French lentils and red lentils)**
- **Navy beans**
- **Pinto beans**

Although the flavor of home-cooked beans is definitely better than anything you can buy from a can, I usually use canned beans for convenience. That's why all of the recipes in this book call for canned beans, but you can certainly substitute home-cooked. (Tip: A cup of dried beans is equal to 3 cups cooked beans, drained.) Cooking dried beans is easy-peasy if you invest in a multicooker such as an Instant Pot, which is much easier to use than the old-fashioned pressure cookers.

If you really get into beans (and I hope you do!), look into experimenting with heirloom beans. Like other heirloom plants, heirloom beans haven't been bred to have characteristics desired for large-scale agriculture, so they remain just as they were generations ago. Not only do heirloom beans have incredible taste, but many offer more nutritional bang than conventional beans. (See page 398 for where to buy heirloom beans online.)

A Note About Canned Beans

When buying canned beans, it is super important to look for BPA-free packaging. BPA, or bisphenol-A, is a toxic chemical and endocrine disruptor. Consumers are now savvier about the dangers of BPA, and some manufacturers have replaced it with bisphenol-S (BPS) or bisphenol-F (BPF), which are also harmful. Most organic brands are packaged in cans without these harmful toxins. Cartons and boxes are also generally nontoxic.

If you want to get rid of the "tin can" taste in canned beans, simply rinse the beans with water and drain well. However, if you want to take things to the next level, you can always simmer canned beans (rinsed and drained) in water for five to ten minutes, then drain once more. This is definitely an extra step, but it makes a big difference in taste.

Whole Grains

We buy only unrefined whole grains. (Refined grains like white rice have the bran removed.) Also, just like with flour, you want to look for sprouted whole grains whenever possible. Not only are they more nutritious and easier to digest, but they cook much faster! If you want to sprout your own whole grains, you can certainly do that, and you'll find plenty of resources online for how to do so.

If you plan on making whole grains a part of your daily diet, it is definitely worth the money to invest in either a rice cooker or multicooker, like an Instant Pot. You can cook any whole grain in either device: simply measure the grain, pour in the water, and set the timer. (The appliance's instruction manual will list the cooking times for all whole grains.) You can make meals in minutes if you have cooked whole grains in your fridge— one of my favorite five-minute lunches is a whole-grain bowl with beans, leftover vegetables, and whatever sauce I have on hand (pesto, marinara, mole sauce, etc.). If you are looking for a nutritious and filling alternative to sugary packaged cereal, give cooked whole grains a try! Top them with fruit, spices, a drizzle of pure maple syrup or raw honey, some chia or flax seeds, and your plant milk of choice, and you've got a nutrient- and fiber-packed breakfast.

You will find it more economical to buy whole grains in bulk either online or at a natural foods store. Some natural foods stores are starting to stock frozen cooked whole grains. You will pay a premium for the convenience, but it's good to have a bag or two on hand in a pinch.

Here are the gluten-free whole grains that I use most frequently:

- **Barley**
- **Black rice.** This variety of rice is especially rich in antioxidants.
- **Brown rice** (preferably sprouted)
- **Buckwheat groats.** Despite the "wheat" in its name, this whole grain is gluten-free.
- **Corn grits**
- **Millet**
- **Old-fashioned rolled oats and steel-cut oats** (avoid processed instant oats)
- **Quinoa** (both white and red)
- **Wild rice** (technically not a grain but the seed of a North American marsh grass)

Unrefined Oils

The healthiest fats are from unrefined whole foods. That's because the whole food comes packaged with all the antioxidants, phytonutrients, vitamins and minerals, and fiber. Having said that, an oil-free diet would be extremely difficult to follow and not nearly as tasty. So the next best thing to eating the whole food is using the highest-quality unrefined oil you can buy.

Choosing a superior-quality oil is crucial for both the taste of your food and your health. Low-quality refined oil is one of the most harmful and pro-inflammatory foods that can be consumed, and unfortunately, it lurks everywhere in packaged convenience foods and restaurant foods.

Seek out oils that have not been exposed to heat, light, and oxygen during processing, which can damage even healthful oils. For olive oil and coconut oil, buy only cold-pressed, extra-virgin oils that are made from the very first pressing and thus have more nutrients, more antioxidants, and superior flavor. Although it's not a perfect test for quality, smelling the oil can be a good indicator of whether it is fresh or not. If an oil smells bad or rancid, then you absolutely do not want to use it, no matter how it was processed.

Finally, it is super important to pay close attention to an oil's smoke point. When used at a temperature above its smoke point, an oil becomes damaged and generates pro-inflammatory free radicals. In general, the less heat you can apply to any oil, the better.

Oils for Higher-Heat Cooking (375°F to 475°F)

- **Unrefined avocado oil.** This is relatively expensive, but it is one of the healthiest oils you can cook with. Avocado oil can be substituted for extra-virgin olive oil in any recipe in this book. It has several advantages over olive oil: it can withstand higher heat; it contains nearly triple the amount of carotenoids (an antioxidant), 25 percent more vitamin E, and ten times more chlorophyll (a potent detoxifying agent); and its high antioxidant level helps fight free radicals and reduce inflammation.

- **Unrefined extra-virgin coconut oil.** In its purest form, unrefined extra-virgin coconut oil has incredible antioxidant and antibacterial properties. It is also one of the few oils that are not damaged by high temperatures. The high amount of saturated fat in extra-virgin coconut oil makes it a great plant-based substitute for butter, especially in baked goods such as pie crusts and cookies. Keep in mind that coconut oil is solid at room temperature and may need to be melted or softened before using.

- **Unrefined macadamia nut oil.** The buttery and subtly nutty flavor of macadamia nut oil is a great complement to a wide number of foods. You can substitute macadamia nut oil for extra-virgin olive oil in any recipe in this book. Like avocado oil, macadamia nut oil has a higher smoke point, so it resists oxidation better than extra-virgin olive oil.

OIL DOS & DON'TS

 Avoid omega-6-rich vegetable oils (such as corn oil, grapeseed oil, regular vegetable oil, soybean oil, sunflower oil, and safflower oil) and instead choose oils rich in omega-3, like flax oil, or in monounsaturated fat, like extra-virgin olive oil. Plant-based saturated fat oils like extra-virgin coconut oil should be used for higher-heat cooking.

 Be choosy and select only the absolute highest-quality oils. You want to look for unrefined and cold-pressed oils that have not been exposed to high heat. Even the bottle the oil comes in makes a difference in the freshness of the oil. For the freshest oils, look for dark glass bottles or cans that block light altogether.

 Use only heat-safe oils when cooking; otherwise you risk damaging the oil and generating toxic by-products. (See the list above and on page 70 for oils that are safe at different temperatures.)

 Always use oil in moderation and use common sense. Less oil is generally better. Zero oil is probably going overboard.

 Do not buy high-oleic oils such as high-oleic safflower or sunflower oil to cook with at home, and eat prepared foods containing these oils only in a pinch and when the other ingredients are healthy. Food manufacturers like to use high-oleic oils because they don't contain trans fats and are very shelf-stable, but high-oleic oils are processed oils, and they do not have the same nutritional profile of an unrefined oil that is *naturally* rich in oleic acid, such as extra-virgin olive oil.

 Avoid any oil that is hydrogenated or partially hydrogenated.

Oils for Moderate-Heat Cooking (250°F to 375°F)

- **Extra-virgin olive oil.** Real, high-quality extra-virgin olive oil has well-researched anti-inflammatory compounds, antioxidants, and numerous heart-healthy macronutrients, which explains why olive oil is known for having so many impressive health benefits. Extra-virgin olive oil's benefits include lowering rates of inflammation, heart disease, dementia, and obesity. But with all of that in mind, unfortunately, not all olive oil is created equally—not even all of the "extra-virgin" kinds are as healthy as you may think. You have to be incredibly careful about which olive oil you buy these days, especially the ones from Italy. In fact, much of the Italian olive oil on shelves is neither Italian nor extra-virgin. Unless you bought it directly from a producer or certified distributor, the olive oil in your kitchen marked "Italian extra-virgin" is very likely a fake. A CBS report found that up to 70 percent of the extra-virgin olive oil sold worldwide is watered down with other oils and enhancers. At worst, it's not olive oil at all but a pro-inflammatory vegetable oil disguised with coloring and aroma. Check out page 399 of the resources section for a list of the extra-virgin olive oil brands we trust.

- **Organic, unrefined red palm oil.** This is an incredibly nutrient-dense oil. One tablespoon contains a whopping 240 percent of the recommended daily amount of vitamin A and 25 percent of the recommended daily amount of vitamin E. However, there is an environmental concern with this oil, so it is very important to look for a reputable brand that is fair trade and says "orangutan safe" on the label.

Oils for No-Heat Recipes

The oils listed below should never be heated—drizzle them on cooked food (especially whole grains and vegetables) or use them to make salad dressings. Store these oils in the refrigerator to prevent oxidation. Buy small quantities, as these oils can easily go rancid after about six months.

- **Unrefined walnut oil.** If you are looking to boost your intake of anti-inflammatory omega-3 fats, then unrefined walnut oil is great. It has a delicious nutty flavor that pairs well with a wide variety of recipes.

- **Unrefined toasted sesame oil.** This is the olive oil of many Asian cultures—the most basic oil used in cooking. It is the only omega-6-rich oil that I use, and since it is high in omega-6, you don't want to use it as your primary oil. Use it sparingly and you'll be fine. You can purchase either toasted or untoasted, but toasted has a richer flavor.

- **Unrefined flax oil.** Just like walnut oil, unrefined flax oil is an excellent source of omega-3 fats. It has a rich, grassy flavor and it is excellent for dipping whole-grain bread in.

SOFTENED VS. MELTED COCONUT OIL

When following the recipes in this book, it is important to be aware of the difference between "softened" and "melted" coconut oil. Unless the room is very warm, coconut oil is usually soft-solid at room temperature, but if it is refrigerated, it can be hard-solid. If you are using coconut oil to sauté, then it doesn't really matter whether it is solid or liquid, but if you are baking a cake, then the consistency of the coconut oil in the batter will change the outcome. So be sure to note if a recipe calls for softened or melted coconut oil.

The consistency of softened coconut oil is similar to that of softened butter. To soften coconut oil, set the jar of coconut oil in a heatproof bowl and pour boiling water into the bowl until it comes up to the level of the oil in the jar. Do not let the water reach more than three-quarters of the way up the jar. Wait about 1 minute, then stir the oil.

To melt coconut oil, follow the softening instructions above but leave the jar in the hot water until the oil is fully melted, 3 to 4 minutes.

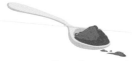

Superfood Powders

Superfoods are so jam-packed with nutrients that they take the idea of "health food" to a whole new level. They supply megadoses of nutrients in a whole-food form that your body can easily utilize. This is in sharp contrast to megadosing with man-made vitamins. The difference is that your body can't necessarily absorb or utilize the nutrients in synthetic vitamins. For example, vitamin C can be absorbed by your body only if it is consumed with the bioflavonoids found within the whole food.

Superfood powders are made from the whole food; it's simply dehydrated and then ground to a powder. I have lots of superfood powders in my pantry, but camu powder, maca root powder, and acai powder are the ones I use most frequently. I add them to smoothies, stir them into almond yogurt, mix them into my morning grain bowl, sprinkle them on popcorn (see page 142), or simply stir them into water. (See page 399 for where to purchase superfood powders.)

- **Camu powder.** This is the whole-food version of the popular Emergen-C supplement. With as much as sixty times more vitamin C per serving than an orange, the camu berry is one of the world's most abundant sources of this important antioxidant. One teaspoon of camu powder delivers more than 700 percent of the recommended daily amount of vitamin C. It's also rich in essential minerals, vitamins, and a wide array of anti-inflammatory phytonutrients. Like most vitamin C–rich fruits, camu has a pleasant tart-and-tangy taste.

- **Maca root powder.** Also known as Peruvian ginseng, maca is a part of a rare group of plants called adaptogens that help the body naturally adapt to environmental stressors, like a busy schedule or a demanding job. Like all superfoods, maca delivers a host of important micronutrients and is jam-packed with antioxidants. It has been shown to improve libido, balance hormone levels, and improve energy, mood, and memory. I look for gelatinized maca because it is easier to digest. Maca tends to have an earthy, slightly nutty taste with a hint of butterscotch and works especially well in oatmeal or breakfast grain bowls.

- **Acai powder.** A dark purple Brazilian superfruit, acai is an incredible source of fiber, phytonutrients, antioxidants, and healthy omega-3 fats. Although it is not easy to find them fresh, freeze-dried and powdered acai berries are available in any natural foods store. With a flavor somewhere between chocolate and wild berries, acai powder is the perfect superfood to add to chocolaty desserts or smoothies.

DRIED FRUITS

We use dried fruits rather frequently, especially for making homemade trail mix, sweetening smoothies, and sprinkling on top of salads or morning whole-grain bowls. One of the best tricks for kicking the candy habit is to substitute dried fruits, which not only are sweet but also have a wide variety of nutrients that help curb food cravings.

When buying dried fruits, take note of the ingredients list: only the fruit should be listed. Avoid added sweeteners (particularly in tart fruits, like cherries and cranberries) and added oils. Look for packages that say "no sulfites," a preservative that maintains color.

Apples	Dates (both medjool and Deglet Noor)	Mulberries (another superfood!)
Apricots	Figs	Pineapples
Blueberries	Goji berries (a superfood!)	Raisins (golden and black)
Cherries	Mangoes	Unsweetened shredded coconut
Cranberries		

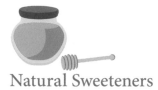

Natural Sweeteners

Unlike refined sugar, natural sweeteners are not empty calories, and they have not been chemically processed. The healthiest and most nutrient-rich natural sweetener is fruit (including dried fruit, such as dates). Although most of the sweeteners here are concentrated sources of calories, they still contain nutrients. Having said that, too much of any type of sweetener is not health promoting. Use these sweeteners in moderation.

- **Blackstrap molasses.** This sweetener is a good source of iron. Did you know that 1 tablespoon of molasses has 0.9 mg of iron?

- **Coconut sugar.** Also known as coconut palm sugar or coconut crystals, this natural sweetener has a flavor very similar to brown sugar. However, unlike brown sugar, it has inulin, a fiber that helps slow the absorption of glucose and prevent blood sugar fluctuations. Inulin fiber also stimulates the growth of beneficial gut bacteria. In addition, coconut sugar contains vitamins, minerals, and phytonutrients—not a lot, but unlike refined white sugar, at least *some*!

- **Dates (medjool and Deglet Noor).** Dates have a delightful sweet flavor with hints of caramel. They also deliver plenty of minerals, vitamins, phytonutrients, and even fiber! With a high-powered blender and a bit of liquid, you can puree dates into a smooth, creamy syrup—and if you use less liquid, you can make a date paste. I bake with them frequently and use them as a sweetener in everything from smoothies to cookies, cakes, pies, muffins, and more.

- **Manuka honey.** If money grew on trees, this is the honey I would use all the time—but it is very pricey. However, manuka honey has incredible medicinal properties, including antibiotic and antimicrobial benefits. I use it primarily in tea, although sometimes I'll do a manuka honey, lemon, and camu powder "shot" if I feel I am coming down with a cold. Manuka honey is graded, so look for a UMF (Unique Manuka Factor) rating of 15+ for optimal therapeutic benefits. It is important not to heat manuka honey or you will destroy the enzymes that give it some of its important healing properties.

- **Pure maple syrup.** Check the ingredients list to confirm that it's made of 100 percent pure maple syrup, not maple "flavor" or high-fructose corn syrup.

- **Raw honey.** Be sure to look for raw honey, as most of the honey at the grocery store is heavily refined during pasteurization, which destroys many vitamins, minerals, amino acids, and enzymes in the honey. Over time, raw honey may crystallize. To return it to a liquid state, place a jar of honey in a bowl of hot tap water, about 100°F. Do not heat it above 95°F to 100°F; higher temperatures will kill the natural enzymes found in raw honey.

- **Stevia.** A native South American herb, stevia is a calorie-free sweetener that is approximately 300 percent sweeter than table sugar. A teeny-tiny bit goes a very long way! I don't bake with stevia because heat alters the flavor a bit, and it can be tricky to get the sweetness just right. I use it mostly to add a touch of sweetness to beverages, especially teas and smoothies. Stevia comes in both liquid and powdered form; I prefer the powdered form. Look for 100 percent pure stevia.

BAKING WITH DATES

Medjool dates are slightly larger than Deglet Noor dates, so when pureed with liquid, they yield a slightly higher volume—and when you're baking, if the volume is not exactly right, then the result will be thrown off, so make sure you use the variety the recipe calls for. Deglet Noor dates have a bit more fiber, but medjool dates are sweeter and softer, so they are better in some recipes. If you don't have a high-powered blender, such as a Vitamix, soak Deglet Noor dates and drier medjool dates in water for 15 to 30 minutes to soften them before pureeing. (Very moist, succulent medjool dates do not require soaking.)

Cupboard Condiments & Canned Items

- **Cacao nibs (raw and unsweetened).** With the same health benefits as raw cacao powder, cacao nibs are a nutrient-dense alternative to chocolate chips.

- **Cacao powder (raw and unsweetened).** Cacao powder is the raw, natural source of one of the most-loved treats of all time: chocolate! Even more exciting, this unprocessed form of chocolate has incredible health benefits, elevating it to superfood status. It's one of the most antioxidant-rich foods on the planet and one of the best plant-based sources of magnesium, a nutrient many people don't get enough of. Cacao is also an excellent source of iron, calcium, and a wide array of anti-inflammatory phytonutrients. Mix it with some dietary fat (such as coconut butter) and a little something sweet (such as maple syrup or date paste), and you've got clean chocolate!

- **Canned artichokes.** Great for pureeing with bean dips. Also, if you rinse and drain the artichokes and then puree them with a bit of extra-virgin olive oil, chopped garlic, and Italian spices, you've got a delightful bread spread!

- **Canned or boxed tomatoes** (whole, crushed, diced)

- **Chipotles in adobo sauce.** Use these anytime you need a spicy kick with a south-of-the-border flavor.

- **Chopped green chiles.** Mild flavored, these are perfect in many Mexican recipes.

- **Coconut butter / coconut manna.** Made from pureed coconut meat, coconut butter / coconut manna is absolutely delicious in smoothies, sauces, desserts, and baked goods. To soften coconut butter, follow the same steps used to soften coconut oil (see page 70). (See Resources, page 400, for brand recommendations.)

- **Dairy-free chocolate chips.** One of the things that makes commercial chocolate unhealthy is that most brands are made with dairy, along with excessive amounts of refined sweeteners. But healthier brands do exist. If you can't yet make the jump to cacao nibs, dairy-free chocolate chips are a good alternative. In the resources section on page 400, you will find the three brands of dairy-free chocolate chips I use; one is sweetened with cane sugar (not optimal), one is sweetened with stevia, and one is unsweetened (but still very decadent and good!).

- **Full-fat coconut milk.** Look for shelf-stable canned coconut milk in the middle aisles of the supermarket, not the coconut milk sold in the refrigerated section, which is typically loaded with added ingredients (not all of which are healthy). I use coconut milk all the time. It's amazing in soups, smoothies, baked goods, and so much more.

- **Marinara sauce.** For both health and taste purposes, I only buy marinara sauces made with extra-virgin olive oil. Many cheaper brands use refined oils, so you really need to read the labels. (See Resources, page 400, for my favorite brands.)

- **Organic broth**—vegetable, chicken, and beef. (See Resources, page 400, for my favorite brands.)

- **Roasted red peppers**

- **Tomato paste**

- **Worcestershire sauce.** Look for an organic Worcestershire sauce for the cleanest option. If you're gluten-free, there are also gluten-free varieties. (See Resources, page 400, for my favorite brands.)

COCOA POWDER IS NOT THE SAME AS CACAO POWDER

Cocoa powder starts the same way cacao powder does: as harvested beans from the plant's seed pods. During processing, however, it's heated to very high temperatures, which degrades all of cacao's awesome antioxidants and nutrients. Dutch-processed cocoa powder (also known as dark cocoa), which is very popular in dessert recipes, undergoes additional processing with an alkalized chemical solution to make the end product richer and less acidic. Unfortunately, further processing only increases the degradation of all those nutrients.

COCONUT CREAM

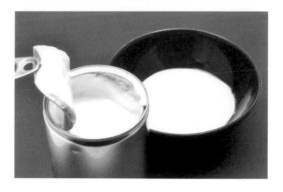

Coconut cream is the thick, rich, and nonwatery part of canned full-fat coconut milk. To get the cream, refrigerate the can of coconut milk for five or six hours or pop it in the freezer for at least an hour, then use a spoon to scoop off the cream that has separated and risen to the top; it will be very thick and stiff. This cream is what you will use for the recipes in this book that call for coconut cream. (You can reserve the remaining liquid for smoothies or post-workout hydration.) One 13.5-ounce can of full-fat coconut milk will yield almost 1 cup of coconut cream. It's important to note, coconut cream doesn't have a coconutty flavor, and you can use it just as you would heavy dairy cream—you can even whip it and make a luxuriously rich whipped cream! Discovering coconut cream is the only thing that allowed me to give up dairy cream in my coffee. I haven't drunk milk in ages, but for years I still had to put just a dash of real cream in my morning coffee because I couldn't find a plant-based option that didn't negatively affect the flavor. Coconut cream has been a total game changer for me!

Nut & Seed Butters

Always look for nut butters made without added sugar, salt, or oil.

- **Almond butter** (raw or roasted)

- **Freshly ground peanut butter.** Many supermarkets have a grind-your-own-peanut-butter station. You can be assured that you are getting nothing but peanuts when you grind your own! Fresh peanut butter always tastes better, too.

- **Macadamia nut butter**

- **Pistachio butter.** This one is not super easy to find, but if you do locate it, you'll want to stock up!

- **Tahini (ground sesame seeds).** Tahini is used to make hummus and baba ghanoush. It's also delicious in sauces, salad dressings, smoothies, and even brownies.

Teas

I probably drink more caffeine-free tea than plain water. That might sound like an unhealthy habit, but sipping tea all day is a super way to get a steady stream of antioxidants. Andy always tells his patients who are concerned with weight loss to start drinking caffeinated tea; many times thirst can be mistaken for hunger, and chances are you will have fewer food cravings once you start drinking tea. On top of that, plenty of studies have shown that teas can help protect your teeth and your heart, as well as possibly help protect against certain types of cancer.

Herbal teas do not have caffeine and can be consumed just like water. Caffeinated teas (such as green tea and black tea) should be consumed earlier in the day so as not to interfere with sleep. You can drink any tea hot or cold; just be sure not to add sugar or dairy milk! Make sure your tea is not made with "natural flavors," which is a vague and poorly regulated term.

I can't possibly list every tea I have on my tea shelf, but below are my top ten favorites.

Caffeinated Teas

- **Black tea.** This has high concentrations of the antioxidant compounds known as theaflavins and thearubigins. Research has shown that people who drink three or more cups of black tea daily may cut their risk of stroke by 21 percent.

- **Matcha.** Premium green tea powder from Japan, matcha tea has tremendous anti-inflammatory benefits. This is one of my absolute favorite teas. I drink at least one cup of matcha tea a day.

- **Oolong.** This has less caffeine than black tea, but enough to give you a noticeable boost. It also has plenty of antioxidants.

- **White tea.** This one often gets overshadowed by green tea, but it has just as many health-promoting benefits.

- **Yerba mate.** The official national drink of Argentina, yerba mate not only enhances cognitive function but also is a nutritional powerhouse loaded with vitamins, minerals, and antioxidants.

Caffeine-Free Herbal Teas

- **Chamomile tea.** I love sipping chamomile in the late evening just before bed.

- **Dandelion root.** This is excellent for enhancing your body's natural detox system.

- **Lemon balm tea.** A mood booster, lemon balm tea is great for lifting the spirits and beating the winter blahs. It's also good for improving concentration.

- **Peppermint tea.** If you have gas, bloating, nausea, or intestinal issues, this is the tea to drink.

- **Rooibos.** Known to relieve stress, nervous tension, and hypertensive conditions, rooibos tea is rich in many minerals, such as iron, calcium, potassium, copper, manganese, zinc, and magnesium.

Spices & Flavor Boosters

As a general rule, I buy seasonings—especially dried herbs and spices—in small amounts because they don't stay fresh forever.

Seasonings

- **Himalayan pink salt.** This delicious unrefined seasoning has some pretty impressive nutritional and therapeutic properties, not to mention incredible culinary uses. Table salt is typically 97.5 percent to 99.9 percent sodium chloride. Himalayan pink salt is only about 87 percent sodium chloride; the rest is minerals, such as calcium, magnesium, potassium, and iron, plus valuable electrolytes. Table salt leaves you with just one mineral (sodium) and some artificially added iodine, along with anticlumping (and health-hazardous) yellow prussiate of soda. Many commercial salts also undergo a bleaching process and contain aluminum derivatives and other toxic substances. If you switch to Himalayan pink salt, your food will taste better (much better), and you'll feel good about knowing you are getting eighty-four minerals!

- **Maldon sea salt.** Also an unrefined salt, this one is not as readily available as Himalayan pink salt, but its taste is pretty amazing! This flake salt is often used as a finishing salt, but you can substitute Maldon sea salt in any recipe that calls for Himalayan pink salt.

- **Bay leaves**

- **Cayenne pepper**

- **Chili powder**

SALT SIZE MATTERS

Believe it or not, the size of the grain of salt you use matters (unless you're seasoning "to taste"). For all of the recipes in this book, I used medium-grind Himalayan pink salt. If you use finely ground salt, you may want to slightly decrease the amount of salt called for in the recipes in this book; if you use coarse salt, you may find you need to add a little more.

- Crushed red pepper
- Dried oregano leaves
- Dried thyme leaves
- **Garam masala.** An essential spice blend for Indian cuisine.
- Garlic powder
- **Ground black pepper.** For the best flavor, use a pepper mill to freshly grind black pepper as needed.
- Ground cinnamon
- Ground cumin
- Ground nutmeg
- Italian seasoning
- **Nutritional yeast (unfortified).** Nutritional yeast gives food an incredible rich and savory cheese flavor. It's also got some impressive health perks! Rich in both fiber and plant protein, unfortified nutritional yeast supplies all eighteen amino acids and a range of minerals (including iron, selenium, and zinc), B vitamins, and immune-enhancing beta-glucans. Seek out unfortified nutritional yeast: it tastes better than the fortified kind, and it does not contain the synthetic vitamins found in conventional nutritional yeast. (See Resources, page 401, for my favorite brands.)
- **Old Bay Seasoning.** A seventy-five-year-old spice blend, this is a must-have seasoning for seafood lovers.
- **Onion powder**
- **Paprika**
- **Saffron threads**
- **Turmeric powder.** This is the one spice I make sure to eat every day, whether in supplement form or food. It is an incredibly potent anti-inflammatory and antioxidant. I also mix it with yogurt and lemon for a daily face mask.

Vinegars & Sauces

- **Balsamic vinegar.** Look for "aceto balsamico tradizionale" on labels for the very best balsamic vinegar. Traditionally made balsamic vinegar is aged for no less than twelve and up to fifty years, and it gets sweeter and more velvety the longer it ages. But superior-quality traditional balsamic vinegar can be a bit pricey. If you want a less expensive (but still tasty!) option, look for one made with a mix of grape must (unfermented pressed grapes) and red wine vinegar. Key ingredients to look for on the label: grape must, aged grape must, or mosta d'uva. (See Resources, page 401, for my favorite brands.)
- **Fish sauce**
- **Gluten-free tamari (Japanese soy sauce).** Made with 100 percent soy and no wheat, tamari has a richer, milder, more complex flavor than regular soy sauce. Use it just as you would traditional soy sauce. (See Resources, page 401, for my favorite brands.)
- **Hot sauce.** My favorite is Tabasco.
- **Liquid aminos.** A salty and gluten-free alternative to both tamari and soy sauce, you can buy either soybean-based or coconut-based aminos. (See Resources, page 401, for my favorite brands.)
- **Nama shoyu (unpasteurized soy sauce).** This sauce is not gluten-free, but if that works for you and you're looking for a healthful substitute for conventional soy sauce, this is a good choice. It is made from cultured soybeans and wheat and is aged for months or even years. Without preservatives and full of enzymes, it has incredible depth of flavor.
- **Sriracha sauce.** This hot sauce has an almost cultlike following. Many different brands exist; look for one made without sugars or additives. (See Resources, page 402, for my favorite brands.)
- **Ume plum vinegar.** A salty/tangy must-have condiment if you love Japanese-inspired dishes. Look for traditionally brewed versions; commercial brands contain red chemical dyes, preservatives, and additives. (See Resources, page 402, for my favorite brands.)

Condiments

- **Barbecue sauce.** See the recipe for my homemade barbecue sauce on page 386, or look for a store-bought one sweetened with dates. (See Resources, page 401, for my favorite brands.)

- **Dijon mustard**

- **Ketchup.** See the recipe for my homemade ketchup on page 390, or look for a store-bought one sweetened with dates. (See Resources, page 401, for my favorite brands.)

- **Mayonnaise.** See page 392 for my homemade egg free mayonnaise recipe or the resources section, page 401, for brand recommendations.

- **Prepared horseradish.** An incredible antioxidant-rich food with potent antibacterial and antimicrobial benefits, prepared horseradish is also great for stimulating healthy digestion. I use it most mixed with ketchup (see recipe, page 390) for shrimp dip, and I love it mixed with my sour cream (see recipe, page 372) for beef and lamb. (See Resources, page 402, for my favorite brands.)

- **Whole-grain mustard**

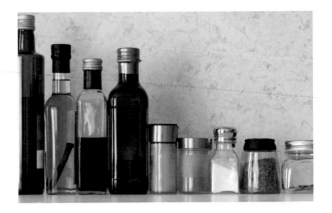

Extracts & Essential Oils

- **Food-grade lemon essential oil.** Essential oils are an excellent (and healthy) way to add incredible flavor to recipes. However, it is very important that you use a high-quality, therapeutic-grade or food-grade oil. An alternative to lemon essential oil is pure lemon extract. When substituting extract for essential oil, use 1 teaspoon extract for 1 to 2 drops of oil. (See Resources, page 401, for my favorite brands.)

- **Pure almond extract**

- **Pure lemon extract.** This is a good substitution for lemon essential oil (see above).

- **Pure peppermint extract.** Food-grade peppermint essential oil works as a substitute; use 1 drop of oil for 1 teaspoon extract. (See Resources, page 401, for my favorite brands.)

- **Pure vanilla extract**

WHAT'S THE DEAL WITH MAYO?

If you use the highest-quality unrefined ingredients, then homemade mayonnaise is actually a healthy food. Most mayonnaise is made with raw eggs, vinegar or lemon juice, salt, mustard, oil, and sometimes a tad bit of sugar. The main reason my recipe for homemade mayo (page 392) is egg-free is that I can't help but worry about the risk of salmonella, one of the most common causes of food poisoning in the United States. Store-bought mayonnaise is made with pasteurized eggs, which are safe from salmonella, but unless it's labeled "pasture-raised," you can be assured the eggs are factory-farmed. That's one reason I avoid it, but also, I'm not particularly fond of eating an egg-containing food that can sit on the store shelf for over a year. The other main problem with most store-bought mayo is that it contains highly refined, pro-inflammatory oils. Having said that, I realize it is not always convenient to make your own mayonnaise; if you want to use store-bought, see the resources section, page 401, for brands that use healthful unrefined oils and pastured eggs.

Canned Seafood

As explained in chapter 2, getting enough omega-3 fats from seafood plays a critical role in the anti-inflammatory benefits of Clean Cuisine, so I always make sure to have the highest-quality canned seafood on hand. Although tuna is probably the most popular canned seafood item, I typically steer away from it because it is high in mercury and relatively low in omega-3. All of the seafood listed below is low in mercury and very rich in omega-3 fats.

- **Anchovies.** Look for wild anchovies packed in olive oil.

- **Anchovy paste.** I use this stuff all the time, just a teeny squeeze in everything from soups to sauces, salad dressings, and pilafs. Made from ground anchovies, salt, and oil, this concentrated paste brings a savory boost to food without revealing itself as an ingredient. Look for wild-caught anchovies packed in olive oil in easy-to-use tubes in the supermarket. (See Resources, page 402, for my favorite brands.)

- **Clam juice** (See Resources, page 402, for my favorite brands.)

- **Fish stock** (See Resources, page 400, for my favorite brands.)

- **Sardines.** Make sure these are packed in olive oil and not a refined vegetable oil. Also, not all canned sardines are equal. The best-tasting ones are wild-caught from Portugal. (See Resources, page 402, for my favorite brands.)

- **Wild salmon**

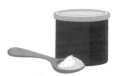

Miscellaneous Items

- **Aluminum-free baking powder.** Conventional baking powder can contain aluminum, which not only has a metallic flavor but has been linked to neurological disorders. Aluminum-free baking powder is easy to find in any natural foods store or online.

- **Arrowroot (aka arrowroot flour / starch).** A nutritionally dense and gluten-free starch, arrowroot is an excellent alternative to highly processed cornstarch. It's perfect for thickening puddings, sauces, and stews. It can also be used to thicken fruit pie fillings or as a binder for veggie burgers or meatloaf.

- **Baking soda**

- **Red curry paste** (See Resources, page 402, for my favorite brands.)

- **Sun-dried tomatoes** (packed in extra-virgin olive oil). (See Resources, page 402, for my favorite brands.)

- **Unsweetened applesauce.** I use this a lot in baking when I am trying to reduce the amount of oil in a recipe. (See Resources, page 402, for my favorite brands.)

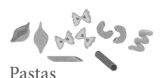

Pastas

I always keep a wide variety of pastas made with different whole grains, seeds, and even beans in the pantry. Read the ingredients carefully, though, as not all "healthy-looking" pastas are made with unrefined ingredients. My favorite gluten-free pastas are made with a combination of corn and quinoa flour or brown rice flour. For Asian-inspired dishes, I love 100 percent buckwheat soba noodles. (Despite its name, buckwheat is not wheat; it's a seed, not a grain, and it's gluten-free.) My favorite grain-free pastas are made with chickpeas. (See Resources, page 402, for my favorite brands.)

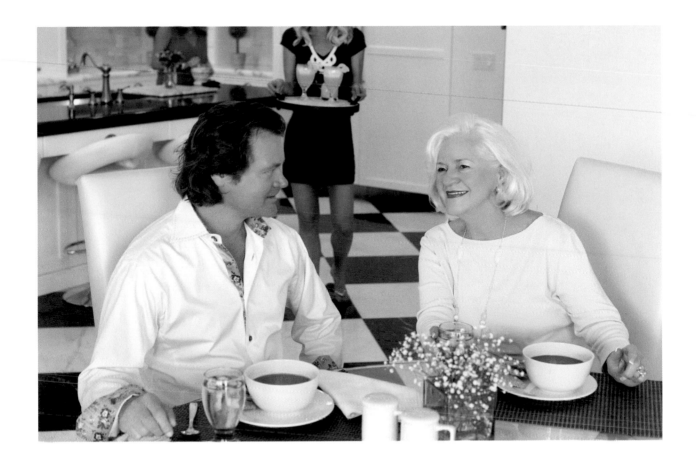

in the freezer

If you have the space and can purchase a freezer for your garage, then you will save money in the long run—as you'll see, there's a lot that keeps best in the freezer! Also, buying meats in bulk and storing them in the freezer is a great way to save money.

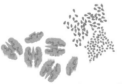

Nuts and Seeds

Space permitting, it is generally best to store nuts and seeds in airtight containers in the freezer or refrigerator. Nuts can go rancid if exposed to too much light and left sitting around too long at room temperature. However, if you use nuts frequently, it is fine to store them in airtight containers in the pantry. It is definitely cheaper to buy nuts and seeds in bulk. If you don't have a natural foods store near you, online is your best bet. Look for raw nuts and seeds and avoid those that have been roasted in unhealthy oils.

Seeds

- **Chia seeds**

- **Flax seeds.** In order to absorb the nutrients in flax seeds, including the super-important omega-3s, we need to eat them ground. For the best flavor, grind small quantities (about ½ cup at a time) in a clean coffee or spice grinder and then store the resulting meal in a sealed container in the freezer and use it within a couple of weeks. You can also purchase ground flax seeds, but be aware that they will go rancid quicker than whole flax seeds. I sprinkle ground flax seeds on everything from nut-based yogurt to smoothies and oatmeal, and I frequently work them into muffins and baked goods.

- **Hemp seeds.** I love to sprinkle hemp seeds on salads (they are kind of like sesame seeds!) and blend them into smoothies, salad dressings (such as my Caesar salad dressing on page 158), oatmeal, and muffins.

- **Raw, hulled sunflower seeds**

- **Raw pumpkin seeds**

- **Raw, unhulled sesame seeds**

Nuts

- **Almonds.** I haven't specified raw almonds for one simple reason: almonds from California are required by law to be pasteurized. At this time, unpasteurized raw almonds can only be bought directly from farmers.

- **Raw Brazil nuts**

- **Raw cashews.** Most cashews labeled as raw are not truly raw because they are heated to remove them from their shells. For superior flavor and nutrition, seek out truly raw cashews from specialty raw food suppliers.

- **Raw hazelnuts**

- **Raw pecans**

- **Raw pine nuts**

- **Raw pistachios**

- **Raw walnuts**

SOAKING NUTS

Although I don't always take the time to do it, it's preferable, for a few reasons, to soak nuts in water and then drain and rinse them before pureeing. The soak-drain-rinse process makes nuts easier to digest and removes any bitter flavors without requiring the nuts to be roasted. In addition, soaked nuts become creamier than unsoaked nuts when pureed, giving you ultra-smooth nut milks, nut creams, and any number of sauces. I have the advantage of owning a powerful Vitamix blender, which allows me to skip this soaking step if I'm pressed for time (using a Vitamix, the texture of sauces and milks made with unsoaked nuts is almost as creamy and smooth as when using soaked nuts). However, please note that it is especially important to soak nuts if a recipe calls for pureeing nuts and you don't have a high-speed blender or you're using a food processor.

The amount of time needed for soaking depends on how dense the nut is. Harder nuts, such as almonds, hazelnuts, and pistachios, are best soaked for four to eight hours. Medium-hard nuts, such as Brazil nuts, pecans, and walnuts, only need to soak for two to four hours. Soft nuts, such as cashews, macadamia nuts, and pine nuts, don't have skins and therefore don't contain phytic acid, so they require less soaking time; in fact, soaking these types of nuts too long can reduce their health-promoting oils. One to two hours is about all that is needed for cashews and macadamia nuts; thirty minutes will do the job for pine nuts. You can soak any medium-hard or hard nuts overnight if that is more convenient, but keep in mind that the more waterlogged the nuts become, the less liquid you will need in a recipe that uses them.

Frozen Fruits & Vegetables

Although many health enthusiasts shun frozen produce for fresh, the cold truth is that frozen fruits and veggies can sometimes be even more nutritious than fresh. Frozen produce is picked at the peak of freshness and then flash-frozen, so nutrients are preserved. With fresh produce, on the other hand, the longer it sits on a supermarket shelf or spends time on a truck, the more its nutrient content declines. So don't feel bad about using frozen fruits and vegetables. However, do keep in mind that not all fruits and vegetables freeze well. The following are the ones I use.

Frozen Fruits

- **Bananas.** Once the bananas on the counter start to get too soft to eat, I peel and slice them and freeze them in zip-top bags for use in smoothies and ice creams.

- **Blueberries.** My favorite is wild blueberries, for both their taste and their incredibly high antioxidant content. (See Resources, page 403, for my favorite brands.)

- **Cherries**

- **Cranberries.** Instead of ice cubes, I pop frozen cranberries in water for extra flavor and vitamin C!

- **Strawberries.** Perfect for smoothies! Once defrosted, they have an undesirable mushy texture, so I only use them frozen.

- **Unsweetened pureed acai packets.** This Amazonian superfood is a great source of omega-fats and is loaded with antioxidants. It's perfect for smoothies and breakfast bowls. (See Resources, page 403, for my favorite brands.)

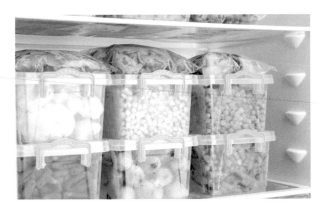

Frozen Vegetables

- **Artichoke hearts.** I drizzle olive oil on still-frozen artichokes and roast them at 400°F for 25 minutes—delicious!

- **Broccoli florets**

- **Cauliflower florets and riced cauliflower**

- **Chopped greens** (kale, broccoli rabe, collards, and spinach)

- **Cubed or pureed butternut squash**

- **Edamame**

- **Mixed vegetables.** One of my son's favorite after-school snacks when he was little was frozen mixed vegetables, steamed and topped with a little pat of grass-fed butter. He still eats it to this day.

- **Petite green peas**

- **Sweet corn**

Miscellaneous

- **Almond tortillas** (See Resources, page 398, for my favorite brands.)

- **Coconut-based ice cream** (See Resources, page 403, for my favorite brands.)

- **Sprouted corn tortillas** (See Resources, page 398, for my favorite brands.)

- **Sprouted whole-grain bread.** There are good gluten-free and non-gluten-free options. See Resources, page 399, for my favorite brands of both types.

- **Veggie burgers** (See Resources, page 403, for my favorite brands.)

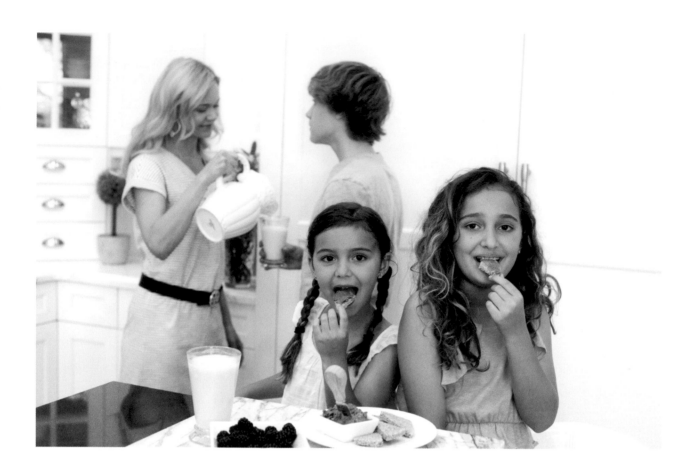

in the fridge

Finally we get to the fridge. Whenever someone comes to our house and hears about Clean Cuisine, the first thing they want to do is take a peek inside the fridge! This is what they would find.

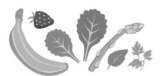

Fresh Fruits, Vegetables & Herbs

Depending on what's in season and what I have planned for our weekly meals, the produce in our fridge varies, but some things are always in there. We eat a salad with our meal almost every night, so I keep a wide assortment of greens on hand.

(Just as with grains, I rotate our greens so we don't eat the same ones day after day.) I also keep fresh garlic, ginger, scallions, onions, lemons, limes, red and green bell peppers, carrots (both whole and shredded), and celery on hand at all times. I buy other fresh vegetables, such as beets, broccoli, asparagus, green beans, squash, and corn, based on what I plan to cook that week. And I keep lots of different olives on hand.

And we always have fresh fruit galore! Depending on the fruit, I'll store some in the fridge and some on the kitchen counter. I buy different fruits depending on what I plan to make that week, but I always have bananas, apples, berries, oranges, and grapes in the house. I buy other fruits, such as peaches, kiwis, pineapples, and cherries, depending on what's in season and what looks good at the store.

Finally, you'll always find at least three different types of fresh herbs in our fridge. I use basil, parsley, and cilantro the most, but I love all fresh herbs, including rosemary, mint, sage, and thyme.

TO PEEL OR NOT TO PEEL

In general, I try to keep the skin on as many fruits and vegetables as I can. That's because the peels are packed with antioxidants, vitamins, and fiber. For example, about one-third of the nutrients in an apple—such as vitamin C, vitamin A, and potassium—can be found in the peel. And as a rule, peels and rinds generally make up around half of a fruit's overall fiber content. So I make foods like mashed potatoes and apple pie without peeling my potatoes or apples. As an added bonus, it saves time too! But that doesn't mean you should eat orange peels, for instance. Use your best judgment: if the fruit or vegetable has a tough exterior, you may be better off peeling it, especially if a smooth texture is desired. For example, when making no-milk shakes and "whole" juices, where smooth texture is what you want, I peel cucumbers. Of course, if you really can't stand eating apples with skins on, then you are better off eating a peeled apple than no apple at all!

Assuming they're organic and grown without pesticides, here is a list of fruits and vegetables that I generally don't bother peeling:

Apples	Nectarines	Potatoes
Cucumbers	Pears	Summer squash
Eggplant	Plums	Zucchini

But if a fruit or vegetable is not organic and is on the "Dirty Dozen" list (see page 64)—and therefore may contain a lot of pesticides—I'll peel it. Unfortunately, research shows that peeling (and washing) alone is not enough to eliminate pesticides, which can penetrate into the underlying flesh of the fruit or vegetable. Just another reason to buy organic whenever possible!

Dairy Alternatives

- **Almond-based yogurt** (See Resources, page 403, for my favorite brands.)

- **Almond milk.** See page 368 for my homemade almond milk recipe. If you're using store-bought, make sure it's unflavored and unsweetened.

- **Nut cheese** (See Resources, page 403, for my favorite brands.)

- **Plain, unsweetened hemp milk.** Look for one that does not contain carrageenan, a common food additive that has been linked to inflammation and stomach problems. (See Resources, page 403, for my favorite brand.)

Plant-Based Proteins

- **Extra-firm and silken tofu** (See Resources, page 403, for my favorite brands.)

- **Tempeh.** A fermented soy food that is rich in probiotics, tempeh is also an excellent source of plant protein and contains high levels of vitamins B_2, B_3, B_5, and B_6. (See Resources, page 403, for my favorite brands.)

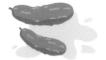

Fermented Favorites

Naturally fermented foods are an excellent source of probiotics. Just one or two small servings of these foods each day will improve digestion, enhance nutrient assimilation, and boost immunity. Plus, their delicious tangy taste adds a burst of flavor to meals.

- **Chickpea miso.** This has a much milder flavor than soy-based miso. (See Resources, page 403, for my favorite brands.)

- **Dill pickles.** Look for naturally fermented pickles in the refrigerated section of your supermarket. (See Resources, page 403, for my favorite brands.)

- **Fermented vegetables.** My favorites are carrots and radishes. (See Resources, page 403, for my favorite brands.)

- **Kimchi.** A spicy, probiotic-rich pickled cabbage, kimchi adds umami to a variety of foods. It's especially good with grilled chicken. (See Resources, page 403, for my favorite brands.)

- **Kombucha.** A naturally fermented sparkling beverage that is loaded with probiotics. (See Resources, page 403, for my favorite brands.)

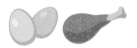

Pasture-Raised Eggs & Chicken

More than 90 percent of US eggs come from caged hens. These birds have a space smaller than a sheet of paper to move around in, and they live in filthy conditions—and unsurprisingly, they (and their eggs) aren't as nutritious as hens raised on pasture.

Pastured hens live outside, where they can do what hens naturally do: roam free and forage for bugs and grass. Studies have found that pastured hens have more vitamins and omega-3 fats than caged hens. Eggs from pastured hens contain twice as much vitamin E and almost three times more omega-3 fats than eggs from caged birds.

In an ideal world, you would purchase your eggs and chicken from a local farm where you could see the chickens roaming on pasture. Your second-best bet is to buy them from a natural foods store where they are clearly labeled "pastured" or "pasture-raised." "Free-range" and "free-roaming" are not as good because the chickens aren't guaranteed any specific amount of time outdoors. Unfortunately, there is no third-party inspection for the use of any of these labels.

USDA-certified organic chickens and their eggs do have third-party inspection, and they are offered access to the outdoors, though that doesn't mean they actually ever go outside. They are, however, fed certified organic feed and are free of antibiotics. But organic is still not as good as pasture-raised.

Ultimately, your best bet is to try to find out exactly where your chicken and eggs come from and what they eat. (See Resources, page 403, for the brand of organic, pasture-raised eggs we buy. They are nationally distributed.)

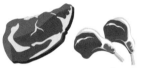

Pasture-Raised Meat

We talked earlier in this chapter about how important an animal's diet is in determining whether a food is healthful (see page 65). Look for 100 percent grass-fed, pasture-raised meats, including beef, lamb, and bison. (We choose not to eat pork because the natural diet of a pig would not be considered "clean food.")

In addition, look for the leanest cuts of meats. Just like humans, animals store toxins in their fat, so if an animal has been exposed to antibiotics, pesticides, exogenous hormones, fungicides, or other dangerous compounds, most of that toxic residue will be found in the animal's fat. (Even if an animal is 100 percent pasture-raised and organic, it will still store toxins in its fat.) For that reason, and because we are trying to limit our consumption of animal-based saturated fat, I always choose the absolute leanest cuts of meat and trim any visible animal fat before cooking. (Kitchen shears make snipping fat a snap!)

EGG WHITE OMELETS ARE NOT ALL THEY ARE CRACKED UP TO BE

Eggs are a nutrient-dense food that happen to also be low in saturated fat. One large egg has just 70 calories and 1.5 grams of saturated fat, and you get a lot of nutrient bang for your paltry calorie buck. In fact, one whole egg has way more to offer nutritionally than 70 calories of chicken. And most of those nutrients are found in the yolk!

Here are just a select few of the nutrients you will get when you eat the whole egg, not just the egg white:

- **Vitamin D:** An anti-inflammatory nutrient that's associated with decreased risk of cancer and heart disease. Importantly, vitamin D is not readily available in many foods other than eggs and fatty fish (the vitamin D in dairy foods is added artificially).

- **Omega-3 fats**

- Lutein: An incredible antioxidant, especially for eye health. Lutein is much better absorbed from egg yolks than from supplements or even spinach.

- Choline: An essential micronutrient that reduces inflammation and supports cardiovascular health and brain function.

- Lecithin: A nutrient that helps the body digest fat and cholesterol.

- **Vitamin A**

- **Vitamin K$_2$:** An important fat-soluble vitamin that plays a critical role in bone and heart health. Pastured eggs are among its very few readily available sources.

Some people are concerned about eating eggs because of their high amounts of cholesterol. But this is a needless concern for several reasons. First, the level of cholesterol in your blood has little to do with cholesterol in the food you eat. The vast majority of blood cholesterol is made by your liver. Second, there is little evidence that dietary cholesterol is a cause of atherosclerosis, heart disease, or stroke. In fact, a large study involving 188,000 people showed those who ate five or six whole eggs a week actually had less heart disease than those who ate less than one egg per week.

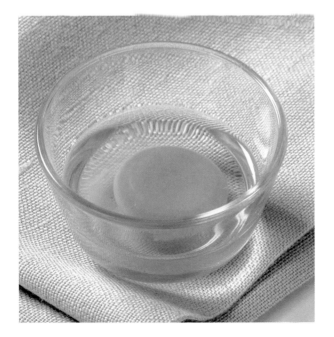

ALLERGIC TO EGGS?

As much as we love eggs, they are one of the "big eight" foods that people are most allergic to. (The others are dairy milk, fish, shellfish, tree nuts, peanuts, wheat, and soy.) If you have an egg allergy or even a sensitivity, here are two ways to replace them in a baked-good recipe, such as for a cake or muffins.

To replace 1 large egg:

Whisk 1 teaspoon chia seeds with ¼ cup water. Set the mixture aside for 15 minutes, or until thickened.

OR

Whisk 1 tablespoon ground flax seeds with ¼ cup water. Set the mixture aside for 5 to 10 minutes, until thickened.

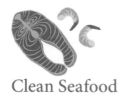

Clean Seafood

The romance associated with a fisherman's life—a life on the sea filled with excitement and peril—has, for the most part, been replaced by fish farms. The reality is there just aren't enough fish in the sea to keep up with demand, so about half the seafood consumed around the world today comes from fish farms.

Unfortunately, farmed seafood can be inferior in taste to wild fish, and the nutritional value is often compromised.

Just like factory-farmed cattle, fish in farms are given antibiotics and other drugs. Then there's the concern about what the fish are eating. Again, just like cattle, if fish don't eat the foods they would naturally consume in the wild, then the fish are not going to be healthy. For example, nature did not intend salmon to be fed soy, poultry litter, and hydrolyzed chicken feathers. As a result of this deviant diet, farmed salmon is lower in vitamin D,

lower in anti-inflammatory omega-3 fats, higher in pro-inflammatory omega-6 fats, higher in saturated fat, and higher in overall contaminants and toxins. It's also disturbing that farmed salmon would be gray in color if it weren't for pink chemical dye. (I feel it is absolutely worth the extra cost for wild salmon, but for a more budget-friendly option, go for sockeye salmon, which is often sold in cans; it cannot be farmed.)

Two other unsettling fishy facts are that only 5 percent of the farmed seafood eaten in the United States comes from domestic fish farms, and only 2 percent of the imported fish consumed in the United States is inspected in this country. Not only does importing seafood leave a big carbon footprint, but most of imported seafood is sourced from locations where health, safety, and environmental standards for raising and catching fish are weak or nonexistent.

Despite all this, we haven't totally ruled out eating farmed fish because it can be safe when done properly. We buy our farmed fish from Cod and Capers (www.codandcapers.com) because we know they set the bar high for quality standards. (See Resources, page 403, for more information.)

WHAT ABOUT THE MERCURY IN SEAFOOD?

While it's absolutely important to be careful not to consume too much mercury, many people avoid seafood altogether because of the mercury concern, and this is going too far. Multiple studies have proven beyond a doubt that fish eaters live longer and suffer fewer heart attacks than people who do not eat fish. Additionally, accumulating evidence suggests that the danger to the fetus of mercury from fish has been overstated, while the danger from missing out on vital omega-3 fats—abundant in fish—has been understated. The largest scientific study performed to date has specifically shown there to be no harmful relationship between either prenatal or postnatal mercury exposure and developmental outcomes in either five-year-olds or nine-year-olds. In these studies, pregnant women ate on average twelve servings of fish weekly. However, there were developmental problems among the children of women who had low levels of omega-3s and high levels of omega-6s during pregnancy. We also know that the effect of ingested mercury by pregnant women from all sources—not just fish—appears to result in a lowering of the child's IQ by less than one point. The effect of an omega-3 deficiency as a result of avoiding fish is far more dramatic: a drop of five or six IQ points.

You can lower your mercury levels over time (it takes months, unfortunately) by avoiding shark, swordfish, king mackerel, and tilefish, all of which have unacceptably high levels of mercury. It's definitely best to choose low-mercury seafood, such as wild salmon, shrimp, sardines, scallops, trout, crab, and haddock—but don't avoid seafood altogether just to avoid mercury.

If you buy farmed fish, make sure you get it from a reputable place and ask the fishmonger what the fish ate and where it swam.

The big picture, of course, is that fish is an important part of a healthy clean diet. People who consume fish on a regular basis have lower risks of cancers of the pancreas, colon, thyroid, and prostate. And it is interesting to note that three populations who consume fish at least three times per week, the Okinawans, Japanese, and Inuit, have very low incidence of breast cancer. Fish consumption is even associated with enhanced weight loss when dieting, and studies on omega-3 fat consumption have linked low fish intake to an increased incidence of depression, bipolar disorder, postpartum depression, and other mood disorders.

Taking all this into consideration, we are left with the question of which fish to eat. Below are some simple guidelines you can follow to choose the best fish. You should also know that the toxin content of many fish depends on size: bigger fish have more toxins, so it's better to eat smaller fish. Sardines and anchovies are particularly good choices because these small fish are not only low in toxins but also rich in omega-3 fat. Here are the guidelines I follow for choosing fish:

- **Go for small, low-mercury fish** (see the sidebar on page 86).

- **Choose local over imported**.

- **Choose wild over farmed fish when possible.**

- **If you do choose farmed fish, find out how it was farmed**—find out where the fish were raised and what they ate.

- **If you are lucky enough to live near the coast, buy locally caught wild fish.**

- **Look for the blue label of the Marine Stewardship Council**, the world's leading certification and ecolabeling program for sustainable seafood.

- **Avoid fish labeled "fresh from frozen"**; it may look fresh, but the taste and texture will have been compromised. Sometimes these fish sit for days before selling.

- **For the best-tasting fish, buy fresh fish from a reputable source.** Frozen fish can also be a good option—many fish are frozen on the boat just minutes after being caught.

- **Avoid fish that have been given antibiotics and added growth hormones.**

- **Avoid fish that have been given feed that contains poultry or mammalian by-products.**

- **Avoid fish that contain preservatives** such as sodium bisulfite, sodium tri-polyphosphate (STP), and sodium metabisulfite.

- **Prepare your fish healthfully!** If you drown your fish in béarnaise sauce or fry it in vegetable oil, you might as well eat a hamburger.

- **Go for quality over quantity.** A total of three to five modest servings per week provides essentially all of the health benefits, so you don't need much.

- **If ordering fish or seafood online, be sure to order from a reputable company** that sells wild, sustainably caught and/or ethical and environmentally friendly farm-raised fish. (See Resources, page 403, for our suggested online sources for seafood.)

kitchen tools and equipment

Ivy again. I can't walk past culinary stores like Williams Sonoma or Sur La Table without wandering in, but I rarely come out with a purchase. (Unless it's a cookbook—my home office is filled to the brim with cookbooks that I have been collecting for almost twenty years now!) I'm just not big on buying every new culinary gadget and gizmo that hits the shelves. However, there are some kitchen essentials that I just couldn't do without; those are described in this chapter.

To come up with the list, I went through my kitchen with a fine-tooth comb. It may look like a lot of items at first, but if you were to come to my kitchen, you would see that it's not at all overstuffed. It does, however, take a bit of time to accumulate everything. If you are just starting to stock your kitchen with appliances and gadgets, my best advice is to save up and invest in the best-quality products. Trust me, in the long run it will save you money. Cheap tools, gadgets, and appliances just never last.

clean cooking starts with green cookware

Many people don't realize that the cookware they use may be leaching toxins into their food. Perfluorooctanoic acid (PFOA), a carcinogen, is widely used in the production of nonstick cookware, and when nonstick cookware is heated to a high temperature or scratched, it can enter food. The use of nonstick cookware could be one reason PFOA can be found in the bloodstreams of 95 percent of American men, women, and children. Other unsafe nonstick cookware is made using polytetrafluoroethylene (PTFE), which deteriorates when the cookware is heated to high temperatures and emits dangerous gases that have been linked to flulike symptoms in humans. For this reason, the only nonstick cookware I use is a crepe pan, and I'm careful to choose a nontoxic, eco-friendly one. Green Pan is a good brand.

Aluminum, which is used in over half of all cookware, is another concern, as some studies have shown that when heated in contact with an acid (like tomato sauce), potentially dangerous aluminum salts can leach into the food.

Finding a Super-Green Pot to Cook In

Let's face it: healthy living and green product lines have become big business. From skincare products to soaps, detergents, and cookware, many products are sold as "green," but that doesn't necessarily mean they are. Sadly, there are no universal standards that have to be met before a product can be called "green."

I have tried all sorts of green cookware over the years, including stainless steel, cast iron, and even copper. All of them have presented some sort of problem. The one I have found to be the "greenest," as well as the most versatile, is 100 percent ceramic. It's nonscratch, nonreactive, and nontoxic. Foods cooked in ceramic cookware even taste better, because they are free from the heavy metals and toxins that can leach out of other cookware and distort the taste of the food. Ceramic cookware is also incredibly versatile and can be used on the stovetop, oven, broiler, and even the microwave. And I can't help but mention how easy ceramic is to clean! The only downside to ceramic cookware is that it is more fragile than other types of cookware and so must be handled appropriately. (Don't worry—if you follow the manufacturer's care instructions, your ceramic ware will last a lifetime.) My favorite brand of 100 percent ceramic cookware is Xtrema by Ceramcor. I use both their skillet and saucepan.

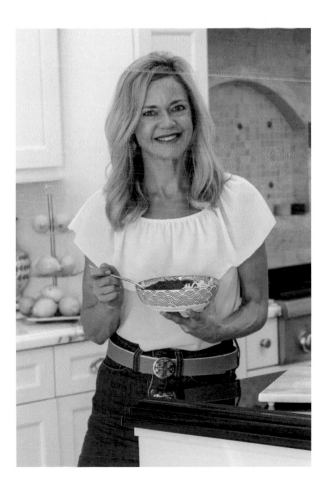

Other Options

My second and third choices are enameled cast iron and stainless steel.

Enameled cast iron is absolutely beautiful with its decorative colors and glossy finishes, but it's not cheap, and not all enamels are created the same. Check for the presence of heavy metals like lead and cadmium in enamel glazes before purchasing. My favorite brand of enameled cast iron is Le Creuset.

Stainless steel is actually a mixture of several different metals, including nickel, chromium, and molybdenum, all of which can trickle into foods from cookware. The upside to stainless steel is that it is extremely long-lasting and won't rust, chip, or break. You can reduce the leaching potential of stainless steel by not using it to cook acidic foods, such as tomato sauce.

Finally, I have to mention cast-iron cookware. Every serious cook should own at least one cast-iron skillet. It will last a lifetime if cared for properly, it can go from stovetop to oven, it's a great heat conductor, and when well seasoned, it is super easy to clean. I can't emphasize enough the importance of having a thick seasoning on your cast-iron skillet, though. Not only does it protect food from sticking to the pan and burning, but it also prevents too much iron from leaching into your food. Excess iron can increase free-radical formation and raise the risks of heart disease, cancer, and accelerated aging. Iron can also cause fat to become rancid faster, so it is not a good choice for high-heat cooking. Although it is not my most frequently used cookware, I do use my cast-iron skillet for moderate-heat cooking.

If you are going to use cast iron, then the most important thing to do is to season it periodically by coating it inside and out with extra-virgin coconut oil and then heating it in a 200°F oven for at least an hour. Seasoning your skillet will make the cooking surface of your pan nonstick, and if you don't season it, the surface will rust every time you wash the skillet.

kitchen essentials

Bakeware

- Glass baking dishes or ceramic casseroles in several sizes: 8-inch square, 9-inch square, 9 by 13-inch
- 8-inch square baking pan
- 9 by 5-inch loaf pan
- 9-inch springform pan
- 9-inch glass or ceramic pie plate
- Ramekins in several sizes: 4-, 6-, and 8-ounce
- Two or three 17 by 12-inch baking sheets, both rimmed and unrimmed
- Muffin tins: standard-size, ½-cup capacity (with 12 wells), and mini, 2-tablespoon capacity (with 24 wells)
- Four individual-sized pizza stones (optional)
- Standard-size donut pan (needed for the recipe on page 112 but otherwise optional)

Blender

I highly recommend you invest in a high-powered blender. They puree ingredients to an ultrasmooth consistency in a matter of moments—even hard or fibrous ingredients, like almonds, cashews, whole garlic cloves, and whole dates.

If you do not own a high-powered blender, a regular blender will work for most uses, and for hard and fibrous ingredients, there are some work-arounds: soak medium-hard or hard raw nuts in water to soften them first (see page 80), and coarsely chop any whole and/or fibrous ingredients, like garlic cloves, fresh ginger, and whole dates, before adding them to the blender. But even with these steps, the result won't be quite as good as it would be with a high-powered blender.

A food processor can be a good alternative to a high-powered blender, just as long as the mixture doesn't need to be too thin (it's not a good idea for shakes or soup, for example).

Mixing Bowls
Having a set of lightweight stainless-steel mixing bowls makes it easy to choose the right size.

Box Grater
A sturdy four-sided grater is the best tool for shredding vegetables. This is also the tool I use for grating citrus zest, using the side with the smallest holes.

Colander
Use a 12-inch colander for draining noodles, greens, and vegetables.

Cutting Boards
Science has validated what many cooks have intuitively known for years: wood is the best surface for cutting. Wooden cutting boards don't dull the blades of your knives like most synthetic materials do, and they're also the most hygienic. Bacteria cannot thrive on natural, untreated wood, while plastic and polyethylene boards breed bacteria and require bleach to keep clean.

Electric Mixer
I use a handheld electric mixer, but many people prefer stand mixers. Either one will get the job done, but a well-stocked kitchen does need an electric mixer.

Food Processor
I have both a large (11-cup) food processor and a mini (3½-cup) one.

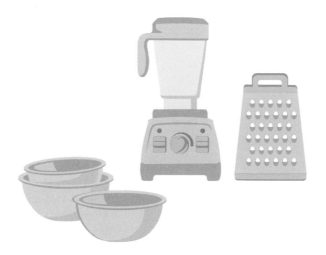

A HIGH-POWERED BLENDER WILL CHANGE YOUR LIFE

Lenore Pinello, the owner of In the Kitchen, my favorite culinary shop in the Palm Beach area, introduced me to Vitamix's high-powered blender in 2009. I was preparing to teach a cooking class at her store, and we had only about 20 minutes before the class was scheduled to begin when I realized I was missing the soy milk I had planned to use in my Grand Marnier chocolate mousse. Lenore suggested I try blending raw cashews and water in the store's Vitamix as a substitute. That suggestion not only saved the day, it completely changed my life in the kitchen. A high-powered blender enables me to make completely dairy-free recipes by pureeing all different types of nuts with water, with zero sacrifice in taste or texture. I also am able to puree dates and other dried fruits (such as prunes, apricots, and pineapple) to use as a sweetener in baked goods, smoothies, pies, custards, and more. I simply would not be able to maintain the nutritional integrity of our recipes and actually make them taste good were it not for a high-powered blender.

I know a high-powered blender can be a pricey purchase, but after using one for almost a decade, I can assure you it is worth every penny. As for which one to buy, I stand firmly by the Vitamix. If you are on a tight budget, consider purchasing a reconditioned Vitamix at about a 25 percent discount. The Vitamix certified reconditioned series is backed by a five-year warranty plus a thirty-day guarantee.

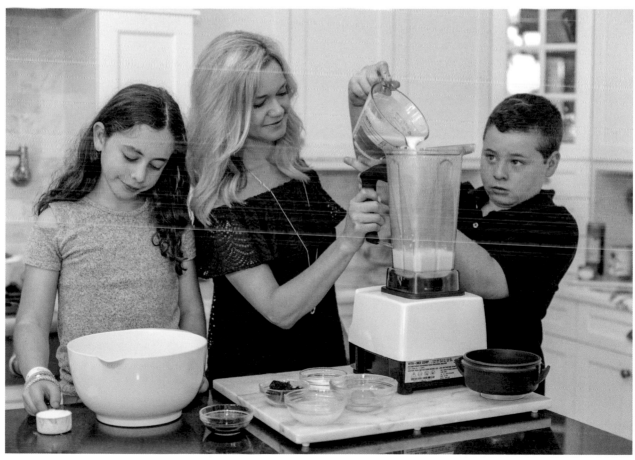

Handheld Stick Blender
(aka Immersion Blender)

This tool is for pureeing soups directly in the pot. I also use it to make mashed cauliflower, sauces, and more. If you do not own a handheld stick blender, you can easily use a jar blender for the same purpose. However, if you're blending something hot, like soup, allow it to cool slightly and blend it in several batches so as not to overfill the blender jar.

Ice Cream Maker

If I were on a tight budget, then an ice cream maker would be one of the last items on my "to buy" list. However, they're certainly nice to have, and you'll need one to make the Key Lime Pie Ice Cream recipe on page 334. Ice cream makers have come a long way, and you can get a superior-quality one for less than $60. I highly recommend the Cuisinart Classic Frozen Yogurt, Ice Cream, and Sorbet Maker, which is perfect for making homemade ice cream in quart-sized portions.

Kitchen Timer

I suppose you could use your smartphone instead, but I still like a good old-fashioned kitchen timer.

Knives

I can't emphasize enough the importance of having a good knife collection. A properly sharpened knife will make your life in the kitchen so much easier and more enjoyable. Knives forged from carbon steel are excellent, but they can rust and stain. Stainless-steel knives will not rust or stain, but they are difficult to sharpen and tend to dull rather quickly. Most chefs use knives made from high-carbon steel, a blend of carbon steel and stainless steel that gives a great sharp edge without the rust.

There are really just four knives that are essential:

- 2- or 3-inch paring knife, for delicate slicing, peeling, and garnishing

- 4- to 6-inch knife with a fine serrated edge, for slicing acidic foods like tomatoes and citrus fruits, which tend to dull straight-edged blades

- 8-inch heavy, all-purpose chef's knife, for most cutting, chopping, and mincing jobs

- 10-inch serrated bread knife

Knife Sharpener

It doesn't make much sense to invest in great knives if they are not kept sharp. A properly maintained knife will make cutting, slicing, and dicing so much more enjoyable. And believe it or not, a super-sharp blade is much safer, since dull knives will not glide through the fibers and tissues of food without some degree of force. I like the manual Chef'sChoice ProntoPro Diamond Hone Knife Sharpener No. 4643.

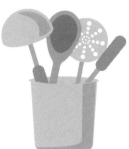

Ladles

It's good to have several sizes of wooden and metal ladles. A 6- to 8-ounce ladle is good for soups and stews, while a 2- to 4-ounce ladle is useful for sauces.

Measuring Cups and Spoons

Look for heavy-duty dry measuring cups and spoons and 1-, 2-, and 4-cup glass measuring cups for liquids.

Parchment Paper

Parchment paper is indispensable; I use it all the time. It's perfect for lining baking sheets because you don't have to grease the pan and cleanup is a breeze. I often use a layer of parchment paper between aluminum foil and food to prevent the aluminum from having direct contact with the acids in the food.

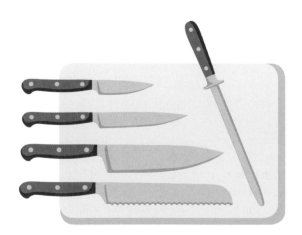

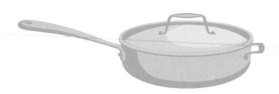

Pots and Pans

Good-quality heavy-bottomed pots and pans are essential. My list of pots and pans includes:

- 7- to 10-inch slope-sided skillet with cover
- 10-inch nonstick skillet (for making crepes, page 118)
- 8- to 10-inch cast-iron skillet
- 10-inch sauté pan with lid (3-quart capacity)
- 1-quart saucepan with lid
- 2-quart saucepan with lid
- 3-quart enameled cast-iron or ceramic pot, for making soups and stews
- 4-quart ovenproof earthenware casserole dish with lid, for baking and oven braising
- 5-quart Dutch oven, for making slow-cooked dishes, soups, and more
- 8-quart stockpot with steamer insert

Rubber Spatula

No tool will empty a bowl or pot more effectively than a rubber spatula. Not to be confused with a plastic spatula, which is brittle, a rubber spatula is heat resistant and extremely flexible. Delicate batters are best folded together gently with a rubber spatula.

Slow Cooker

As a set-it-and-forget-it way to cook, a slow cooker is a must-have for my kitchen. However, just like pots and pans, not all of the inserts in slow cookers are "clean." In fact, most slow cooker manufacturers do not conduct third-party testing for heavy metals on their glazed ceramic inserts. The safest slow cooker is one with a clay pot insert. Clay is free of both heavy metals and flame retardants. My favorite slow cooker brand is VitaClay (which is actually a multicooker with steaming and yogurt-making capabilities).

Spiral Slicer

Many supermarkets now offer vegetables already spiral-sliced into noodles, so a spiral slicer may not be a necessity. However, fresh is still best. I love my Spiralizer 5-Blade Vegetable Slicer, which is incredibly durable. It's also not very pricey. You should be able to pick one up for around $25.

Wooden Spoons

Unlike metal spoons, smooth wooden spoons feel good in your hands, and since they don't transfer heat as metal does, their handles stay cool. Spoons made of metal tend to have thin, straight edges that can tear and bruise delicate foods as well as damage the surfaces of stainless-steel and enamel-coated pots and pans.

Glass Storage Containers

We are big on leftovers, so I keep a variety of 1-cup, 1-quart, and 2-quart glass storage containers with tight-fitting lids.

Tongs

Spring-action stainless-steel tongs give you great dexterity when handling hot foods. They are perfect for plucking herb sprigs and bay leaves from simmering stews and for turning roasted and grilled vegetables. The 8- to 10-inch tongs are the easiest size to use.

Vegetable Peeler

Look for a carbon-steel swivel peeler; stainless-steel peelers tend to dull quickly.

Whisks

Stainless-steel whisks are used to smooth and homogenize mixtures such as vinaigrettes, sauces, and polenta. They are also great for combining dry ingredients for batters and doughs.

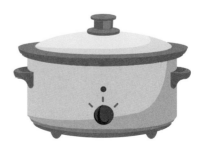

clean cuisine meals

We have tried our best to make the recipes in this book not only easy to follow, no matter your cooking experience, but also as modifiable as possible for people with a wide variety of food restrictions. If you need to avoid a certain food or you follow a specific diet regimen (such as Paleo), hopefully this section will answer any questions you may have and help make using this book easier and more enjoyable!

what you won't find in the recipes

All of the recipes in this book are gluten-free. Every recipe is also dairy-free. That's right—no butter, milk, cheese, or cream. Not a single recipe contains a refined ingredient, either. That means no refined oils, no refined flours, nothing processed.

When possible, we've included ingredient substitutions or omissions to make the recipes suitable for as many eating styles and dietary requirements as possible. Whether you are Paleo, vegan, or a "flexitarian" who is somewhere in between, there should be plenty of recipes in this book that will work for you.

what you will find in every recipe: a fruit, vegetable, and/or superfood

When developing recipes, our biggest goals (aside from making a dish that tastes delicious!) are to have an exceptionally high nutrient-to-calorie ratio and to incorporate a wide variety of phytonutrient-rich ingredients that have intrinsic healing and detoxifying properties.

All of the recipes in this book have a definite "plant slant." That means you will find an abundance of unrefined whole plant foods, such as nuts, seeds, vegetables, beans, whole grains, legumes, and fruits, worked into the recipes in each and every chapter—including the cocktails and desserts! But in addition, we've made sure that every recipe has at least one fruit, vegetable, or superfood, each of which can be considered a nutritional booster. Adding more nutritionally dense fruits, vegetables, and superfoods to your recipes not only reduces inflammation but also helps optimize the overall nutrient, antioxidant, and fiber content of the dish.

what makes it a "clean cuisine" recipe?

Since our way of eating does not fit into any popular diet categories, it's helpful to have an at-a-glance overview of what constitutes a Clean Cuisine recipe. First and foremost, our recipes are based on unrefined whole foods in their most natural and nutrient-rich state.

Even though we are not vegan, many of the recipes have no animal foods at all. Whether vegan or not, all the recipes are rich in plant-based foods (especially from nutrient-dense fruits and vegetables), with animal foods used in moderation. Fish and seafood are the exception to the Clean Cuisine reduced-animal-food guideline; the consumption of these omega-3-rich foods is encouraged.

At first glance, the recipes might not appear to be as plant-rich as they really are, but once you look closely at the ingredients, you'll see that the ratio of vegetables to meat is much greater than in traditional recipes. For example, our burger recipe on page 188 sneaks in a full 2½ cups of vegetables. (But keep in mind that meat-based meals are always served with a great big salad and extra vegetables, too. The meat is never the main attraction on our dinner plate.)

With few exceptions, Clean Cuisine recipes all have the following features:

- Rich in vitamins and minerals, plant phytonutrients, and antioxidants

- Anti-inflammatory

- Exceptionally rich in fruits and vegetables

- Abundant in unrefined whole foods

- Free of refined, omega-6-rich vegetable oils (corn oil, soybean oil, canola oil, etc.)

- Rich in fiber

- Dairy-free

- Gluten-free

- Free of refined sugar, refined flour, and trans fats

- Optimally balanced between omega-6 and omega-3 fats

- Low in animal-based saturated fat

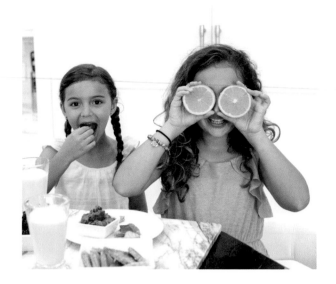

clean remakes of classic favorites

You won't find exotic or ultra-imaginative recipes in this book. Instead, we have taken classic favorites and cleaned them up. For example, in a cake recipe, cassava flour might be used instead of refined all-purpose flour. Or maybe we've snuck in extra vegetables, fruits, and superfoods. But even though the ingredients used to make the recipes might not all be conventional ones, you will probably be familiar with just about every dish in the book.

This book is meant to be an everyday, family-friendly cookbook, not a special-occasion or gourmet cookbook. I have a collection of literally hundreds of cookbooks, and the ones I use most frequently are the ones that have basic recipes. My hope is that even if you just learn how to clean up a handful of your favorite classics, this cookbook will be worthy of a spot on your shelf, and that you will reach for it again and again (fingers crossed!).

You may be wondering why we don't include nutrition facts with our recipes. One big reason is that nutrition facts can be very misleading—while they include a breakdown of the macronutrients (carbohydrate, fat, and protein), they tell you nothing about the nutritional quality of each, if it's from an unhealthy processed or refined food or from a nutritious whole food. Nutrition facts don't even distinguish between saturated fat from plants and saturated fat from animals.

Also, we don't encourage restricting calories, eating "low carb" or "low fat," or tallying up carbohydrate, fat, and protein grams. Counting calories, carbs, fat grams, points, or anything else overly complicates things. In fact, we don't even encourage reading the nutrition facts on packaged foods. (We do, however, encourage reading the list of ingredients.)

Another serious issue we have with the nutrition facts is that they encourage the idea that all foods are okay in moderation. We don't agree. And we aren't the only ones dispelling the conventional wisdom to simply eat everything in moderation. One study published in the prestigious *New England Journal of Medicine* showed that some foods clearly cause people to put on more weight than others. The foods that cause the most weight gain are the ones that have the most calories with the fewest nutrients—french fries, potato chips, sugary drinks, sweets. It should be no surprise that the foods that cause the most weight loss are the ones with the most nutrients per calorie, all of which happen to be anti-inflammatory—nuts, whole grains, fruits, and vegetables.

In the lab, there is no difference between 500 calories of carrots and 500 calories of carrot cake. But don't be fooled. Carrots and carrot cake are absorbed into the bloodstream at completely different rates and have totally different amounts of nutrients, fiber, antioxidants, carbohydrates, fat, and protein, all of which affect health, weight, oxidative stress, hunger, and metabolic rate. The more nutrients per calorie you eat, in this case by choosing carrots over carrot cake, the better protection you'll have against disease and the slower you'll age. You'll also weigh less and be less hungry. But reading the nutrition facts won't tell you much of this.

That's a long-winded explanation for why we don't include nutrition facts in our recipes. Here's the main point: try to make your food count nutritionally rather than count your food!

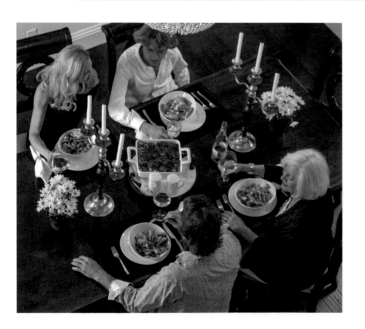

on meal planning

Just as we aren't into counting calories or monitoring nutrition facts, we aren't too big on following strict meal plans, either. We do plan our weekly dinner menus in advance just so we can do one big grocery shopping trip a week, but breakfast and lunch are rarely planned. However, we do follow a few basic meal-planning guidelines.

Breakfast

 Don't eat until you are hungry. (See page 44 for the benefits of waiting twelve hours between dinner and breakfast.)

 Add a fruit and/or vegetable. A rule of thumb: Add a fruit or vegetable serving that is just about equal in size to whatever else is on your plate. For example, if you're having waffles, eat one waffle plus a cup or so of fresh fruit.

 No animal foods other than eggs. The only reason for this is that it's a simple way to keep your plant-food intake high and reduce your animal-food intake without having to worry about portion sizes.

 Drink coffee with healthy additions. A 2002 study found that people who drink coffee have a reduced risk of dying from all causes. It's what you add to your coffee that can be problematic. Skip the sweetener if you can and use coconut cream instead of dairy cream—it doesn't have a coconutty flavor, and it delivers the same richness and creaminess as dairy cream. (See page 74 for more on coconut cream.) Of course tea is also a completely acceptable option.

Lunch

 No animal foods other than eggs. Just like at breakfast, this is a simple way to keep your plant food intake high and your animal-food intake low.

 Add some plant protein. In addition to whatever else you might be eating, include some beans, tofu, or nuts.

 Add a very big salad or one or two vegetables. It's important to get a big serving of greens once a day, even if it's as simple as raw greens drizzled with avocado oil and lemon juice. If you pick vegetables now, try to have a raw green salad at dinner.

 Have fruit for dessert. If you are still hungry after the main dish and want something sweet, then make fruit your go-to. Sometimes just a few bites of dried fruit can totally satisfy your sweet tooth.

 Drink water or tea.

Snack

 Don't eat if you are not hungry. It's never a good idea to eat when you are not hungry. Having said that, a lot of times a small snack later in the afternoon can be helpful, especially on workout days.

 Include a fruit and/or vegetable. Regardless of what the snack might be, try to work in a fruit or vegetable, or both—maybe simply an apple or pear or some carrot sticks with hummus.

 Drink water or tea.

Dinner

 Have a moderate-sized portion of fish, chicken, beef, or lamb. We have Meatless Monday, but otherwise, dinnertime is when we generally have our animal protein for the day. To get enough omega-3s, we try to have fatty fish or seafood at least three times a week.

 Drink a glass of organic natural wine. This is most definitely not something we recommend if you have any tendency to drink in excess. But if you're fine stopping after one glass, wine can enhance the flavor of your food, and organic natural wine has beneficial probiotics and prebiotics. (See page 44 for more.)

 Add a very big salad or one or two vegetables. Just like at lunch, add extra vegetables to your plate. If you didn't have one at lunch, have a large raw green salad with dinner. Otherwise, add vegetables for side dishes.

 Eat a small something sweet. It can be as simple as fresh fruit with a little bit of store-bought coconut-based ice cream (see Resources, page 403, for brand recommendations) or a small serving of a dessert recipe. None of our desserts have refined sugar, refined oil, dairy, or refined flour. #AlmostGuiltFree

 Drink water or tea.

how to use the recipes in this book

The recipes in this cookbook are pretty straightforward and none are particularly complicated. However, if you are new to both cooking and clean eating, it can be a lot to learn all at once. If you start to get frustrated, just remember what Julia Child said: "No one is born a great cook." But whether you are a seasoned chef or newbie, here are a few things to know about the recipes and how they're presented.

Yields
The recipe yield is stated at the top of each recipe. On average, they feed a family of four people, sometimes with leftovers.

Prep and Cook Times
The approximate prep and cook times are stated at the top of each recipe. Please note that when a recipe requires hands-off preparation time, such as the time to marinate meat or freeze something to allow it to set, that time is noted, as a friendly time-planning reminder, following the preparation time.

Please note that time to complete any required subrecipes (such as broth for a soup) is not factored into the prep and cook times.

Storage Information
You will find storage information, and sometimes reheating instructions, for recipes that are likely to leave you with leftovers, depending on the size of your household, as well as for those that make a fair number of multiples, like a muffin recipe, and those that are considered staples, like mayonnaise and salad dressing.

resources

At the back of the book, you'll find helpful information about recommended brands and places to find more information about clean eating. There's also a chart for food allergens and eating protocols for each recipe. It tells you whether a recipe is:

 BEAN-FREE (green beans and green peas allowed)

 DAIRY-FREE

 EGG-FREE

 GLUTEN-FREE

 GRAIN-FREE

 NUT-FREE

 PALEO-FRIENDLY (grain-free, gluten-free, dairy-free, and bean-free)

 SOY-FREE

 VEGAN

 VEGETARIAN

Additionally, many recipes have modifications to make them allergen or diet compliant. These are marked with an asterisk in the chart; look for the instructions for making the necessary modifications at the end of the recipe.

final thoughts

Finally, if you are new to clean eating, we strongly encourage you to read the first four chapters of this book before you begin cooking. This will give you the fundamental building blocks and nutritional goals behind Clean Cuisine. However, do keep in mind this is meant to be a cookbook, not a nutrition book. If you are looking for more in-depth information, including more of the science and research behind our recommendations, then we encourage you to visit our website, CleanCuisine.com, and/or read our book *Clean Cuisine: An 8-Week Anti-Inflammatory Nutrition Program That Will Change the Way You Age, Look, and Feel.*

But most of all, we encourage you to get cooking— and have fun!

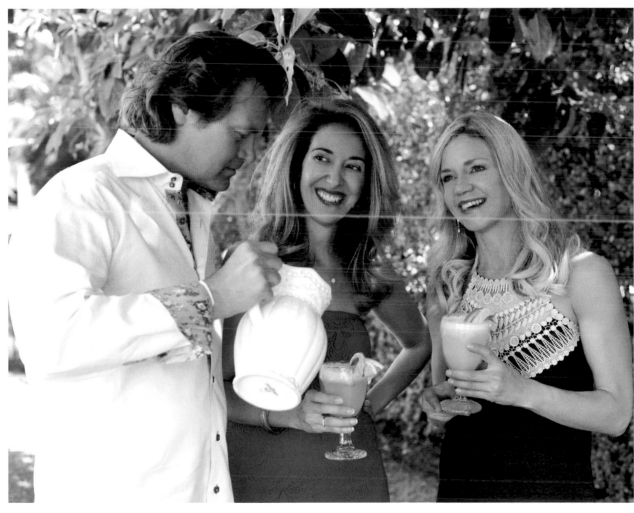

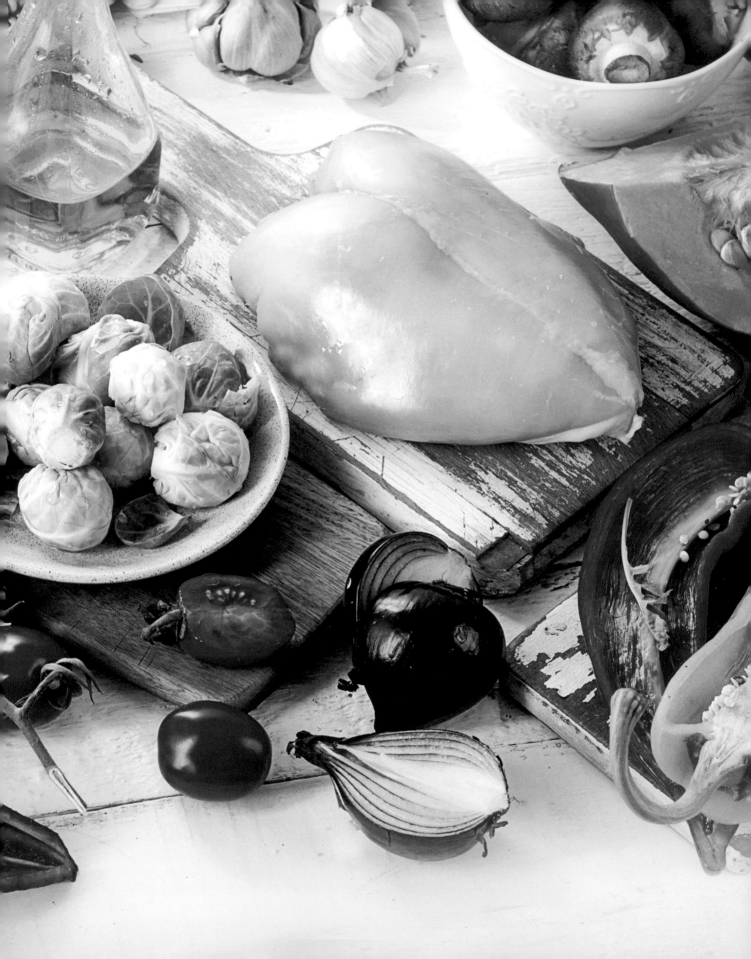

Part 3

clean·cuisine
RECIPES

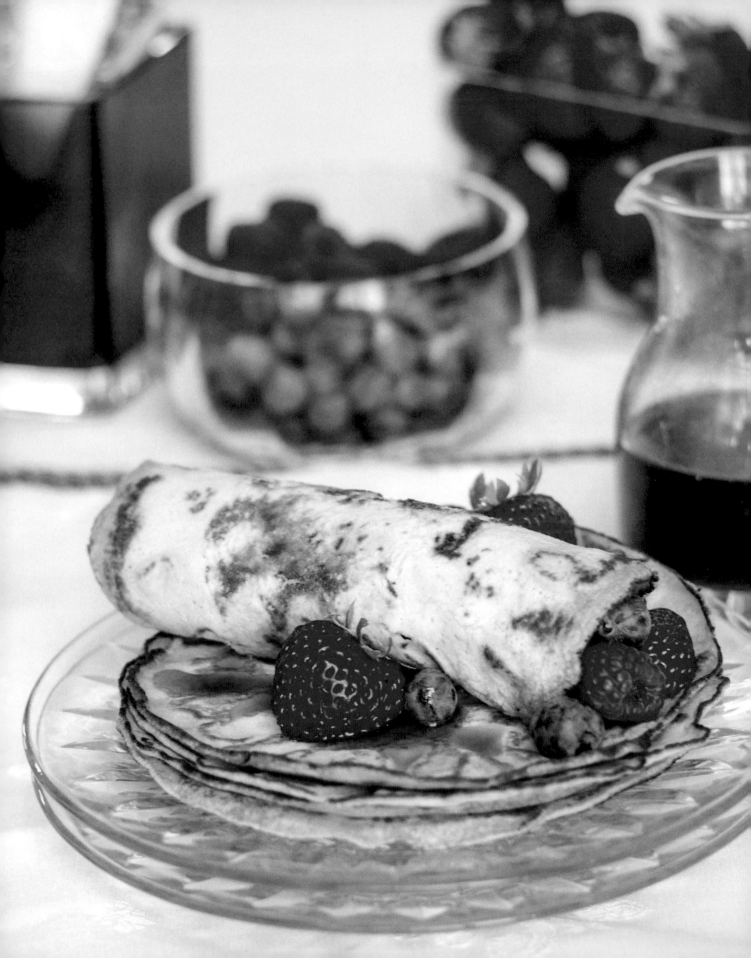

CHAPTER 8

start of the day

---

banana oat muffins

MAKES 1 dozen muffins   PREP TIME: 15 minutes   COOK TIME: 25 to 28 minutes

This is one of my go-to muffin recipes, especially during the hectic school year. They make the perfect grab-and-run breakfast, lunchbox item, or afternoon snack. And they are super quick and easy to make, too. If you've got little kids at home, muffins are the perfect mix-and-measure, no-knife-work recipe for them to help with.

⅓ cup plus 2 tablespoons almond milk, homemade (page 368) or store-bought, or hemp milk

⅓ cup melted extra-virgin coconut oil

¼ cup pure maple syrup

1 tablespoon pure vanilla extract

2 large eggs

5 Deglet Noor dates, pitted (see Note)

3 very ripe bananas, mashed

1 cup cassava flour (or sprouted spelt flour if not gluten- or grain-free)

½ cup gluten-free oat flour

⅓ cup gluten-free old-fashioned rolled oats

¼ cup brown rice flour

1 teaspoon baking soda

1 teaspoon ground cinnamon

½ teaspoon Himalayan pink salt

¾ cup chopped raw walnuts

For the topping:

¾ cup gluten-free old-fashioned rolled oats

2 tablespoons coconut sugar

¾ teaspoon ground cinnamon

1. Preheat the oven to 325°F. Line a standard-size 12-well muffin tin with paper liners.

2. In a blender or food processor, blend the almond milk, coconut oil, maple syrup, vanilla extract, eggs, and dates on high speed until smooth and creamy. Add the bananas to the blender or food processor and pulse until the bananas are pureed.

3. In a large mixing bowl, whisk together the cassava flour, oat flour, rolled oats, rice flour, baking soda, cinnamon, and salt until well blended.

4. Make a well in the center of the flour mixture. Pour the wet banana mixture into the center of the well and use a wooden spoon to mix until the ingredients are just combined. Fold in the nuts.

5. Divide the batter evenly among the muffin wells, filling each about two-thirds full. Sprinkle the top of each muffin with about 1 tablespoon of oats, followed by a light sprinkling of sugar (about ½ teaspoon per muffin) and finally a pinch of ground cinnamon. Bake the muffins for 25 to 28 minutes, until a toothpick inserted into a muffin comes out clean.

6. Place the muffin tin on a cooling rack. Allow the muffins to cool completely before removing them from the pan.

NOTE _____

If you're using a conventional blender rather than a high-powered one or a food processor, soak the dates in water for 15 to 30 minutes to soften them before pureeing.

STORAGE INFORMATION _____

These muffins will keep at room temperature for up to 2 days or in the refrigerator for up to 4 days. They keep well in the freezer in a freezer-safe bag for up to 1 month (just defrost individual muffins as needed).

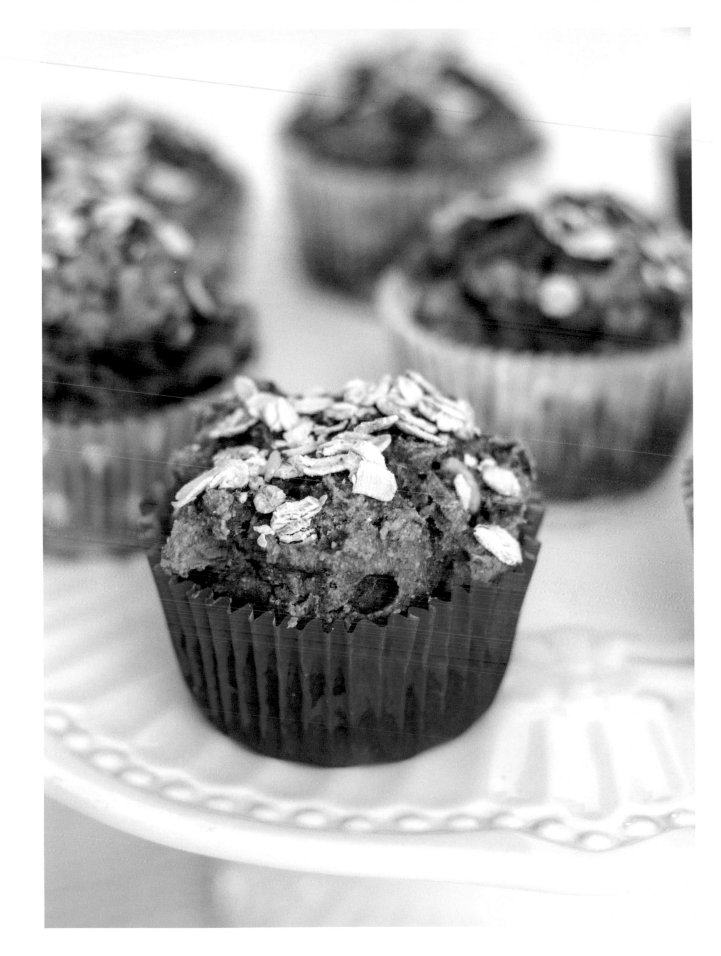

weekend waffles

MAKES 6 waffles   PREP TIME: 15 minutes   COOK TIME: 12 minutes

Waffles are one of my son's absolute favorite weekend breakfast treats. Since our family is not gluten-free, Blake grew up eating (and loving!) whole-grain waffles. However, since so many of our blog readers ask for gluten-free recipes, I have experimented with a number of gluten-free waffles over the years. Let's just say, Blake has not been a super-big fan. But this recipe is different. These waffles are crazy good! I think Blake may even prefer them over traditional waffles. And they sneak in a full serving of butternut squash, which provides moisture as well as nutrients, particularly antioxidants and phytonutrients. And I promise, you won't taste it.

¾ cup cassava flour (or sprouted spelt flour if not gluten- or grain-free)

½ cup brown rice flour

2 teaspoons baking powder

⅛ teaspoon Himalayan pink salt

¾ cup almond milk, homemade (page 368) or store-bought

¾ cup cubed and cooked butternut squash, thawed if frozen

¼ cup melted extra-virgin coconut oil

1 tablespoon pure vanilla extract

2 large egg yolks

3 medjool dates, pitted (see Note)

4 large egg whites

For serving (optional):

Fresh berries or sliced fruit

Pure maple syrup

1. In a large mixing bowl, whisk together the cassava flour, brown rice flour, baking powder, and salt until well blended, then make a well in the center of the mixture.

2. Put the almond milk, butternut squash, coconut oil, vanilla extract, egg yolks, and dates in a blender or food processor. Process on high speed until the mixture is smooth and creamy. Pour the wet ingredients into the well in the center of the dry ingredients. Stir together thoroughly but briefly, until just combined; do not overmix the batter.

3. Preheat a waffle iron to medium heat.

4. Wash the blender or food processor and dry it. Put the egg whites in the blender or food processor and process on high for 1 full minute, or until foamy. Stir the egg whites into the batter and stir gently to combine.

5. Pour about ⅓ cup of the batter into the preheated waffle iron. (The exact amount of batter per waffle will vary according to the iron; check the manufacturer's instructions for the correct amount for your iron.) Cook the waffle for about 2 minutes, until it is lightly browned. (The exact cooking time may vary according to the waffle iron.) Repeat with the remaining batter. Serve warm with fresh fruit and syrup, if desired.

NOTE

If you're using a conventional blender rather than a high-powered one or a food processor and your dates are on the dry side, soak them in water for 15 to 30 minutes to soften them before pureeing (very moist, succulent medjool dates do not require soaking).

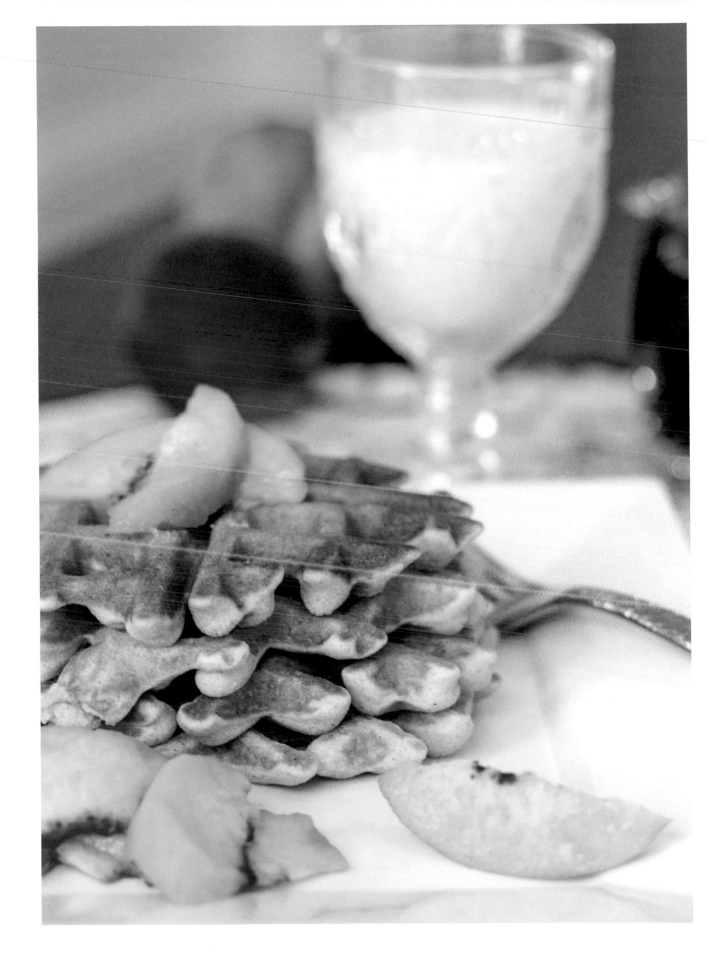

dutch apple pancakes

MAKES 4 medium pancakes   PREP TIME: 15 minutes   COOK TIME: 25 minutes

In our house, we call these pillowy pancakes "Jersey cakes" because I used to make a version of this recipe all the time when we lived in New Jersey. That was in the first five years of our marriage, while Andy was in residency. Back then, he often worked over one hundred hours a week and spent the night at the hospital every third night. When he'd come home in the morning, he would be starving, and Dutch apple pancakes were one of his favorite post-call breakfasts. Even if you haven't been working all through the night, "Jersey cakes" always hit the spot!

For the apples:

1 apple, cored and sliced into thin rings (leave skin on)

½ teaspoon ground cinnamon

3 teaspoons extra-virgin coconut oil

¼ cup almond milk, homemade (page 368) or store-bought, or hemp milk

¼ cup unsweetened applesauce

1 tablespoon extra-virgin coconut oil, melted (but not hot), plus more for the pan

2 teaspoons pure vanilla extract

2 large eggs

¼ cup cassava flour (or sprouted spelt flour if not gluten- or grain-free)

3 tablespoons coconut sugar

3 tablespoons sorghum flour

2 tablespoons ground flax seeds

2 tablespoons medium-grind cornmeal

½ teaspoon baking powder

¼ teaspoon baking soda

Pure maple syrup, for serving (optional)

1. Arrange the apple slices on a large plate and sprinkle both sides with the cinnamon.

2. Heat 1 teaspoon of the oil in a large skillet over medium heat and add 3 or 4 apple slices to the skillet. Cook the apples for about 2 minutes per side, until soft. Repeat with the remaining 2 teaspoons of oil and apple slices. Set the cooked cinnamon apple slices aside.

3. In a medium-sized bowl, whisk together the almond milk, applesauce, the 1 tablespoon of oil, vanilla extract, and eggs.

4. In a large bowl, whisk together the cassava flour, coconut sugar, sorghum flour, ground flax seeds, cornmeal, baking powder, and baking soda. Make a well in the center of the flour mixture and pour in the wet ingredients. Whisk together until just combined; do not overmix.

5. Generously oil the bottom of a skillet and set it over medium heat. When the skillet is hot, put 1 apple slice in the skillet and pour ⅓ cup of the batter on top of it. Cook the pancake for about 2 minutes, until very small bubbles start to form. Use a spatula to gently flip the pancake and cook for another 2 minutes or so, until light brown on both sides. Repeat with 3 more apple slices and the remaining batter.

6. Serve the pancakes with the remaining cooked cinnamon apple slices and maple syrup, if desired.

MAKE IT NUT-FREE

Use hemp milk instead of almond milk.

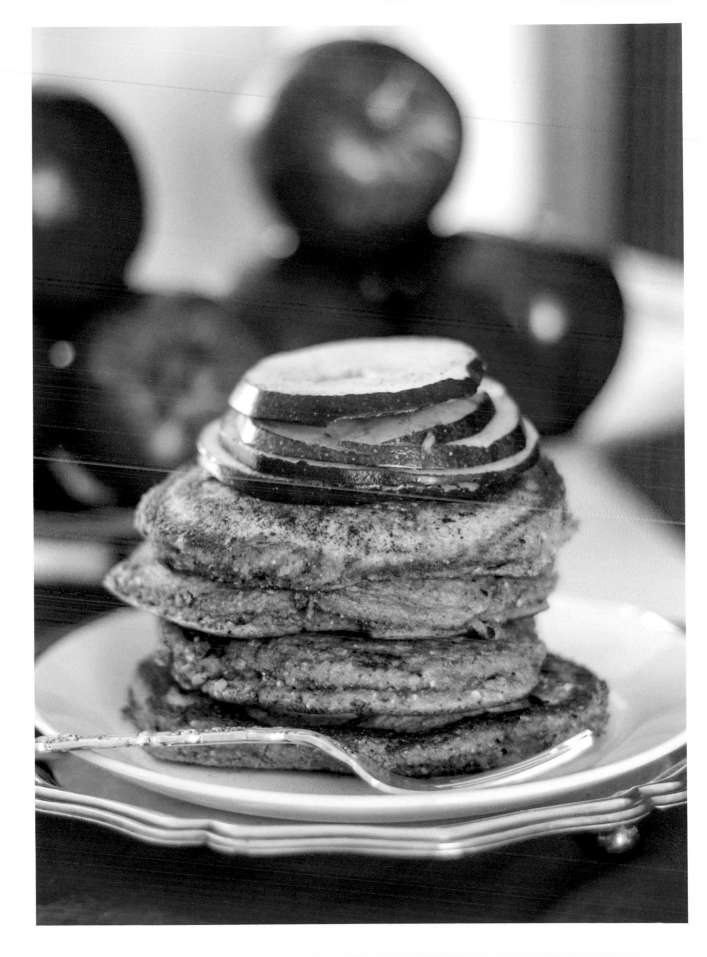

baked oatmeal with wild blueberries & crunchy almond topping

SERVES 6 to 8   PREP TIME: 15 minutes   COOK TIME: 40 minutes

Start your day right! I promise this one recipe will change your whole morning. Because let's face it: breakfast time arrives way too early in the morning for most of us. Cooking a delicious and well-balanced hot breakfast sounds great, but it's often just not possible if you work outside of the home or have small children. Even pulling out all the ingredients to make a smoothie can sometimes be too stressful. Make-ahead breakfasts like this one will save your sanity and help you start the day on the right foot—just bake the night before and reheat in the morning!

3 cups frozen wild blueberries (see Note)

2 cups gluten-free old-fashioned rolled oats

1 teaspoon baking powder

¼ teaspoon Himalayan pink salt

2 large eggs, beaten

2¼ cups almond milk, homemade (page 368) or store-bought

¾ teaspoon pure almond extract

¼ cup pure maple syrup

1 tablespoon unrefined coconut oil, plus more for the pan

1 cup raw almonds

Ground cinnamon, for dusting

1. Preheat the oven to 375°F. Lightly grease the bottom and sides of an 8 by 10-inch baking dish with coconut oil and spread the frozen blueberries in an even layer in the dish. Set aside.

2. Combine the oats, baking powder, and salt in a large mixing bowl. In a separate bowl, whisk together the eggs, almond milk, and almond extract. Pour the egg mixture over the oat mixture and use a wooden spoon to gently stir the ingredients together until just blended. Spoon the mixture over the frozen blueberries and set aside.

3. To create the crunchy almond topping, put the maple syrup, coconut oil, and almonds in a food processor and process until the almonds are finely chopped and coated in the syrup and oil.

4. Spoon the almond topping over the oats, spreading it with the back of a spoon for even distribution. Bake for 35 to 40 minutes, until the liquid is absorbed and the oats are firm. Serve warm.

5. To reheat, place 1 slice of oatmeal on a microwave-safe plate and microwave on high for 1 minute.

NOTE _____

There is no need to thaw the blueberries for this recipe. Don't worry, they will thaw perfectly in the oven.

STORAGE INFORMATION _____

Store leftover baked oatmeal in a covered container in the refrigerator for up to 4 days.

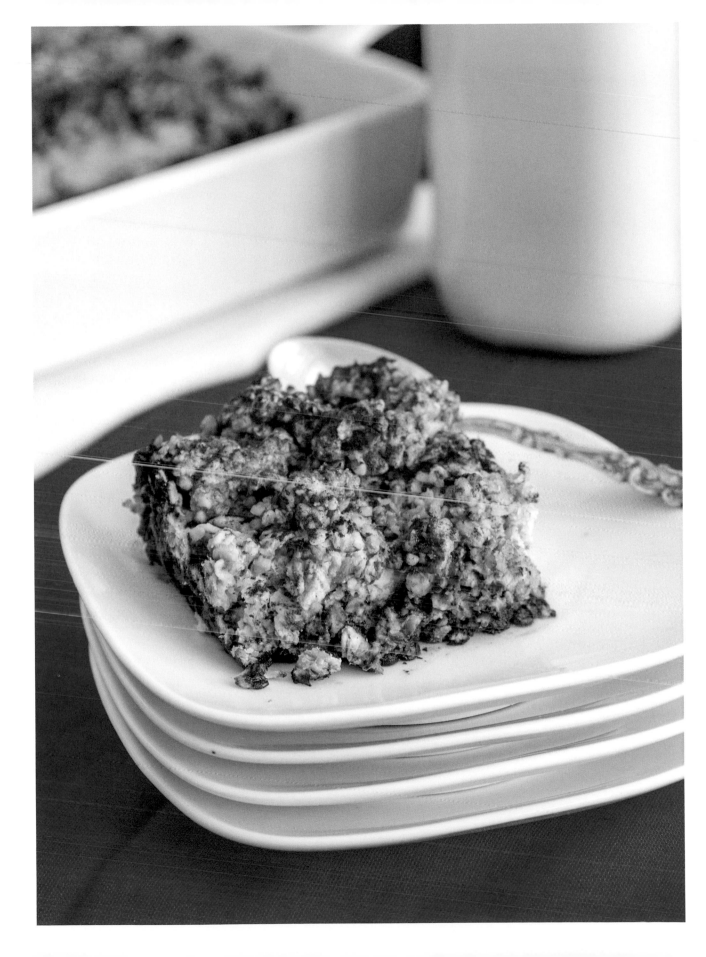

donuts two ways

MAKES 4 donuts   PREP TIME: 15 minutes   COOK TIME: 18 minutes

If you love donuts (and who doesn't?), then you must try this recipe. Believe it or not, clean donuts are truly a "hole" lot easier to make than you might think. And did I mention there are two delicious topping options, chocolate glaze and pecan crumble? You do need a special donut pan, but you can pick one up for about ten dollars at any cooking store. (I use Wilton's six-cavity donut pan.)

For the donuts:

1 cup cassava flour (or sprouted spelt flour if not gluten- or grain-free)

½ teaspoon baking powder

¼ cup pure maple syrup

¼ cup unsweetened applesauce

1 tablespoon coconut oil, melted, plus more for the pan

1 tablespoon pure vanilla extract

2 large eggs

For the chocolate glaze:

3 tablespoons cacao powder

3 tablespoons coconut sugar

1 tablespoon plus 1 teaspoon coconut oil

Pinch of Himalayan pink salt

For the pecan crumble:

¼ cup plus 2 tablespoons raw pecans

3 tablespoons pure maple syrup

½ teaspoon ground cinnamon

Pinch of Himalayan pink salt

TO MAKE THE DONUTS:

1. Preheat the oven to 300°F. Generously grease the bottom and sides of 4 cavities of the donut pan with coconut oil.

2. In a medium-sized bowl, whisk together the cassava flour and baking powder. Make a well in the center of the flour mixture.

3. In a small bowl, whisk together the maple syrup, applesauce, melted coconut oil, vanilla extract, and eggs. Pour the wet ingredients into the well in the flour mixture and mix with a large spoon until well combined.

4. Pour ⅓ cup of the batter into each greased donut cavity. Bake for 18 to 19 minutes, until a toothpick inserted in a donut comes out clean. (Note: If you are using sprouted spelt flour, bake the donuts for 20 minutes.)

5. Allow the donuts to cool for at least 10 minutes before removing them from the pan. To remove the donuts, run a knife around the edges, then flip the pan over and tap the bottom of the pan until the donuts loosen and fall out.

TO MAKE THE CHOCOLATE GLAZE:

1. Put the cacao powder, coconut sugar, coconut oil, and salt in a small microwave-safe bowl. Microwave on high for 45 to 60 seconds, until the coconut oil is melted and hot. Use a fork to whisk the ingredients into a smooth paste.

2. Spread the hot chocolate glaze on all 4 donuts, or on just 2 (if you want to make half the donuts chocolate and half pecan crumble). Serve at once.

SPECIAL TOOLS

Standard-size nonstick donut pan

Mini food processor

MAKE IT NUT-FREE

Use the chocolate glaze topping instead of the pecan crumble.

TO MAKE THE PECAN CRUMBLE:

1. Put the pecans, maple syrup, cinnamon, and salt in a mini food processor. Process until the ingredients are well combined and the nuts are finely chopped.

2. Spread the pecan crumble on all 4 donuts, or on just 2 (if you want to make half the donuts chocolate and half pecan crumble). Serve at once.

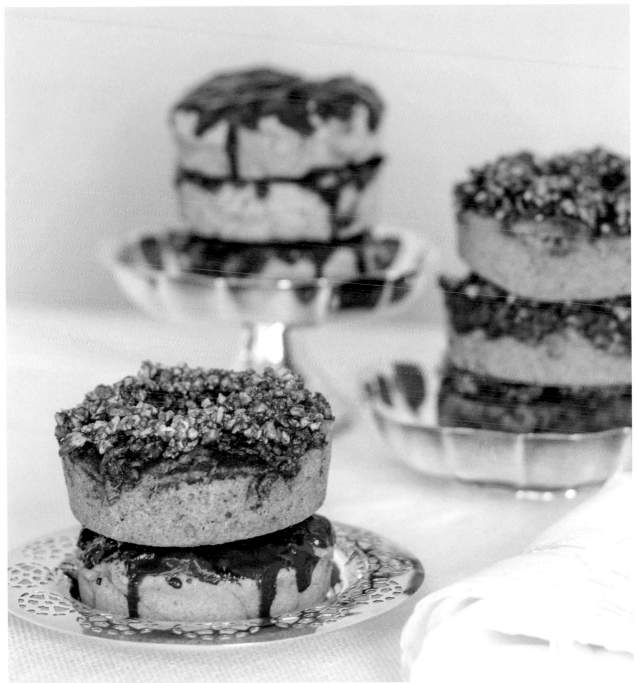

lemon-blueberry scones

MAKES 8 scones   PREP TIME: 20 minutes   COOK TIME: 25 to 30 minutes

I developed this recipe after we returned from a family trip to England, where our son had his first scone, which was not exactly "clean cuisine." He loved it so much that I had to try to create a healthy one back home. Making a clean scone turned out to be a bit tricky, but after multiple tries I finally got it right! I use wild blueberries, which not only are better for baking—they're smaller, so they stay whole when you bake them—but also pack a much bigger nutrition punch than cultivated blueberries. Small but mighty, wild blueberries have more antioxidants than most other fruits and vegetables, and considerably more than cultivated blueberries. The more antioxidants a food has, the more powerful it is for slowing the aging process, fighting disease, reducing inflammation, and optimizing health.

I definitely suggest eating these scones with black tea. There's just something about tea that makes everything about scones better!

1½ cups cassava flour (or sprouted spelt flour if not gluten- or grain-free)

1½ cups gluten-free oat flour

¼ cup plus 2 tablespoons coconut sugar, divided

2 tablespoons arrowroot

1 tablespoon baking powder

½ teaspoon Himalayan pink salt

¼ cup plus 2 tablespoons extra-virgin coconut oil, softened

1 cup coconut cream (see page 74)

2 tablespoons pure maple syrup

2 teaspoons grated lemon zest

3 to 4 drops food-grade lemon essential oil, or 2 teaspoons pure lemon extract

1 cup frozen wild blueberries (see Note)

1 large egg white, whisked

1. Preheat the oven to 425°F. Line a baking sheet with parchment paper.

2. In a large bowl, whisk together the flours, ¼ cup of the sugar, the arrowroot, baking powder, and salt. Using a pastry blender, cut in the coconut oil. Stir to mix the ingredients together until crumbly. Stir in the coconut cream, maple syrup, lemon zest, and lemon oil. Fold in the frozen blueberries.

3. Transfer the dough to a large work surface and gently pat it into a large circle about 9 inches in diameter and about 2 inches thick. Transfer the dough to the prepared baking sheet, then slice it into 8 wedges, but do not pull the wedges apart. Sprinkle with the remaining 2 tablespoons of sugar and brush the whisked egg white over the top.

4. Bake for 25 to 30 minutes, until lightly browned. Allow to cool on the pan for at least 15 minutes before serving.

NOTE

Frozen blueberries work best for this recipe because they stay firm when mixing. I use Wyman's brand frozen wild blueberries, and they are available nationwide. (They even sell them in bulk at Costco!) If you cannot find frozen wild blueberries, you can always purchase fresh wild blueberries and freeze them for the purpose of this recipe. However, if you cannot find wild blueberries, fresh or frozen, substitute frozen cultivated blueberries.

STORAGE INFORMATION

Scones will keep in an airtight container in the refrigerator for up to 3 days or in the freezer for up to 2 weeks. To reheat, microwave for 30 to 45 seconds, until soft.

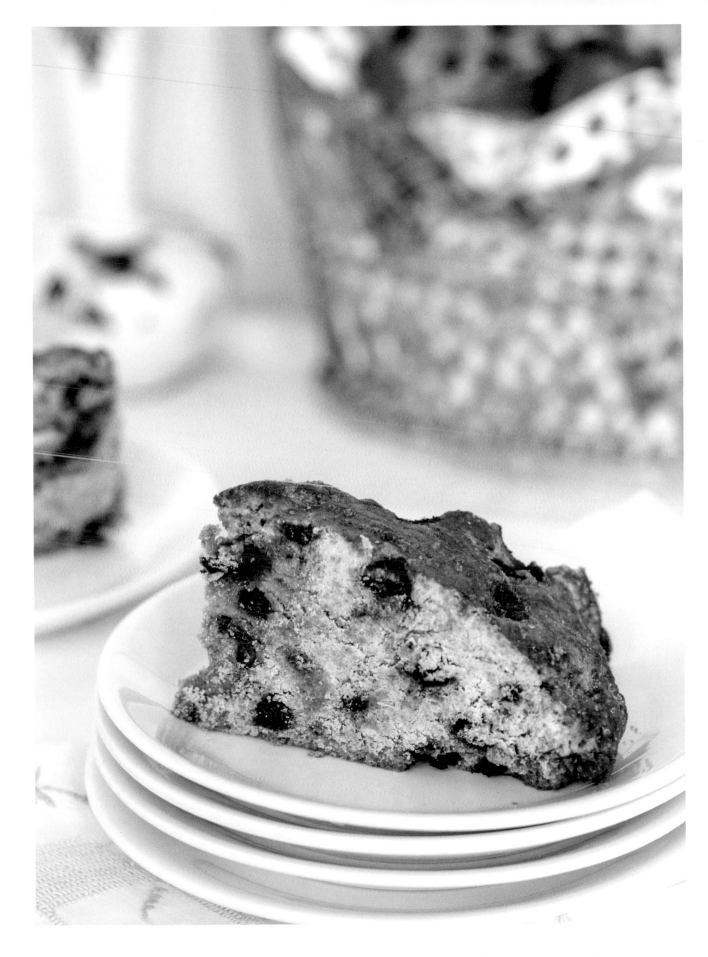

nut butter granola

MAKES 3 cups   PREP TIME: 10 minutes   COOK TIME: 35 minutes

I really wish I had started making granola years ago. It's so incredibly easy, and unlike the vast majority of store-bought brands, homemade granola can have very little sweetener and oil. In fact, I use almond butter as a more nutrient-dense option than oil. In addition to the nutrition benefits, the almond butter gives the granola a better texture, so it's tastier and healthier. A win-win! My favorite way to eat granola is over plain almond milk–based yogurt with fresh berries and maybe a sprinkling of cinnamon. And if you have kids, it makes the perfect after-school snack or lunchbox treat. It sure beats chips or cookies!

2 cups gluten-free old-fashioned rolled oats

¾ teaspoon ground cinnamon

¼ teaspoon Himalayan pink salt

¼ cup pure maple syrup

¼ cup unsalted, unsweetened smooth almond butter or peanut butter

1 teaspoon pure vanilla extract

1 egg white

1 cup raisins, or any chopped dried fruit

1. Preheat the oven to 300°F. Line a rimmed baking sheet with parchment paper.

2. Mix the oats, cinnamon, and salt together in a medium-sized mixing bowl.

3. Microwave the maple syrup and almond butter in a microwave-safe bowl on high for about 45 seconds, or just until the almond butter is soft enough to mix well with the syrup. (Alternatively, gently heat them in a small saucepan on the stovetop over medium heat.) Stir in the vanilla extract and mix well. Beat in the egg white.

4. Stir the wet ingredients into the dry ingredients.

5. Spread the oat mixture out evenly onto the parchment-lined baking sheet. Bake for 20 minutes, stir, and bake for an additional 15 minutes, or until the granola is golden brown. Remove from the oven and stir in the raisins. Set the granola aside to cool before serving or transferring to containers for storage.

STORAGE INFORMATION

The granola will keep in an airtight container in the refrigerator for up to 3 weeks or in the freezer for up to 2 months.

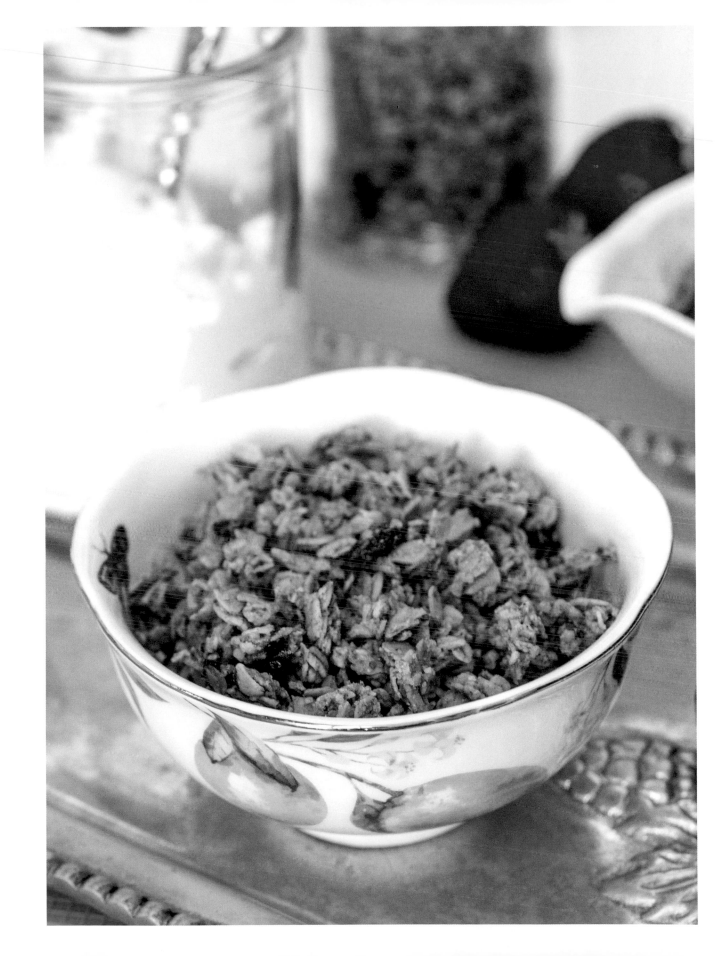

sweet crepes

MAKES about 8 crepes (4 servings)   PREP TIME: 10 minutes   COOK TIME: 15 minutes

They may sound fancy, but crepes are easier to make than you might think. I love them for breakfast—think of them as French pancakes! They are irresistibly delicious with the homemade strawberry sauce on page 384 and make a great dessert option, too. For Meatless Monday, I make a savory version of the crepes (see below) and use them as a substitute for tortillas, rolling them into tasty burritos with salsa, black beans, cilantro, corn, and lettuce. It might sound like an unconventional dinner, but they really are surprisingly good. And filling! FYI: The crepe batter can be made in advance and stored in a large mason jar in the refrigerator for up to three days.

2 large eggs

1 large egg white

1¼ cups plus 3 tablespoons water

2 tablespoons hemp seeds

1 tablespoon extra-virgin coconut oil, melted, plus more for the pan

1 tablespoon plus 1 teaspoon pure maple syrup

½ teaspoon pure vanilla extract

⅛ teaspoon Himalayan pink salt

⅔ cup cassava flour (or sprouted spelt flour if not gluten- or grain-free)

⅓ cup brown rice flour

Fresh berries or Fresh Strawberry Sauce (page 384), for serving (optional)

SPECIAL TOOLS _____

10-inch nontoxic, nonstick skillet (see facing page)

1. Put the eggs, egg white, water, hemp seeds, coconut oil, maple syrup, vanilla extract, and salt in a blender; process on high speed for 1 full minute, or until the mixture is smooth and free of lumps. Add the cassava flour and rice flour to the blender and process again until the mixture is smooth and creamy. (Note: The batter can be made in advance and refrigerated in a covered container for up to 72 hours.)

2. Lightly grease the bottom of a 10-inch nonstick skillet with extra-virgin coconut oil and heat over medium heat until very hot. Pour in ¼ cup of the batter and quickly tilt the pan to cover the bottom with the batter. Return the pan to the burner and cook until the top of the crepe looks dry and the underside is light golden, about 1½ minutes. Use a spatula to carefully flip the crepe and cook for a few seconds more. The underside does not need to be browned, but it should be dry. Immediately flip the crepe out of the pan and onto a plate. Lay a square of parchment paper on top of the crepe to separate it from the next finished crepe. Repeat with the remaining batter, stacking the crepes on top of each other with parchment paper in between.

3. To keep cooked crepes warm, place them on a wire rack on a baking sheet and tuck them inside a 250°F oven. Serve with fresh berries or strawberry sauce, if desired.

STORAGE INFORMATION _____
Store leftover crepes, separated by pieces of parchment paper, in a zip-top bag in the refrigerator for up to a week or in the freezer for up to 4 weeks. To reheat, microwave one at a time for about 30 seconds.

VARIATION: SAVORY CREPES _____
Follow the recipe as written but reduce the amount of maple syrup to ¾ teaspoon and omit the vanilla extract.

As a general rule, because of concerns about toxic components (see page 88 for more on that), I do not cook with nonstick cookware—except when I am making crepes. If you are not a seasoned crepe maker, you will have the best results using a nonstick skillet. Look for a nontoxic, eco-friendly nonstick skillet manufactured without PFAS, PFOA, lead, or cadmium. GreenPan is a good brand.

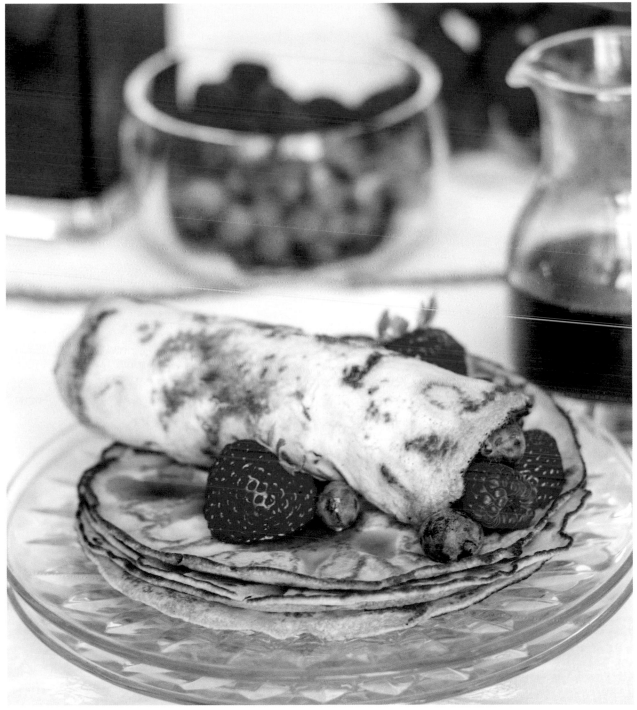

cinnamon "butter"

MAKES about ¼ cup   PREP TIME: 5 minutes

I came up with this recipe one afternoon when my nephew, Ryan, was at our house. He asked for a snack and I happened to be very low on food that day, so I made buttered cinnamon toast, with coconut butter, honey, and coconut oil replacing dairy butter. He liked it so much he practically ate all of the "butter" before I even had a chance to spread it on his toast! It makes a great dip for apples and other sliced fruit, too.

¼ cup coconut butter or coconut manna, softened

1 tablespoon plus 1 teaspoon manuka honey or raw honey

2 teaspoons extra-virgin coconut oil, softened

1 teaspoon ground cinnamon

Place all of the ingredients in a small mixing bowl and use a fork to whisk for about 2 minutes, until smooth and creamy.

STORAGE INFORMATION

Store in the refrigerator for up to a week. It will harden when chilled, so allow it to come to room temperature before using so it becomes spreadable. Alternatively, it can be stored in an airtight container at room temperature for 3 days.

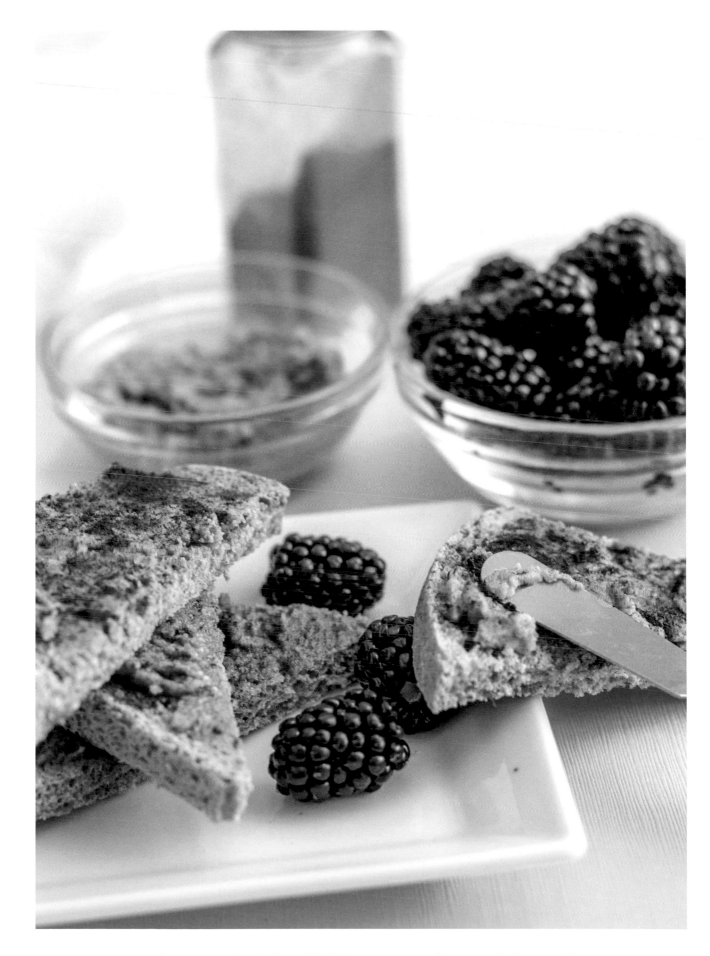

the world's easiest & healthiest blackberry jam

MAKES ¾ cup   PREP TIME: 5 minutes, plus time to set in the freezer

This is not made at all like traditional blackberry jam. In fact, it's so easy to make that I was hesitant to even call it a recipe at first. But it is so simple and so good that I just had to share! Traditional jam recipes require a lot of time, stovetop cooking, and sugar—lots and lots of sugar, typically 1 cup for every 2 cups of fruit. My blackberry jam is a no-cook, no-refined-sugar version that takes no time to whip up.

1¼ cups fresh blackberries

2 tablespoons manuka honey or other raw honey

2 teaspoons very hot water

2 teaspoons unflavored gelatin, divided (see Note)

SPECIAL TOOLS _____ _____
Mini food processor

1. Put the blackberries and honey in a mini food processor and process until smooth. Turn the machine off and set aside.

2. Put the hot water in a small bowl and whisk in 1 teaspoon of the gelatin. Mix until smooth. Immediately pour the gelatin mixture into the blackberry mixture in the food processor and process again until well blended. Pour the jam into a medium-sized bowl, add the remaining teaspoon of gelatin, and stir until dissolved.

3. Transfer the jam to a freezer-safe container and put in the freezer to set for 10 minutes.

STORAGE INFORMATION _____
Store in a jar in the refrigerator for up to 1 week.

NOTE _____
Not all gelatin is "clean," but Vital Proteins is a very good brand: 100 percent pure, pasture-raised, and grass-fed. The amino acids in gelatin are therapeutic and are identical to the protein found in skin, nails, hair, bones, cartilage, and joints.

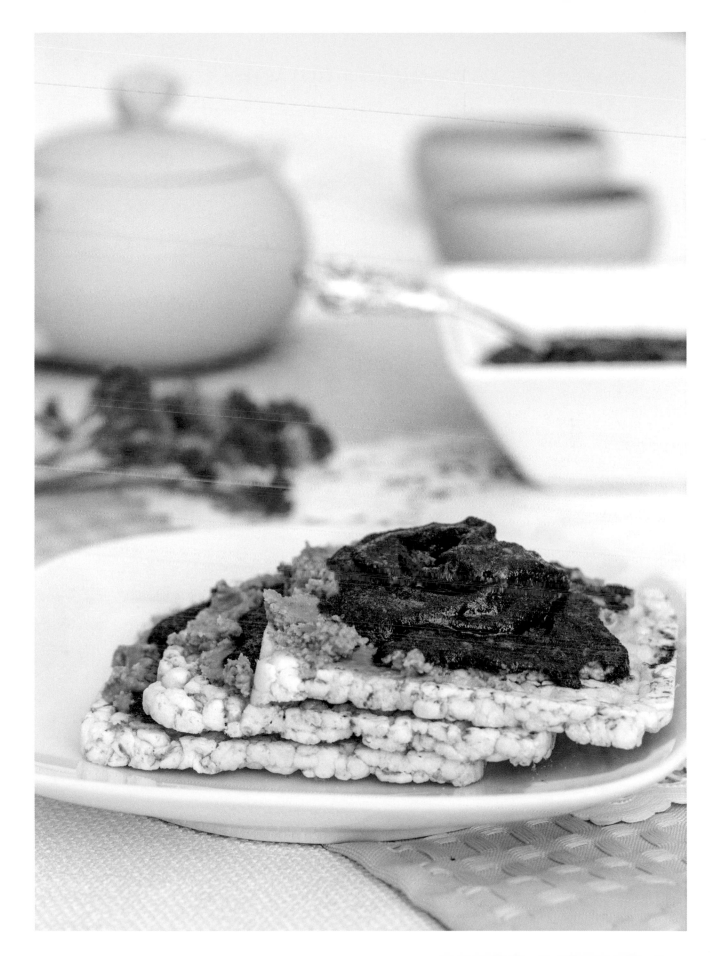

cornbread muffins with kale

MAKES 1 dozen muffins   PREP TIME: 15 minutes   COOK TIME: 28 minutes

I know muffins typically get a bad rap with the clean-eating crowd, but you can definitely bake better-for-you muffins, which these most definitely are. I even managed to sneak in some greens! And don't feel that you have to limit yourself to kale; parsley works great, too (see variation below). My family eats these savory muffins most frequently for breakfast—they are delicious served with sliced tomato, avocado, and kimchi. But I also use them in my Skillet Meat & Bean Casserole with Cornbread Topping (page 222), and many a night I serve them as a starchy side for dinner. You can't go wrong having a batch of these in your refrigerator at all times, especially if you have hungry kids who like to snack a lot.

1½ cups chopped kale

¾ cup masa harina corn flour

¾ cup gluten-free oat flour

½ cup cassava flour (or sprouted spelt flour if not gluten- or grain-free)

2 teaspoons baking powder

1 teaspoon Himalayan pink salt

1 cup almond milk, homemade (page 368) or store-bought

2 large eggs

¼ cup extra-virgin olive oil

2 tablespoons raw honey

1 cup frozen corn kernels, thawed

1. In a steamer basket set over a pot with an inch of boiling water, steam the kale until bright green and just tender, about 5 minutes. Set aside to cool completely. Once cool, use paper towels to squeeze excess moisture from the kale.

2. Preheat the oven to 375°F. Line a standard-size 12-well muffin tin with paper liners and lightly oil the inside of each paper liner. (Alternatively, you may omit the liners and instead generously oil the bottom and sides of each well in the muffin tin.)

3. In a medium-sized bowl, whisk together the masa harina, oat flour, cassava flour, baking powder, and salt.

4. In a blender, blend the almond milk, eggs, oil, and honey until well combined. Pour the wet ingredients into the dry ingredients and stir until just combined. Fold in the kale and corn.

5. Divide the batter evenly among the muffin cups, filling each about three-quarters full. Bake until golden and the tops spring back when lightly touched, about 23 minutes. Let cool for 5 minutes in the pan before serving. Serve warm.

VARIATION: CORNBREAD MUFFINS WITH PARSLEY _____
Replace the kale with 1 cup chopped parsley. Steam just until wilted, about 3 minutes. Complete steps 2 through 5 as written.

STORAGE INFORMATION _____
Muffins can be stored in a zip-top bag in the refrigerator for up to 4 days or in the freezer for up to a month. To reheat, microwave for 30 to 45 seconds, until soft.

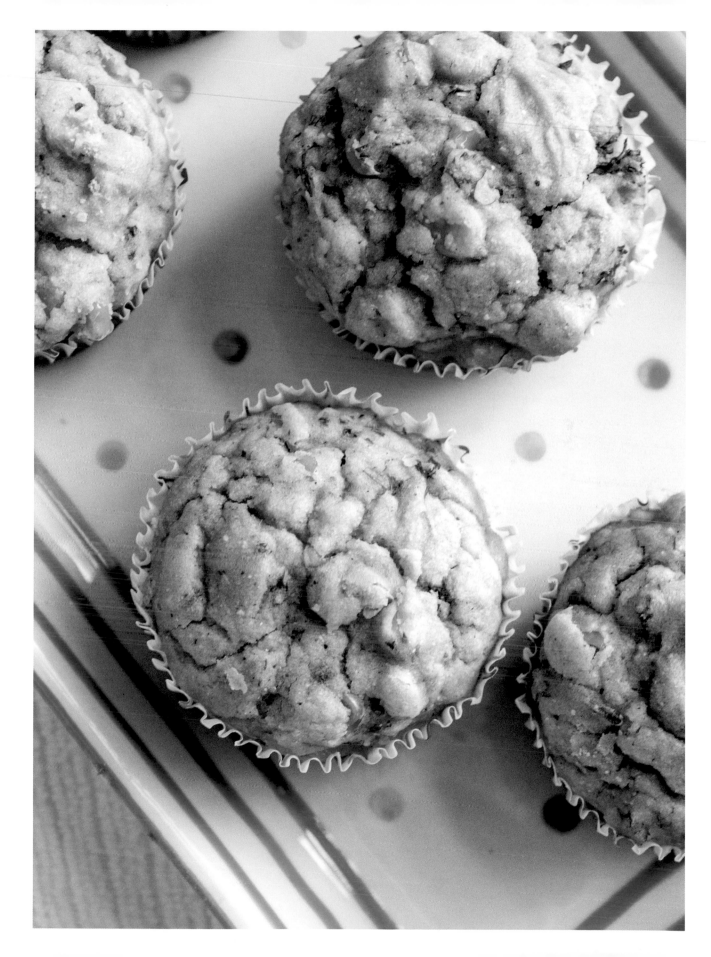

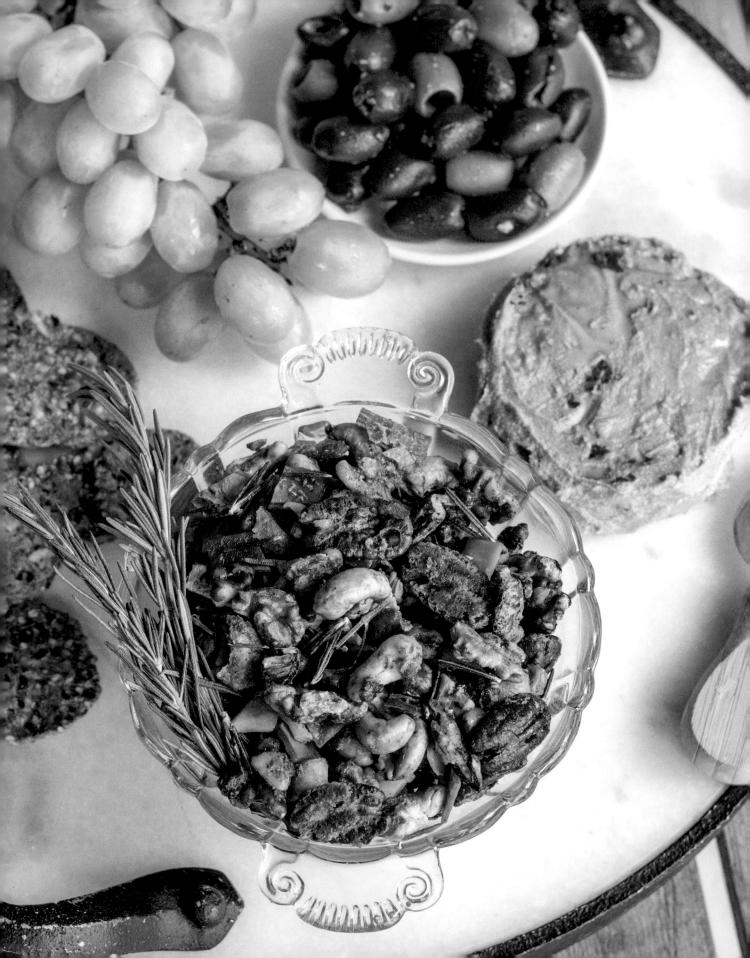

CHAPTER 9

snacks and such

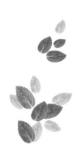

chocolate hazelnut spread

MAKES ¾ cup   PREP TIME: 10 minutes   COOK TIME: 10 minutes

Before my clean-eating days, I studied abroad in London, where I fell in love with Nutella, a divine chocolate-hazelnut spread. (Nutella is available in the United States, too, but for some reason I never had it until I moved abroad.) Spread on toast and topped with sliced banana, it became one of my go-to breakfasts. And no wonder—it tasted like dessert! Now I know that Nutella is loaded with sugar. Luckily, making your own clean chocolate-hazelnut spread is a piece of cake!

½ cup raw hazelnuts

¼ cup plus 1 tablespoon water

3 tablespoons extra-virgin coconut oil, softened

6 medjool dates, pitted (see Note)

3 tablespoons plus 1 teaspoon cacao powder

½ teaspoon pure vanilla extract

⅛ teaspoon Himalayan pink salt

1. Preheat the oven to 375°F. Spread the hazelnuts in a single layer on a rimmed baking sheet and toast in the oven until the skins have become dark brown (but not black!) and are mostly split and the nuts are light golden-brown and fragrant, about 10 minutes. Be careful not to toast too long or the hazelnuts will become bitter. Remove the nuts from the oven and wrap them in a clean dish towel. Allow the nuts to sit for 5 to 10 minutes to cool, then vigorously rub them in the towel to remove as much of the skin as possible. Try to get at least half of the skin off of each nut.

2. Place the roasted and peeled hazelnuts, water, and coconut oil in a high-powered blender or food processor and process for about 2 minutes, until the mixture is smooth, creamy, and lump-free. Add the dates, cacao powder, vanilla extract, and salt and process again until ingredients are well blended. (Note: You may need to stop the blender or food processor several times to mix the ingredients with a spoon to ensure even blending.)

NOTE _____

If you're using a food processor instead of a high-powered blender and your dates are on the dry side, soak them in water for 15 to 30 minutes to soften them before pureeing (very moist, succulent medjool dates do not require soaking).

STORAGE INFORMATION _____

This spread will keep in an airtight container in the refrigerator for up to a week.

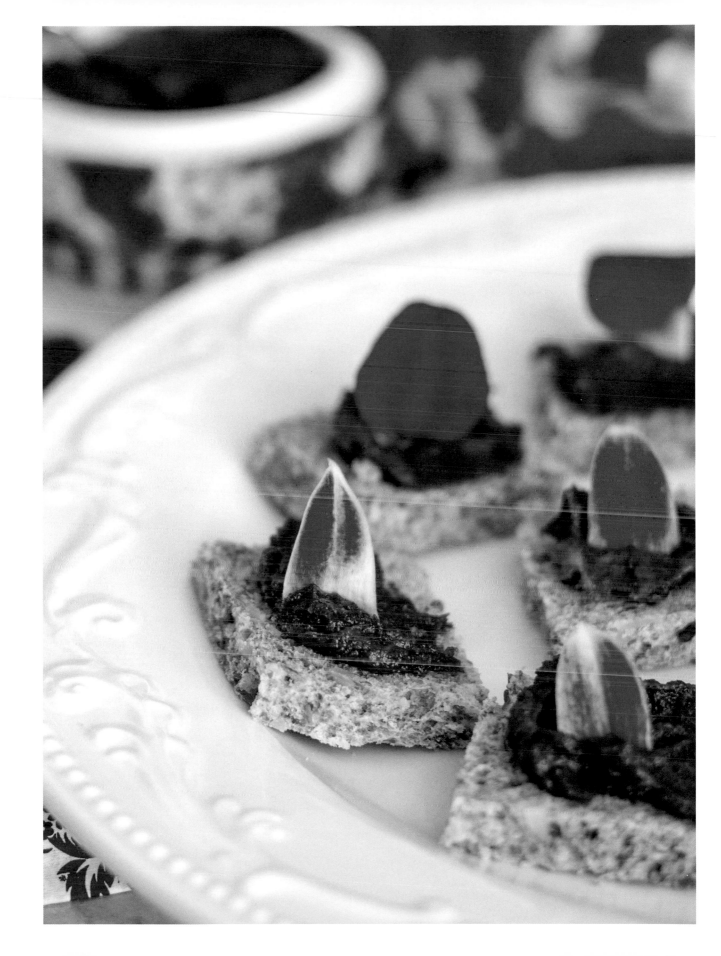

kim's spiced party chickpeas

MAKES 1½ cups   PREP TIME: 15 minutes   COOK TIME: 55 minutes

My sister-in-law, Kim Larson, was the first one to introduce me to the idea of spiced chickpeas as a snack. I've tweaked the recipe a bit from the original one Kim gave me, but what a hit they have been with everyone in the family! For a while, this was all my son wanted to eat for a snack, and they have definitely become a go-to party appetizer. Whether it's a baby shower, Thanksgiving, Christmas, or just a dinner party with friends, these spiced chickpeas are always just the thing to serve. And they're so easy to make, too!

2 (15-ounce) cans chickpeas

3 tablespoons unfortified nutritional yeast

1 tablespoon coconut sugar

½ teaspoon chili powder

½ teaspoon ground cumin

½ teaspoon Himalayan pink salt

½ teaspoon smoked paprika

¼ teaspoon baking soda

¼ teaspoon cayenne pepper

2 tablespoons extra-virgin olive oil

1 clove garlic, crushed to a paste

1. Preheat the oven to 350°F.

2. To prepare the chickpeas, drain the cans, then rinse the chickpeas with water and drain them again thoroughly. Transfer the drained chickpeas to a paper towel and gently pat as dry as possible. (It is very important that the chickpeas be as dry as possible for this recipe.) Spread the chickpeas out on a separate paper towel and let them air dry for at least 10 minutes. Meanwhile, make the spice blend.

3. In a small bowl, mix together the nutritional yeast, coconut sugar, chili powder, cumin, salt, paprika, baking soda, and cayenne pepper.

4. When the chickpeas are dry, use a kitchen towel to gently rub off the thin layer of skin covering each one. Be careful not to smash the chickpeas!

5. Put the chickpeas in a medium-sized bowl, then add the oil, garlic, and spice blend. Gently toss the chickpeas to evenly coat them in the oil, garlic, and spices.

6. Transfer the chickpeas to a rimmed baking sheet. Bake for 50 minutes, until they are slightly browned. Turn on the broiler and broil for about 2 minutes, until they're crispy but not burned. Remove from the oven and allow to cool for 10 to 15 minutes before serving. Serve at room temperature.

STORAGE INFORMATION

Spiced chickpeas are best served the day they are prepared; however, they will keep in an airtight container in the refrigerator for up to 1 day.

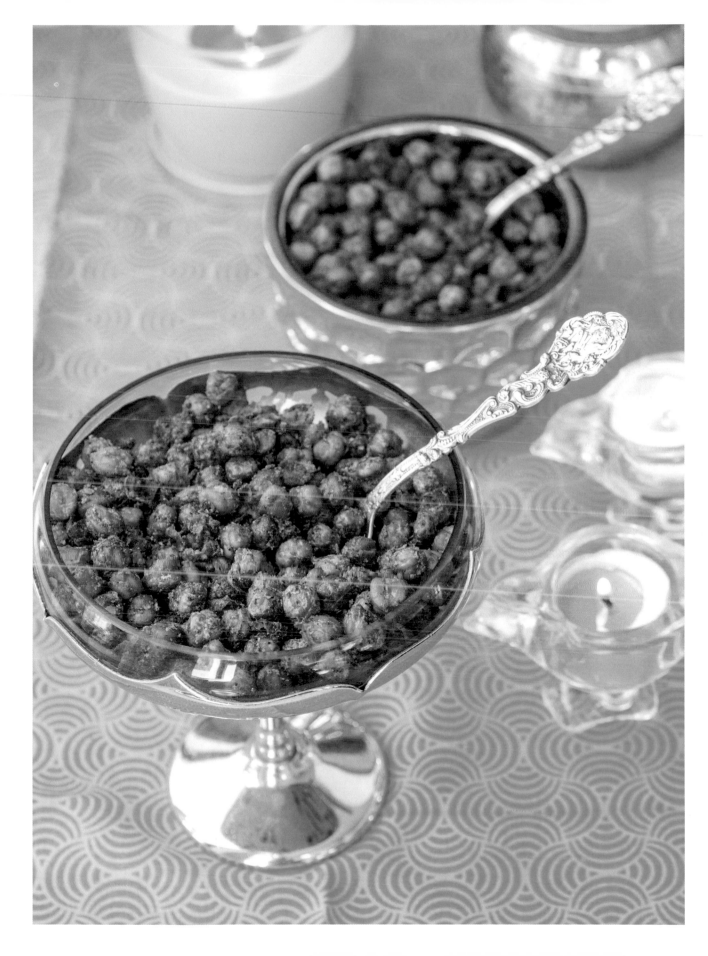

sweet & savory party nuts

MAKES 3 cups   PREP TIME: 7 minutes   COOK TIME: 25 minutes

Whether you are hosting a holiday party or just having some friends over to hang out, this is the nut mix to make! Everyone always goes crazy for the addictive blend of salty, savory, and slightly sweet flavors. It's also got to be one of the easiest recipes in the world to make, and it can be made up to a month in advance and stored in the freezer for all of your impromptu entertaining needs. I usually serve these party nuts with a cheese plate. (By the way, you can create a delicious dairy-free and gluten-free cheese plate using high-quality nut milk–based cheeses and gluten-free crackers—for recommended brands, see pages 398 and 403. We have plenty of friends who are neither dairy-free nor gluten-free, and nobody ever complains when we serve a dairy-free and gluten-free cheese plate with these party nuts!)

2 large egg whites

1 teaspoon coconut sugar

1 teaspoon Himalayan pink salt

¼ teaspoon cayenne pepper

¾ cup raw cashews

¾ cup raw pecans

¾ cup raw walnuts

1 cup chopped dried pineapple or dried mango, or a combination of both

1 tablespoon chopped fresh rosemary

Sprigs of rosemary, for garnish (optional)

1. Preheat the oven to 350°F. Line a rimmed baking sheet with parchment paper.

2. In a large bowl, whisk together the egg whites, coconut sugar, salt, and cayenne pepper. Add the nuts and toss to coat evenly in the seasoned egg mixture.

3. Spread the nuts out in an even layer on the parchment-lined baking sheet. Bake for 20 minutes. Add the chopped dried fruit and chopped rosemary. Return the nuts to the oven and bake for 5 minutes more. Remove the nuts from the oven and set aside to cool for at least 10 minutes before serving. Garnish with sprigs of rosemary, if desired.

STORAGE INFORMATION

Store leftover party nuts in an airtight container in the refrigerator for up to 1 week or in the freezer for up to 1 month.

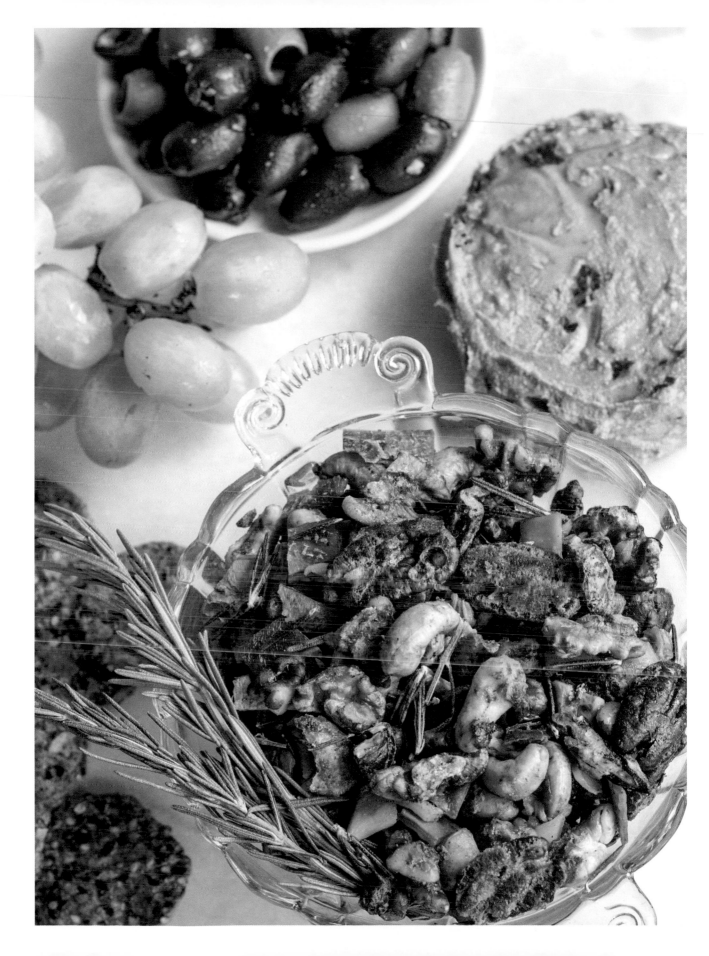

deviled eggs

MAKES 20 deviled eggs   PREP TIME: 15 minutes

This recipe was inspired by the egg "pumpkins" I made for our huge annual Halloween party. I added a dusting of turmeric (instead of cayenne or paprika) at the very end to make the filling orange and put a fresh sage stem at the top of each egg half, so they resembled mini pumpkins. I thought it was a fun and cute idea, but I kind of lost my enthusiasm around the time I started stuffing deviled egg number fifty. If you're having a hundred people to your house, you might not want to serve deviled eggs—even this super-easy version, which skips the pumpkin appearance. As for the flavor, don't worry about the addition of pumpkin puree—the eggs do not taste one bit pumpkin-y. Just like a conventional deviled egg recipe, this one has a very mild flavor.

---

10 hard-boiled eggs

½ cup raw cashews, preferably soaked in water for 1 to 2 hours, then rinsed and drained (see Note)

¼ cup pumpkin puree

2 to 3 tablespoons water

1 teaspoon fresh lemon juice

¾ teaspoon Dijon mustard

¼ teaspoon gluten-free Worcestershire sauce

¼ teaspoon Himalayan pink salt

Cayenne pepper or paprika, for garnish (optional)

Baby spinach leaves, for serving (optional)

1. Peel the hard-boiled eggs and carefully slice each one in half lengthwise. Use a small spoon to remove the yolks. Set the egg white halves aside and transfer the yolks to a blender or food processor.

2. To the blender or food processor, add the remaining ingredients, except for the cayenne pepper and spinach. Process on high until smooth and creamy.

3. Carefully fill each egg white half with the pumpkin–egg yolk mixture. Dust the filling with cayenne pepper (if using). Cover and refrigerate until ready to serve. If desired, serve each egg on a few baby spinach leaves.

NOTE

If you're using a high-powered blender, soaking the cashews is optional, but it does create a creamier texture. If you're using a conventional blender instead of a high-powered one, soaking the cashews is necessary to get the right texture.

STORAGE INFORMATION

Store leftover deviled eggs in an airtight container in the refrigerator for up to 3 days.

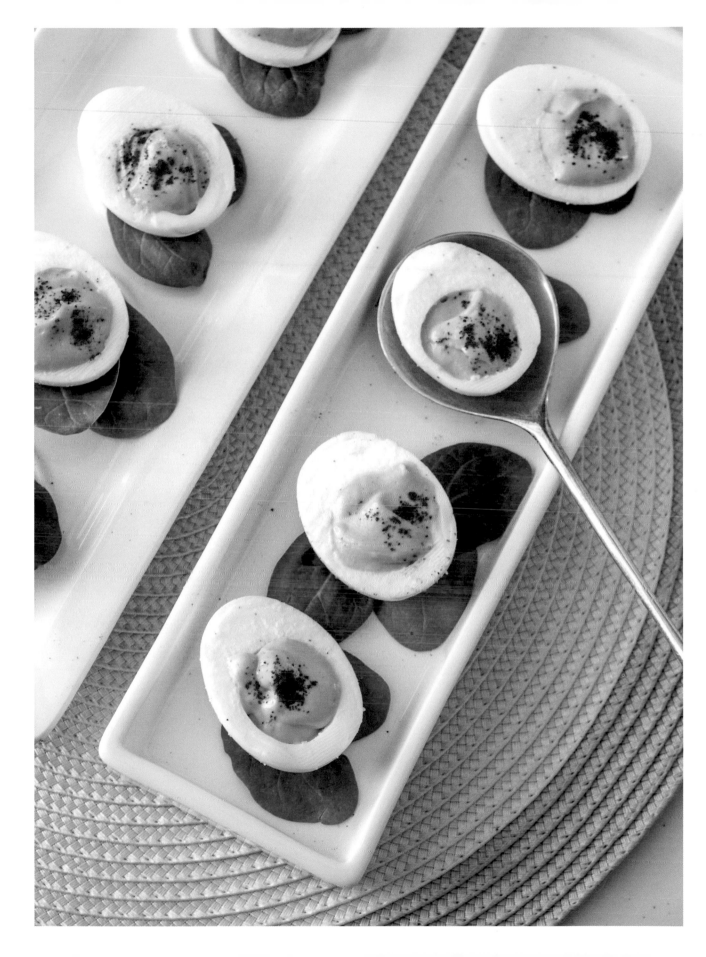

smoked salmon dip

MAKES about 1 cup   PREP TIME: 10 minutes, plus time to chill the dip

I have to be honest, I did not think I was a fan of fish dip until recently. Conventional fish dip is made with ingredients like cream cheese, sour cream, and low-quality mayonnaise, so I always just avoided it. But after my brother-in-law, Mike, brought a smoked salmon dip to our house for Thanksgiving, I totally changed my mind. Mike kept spreading the dip on cracker after cracker and raving about how amazing it was, so I finally caved in and had a bite. Wow! I'd been missing out! Luckily, with a good-quality mayonnaise, you can create an incredibly delicious and authentic-tasting clean fish dip. And if you are wondering whether smoked salmon is healthy, don't worry: not only does smoking the fish not damage its omega-3 fats, but it even boosts the antioxidant profile. So no need to feel guilty about fish dip—at least, not this one! Serve with crudités or gluten-free crackers—my favorite is Suzie's Thin Puffed Cakes made with brown rice and lightly salted.

½ cup mayonnaise, homemade (page 392) or store-bought

4 ounces hot-smoked wild salmon

1 tablespoon fresh lemon juice

½ teaspoon Dijon mustard

2 tablespoons chopped shallots

2 tablespoons minced fresh chives

1 tablespoon minced fresh dill

1½ teaspoons prepared horseradish, drained

Himalayan pink salt

Sprig of dill, for garnish (optional)

Place the mayonnaise, smoked salmon, lemon juice, and Dijon mustard in a food processor and process until the ingredients are well mixed. Add the shallots, chives, dill, horseradish, and a pinch or two of salt and process again until smooth and creamy. Transfer to a serving plate and garnish with a sprig of dill, if desired. Serve chilled.

MAKE IT EGG-FREE
Use Egg-Free Mayonnaise (page 392).

STORAGE INFORMATION
Store this dip in an airtight container in the refrigerator for up to 3 days.

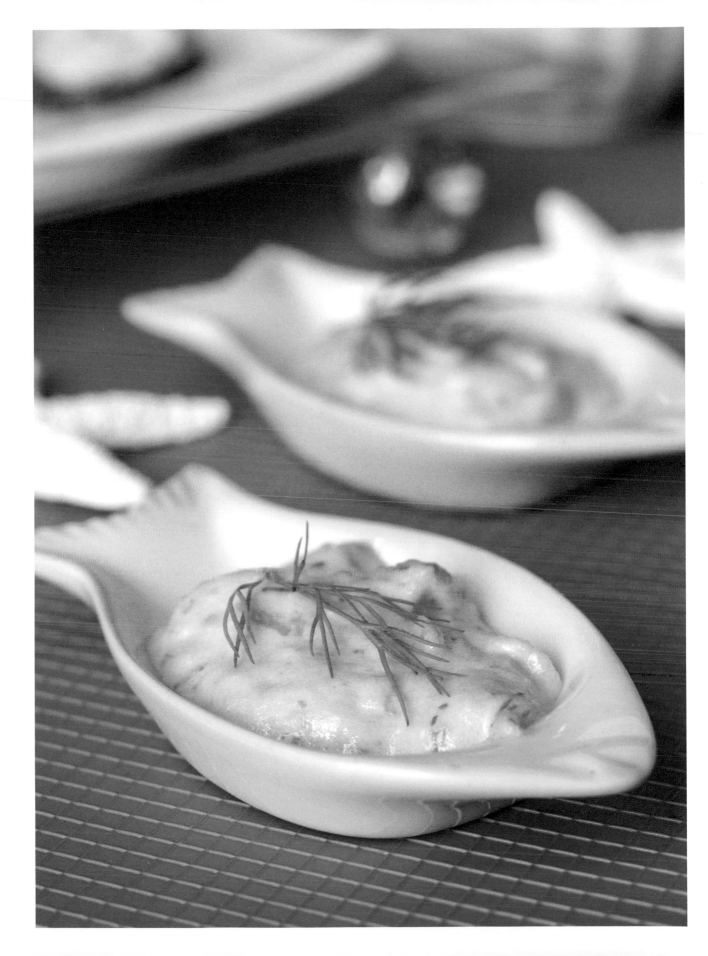

strawberry-banana chia pops

MAKES 4 pops   PREP TIME: 7 minutes, plus time to freeze the pops

When my friends come to visit with their young kids, these strawberry-banana pops are the go-to treat I find myself making again and again. The ingredients take no time to whip together, and since I have a Zoku Quick Pop Maker that freezes ice pops in 7 minutes flat, it's a speedy treat. (It takes longer in a regular freezer, about 4 hours, so if that's what you're using, you'll want to plan ahead.) The kids always love to help make them, too! These pops also make a great alternative to sugary yogurt breakfast pops and are perfect for dessert.

1 frozen banana, chopped

3 medjool dates, pitted (see Note)

1¼ cups frozen strawberries

½ cup plus 2 tablespoons coconut cream (see page 74)

½ cup water

1 teaspoon pure vanilla extract

¼ cup chia seeds

SPECIAL TOOLS _____
4 (2-ounce) ice pop molds

1. Place all the ingredients except the chia seeds in a blender. Process on high speed until smooth and creamy.

2. Stir in the chia seeds. Pour the mixture into four 2-ounce ice pop molds and freeze until set, about 4 hours.

NOTE _____

If you're using a conventional blender rather than a high-powered one and your dates are on the dry side, soak them in water for 15 to 30 minutes to soften them before pureeing (very moist, succulent medjool dates do not require soaking).

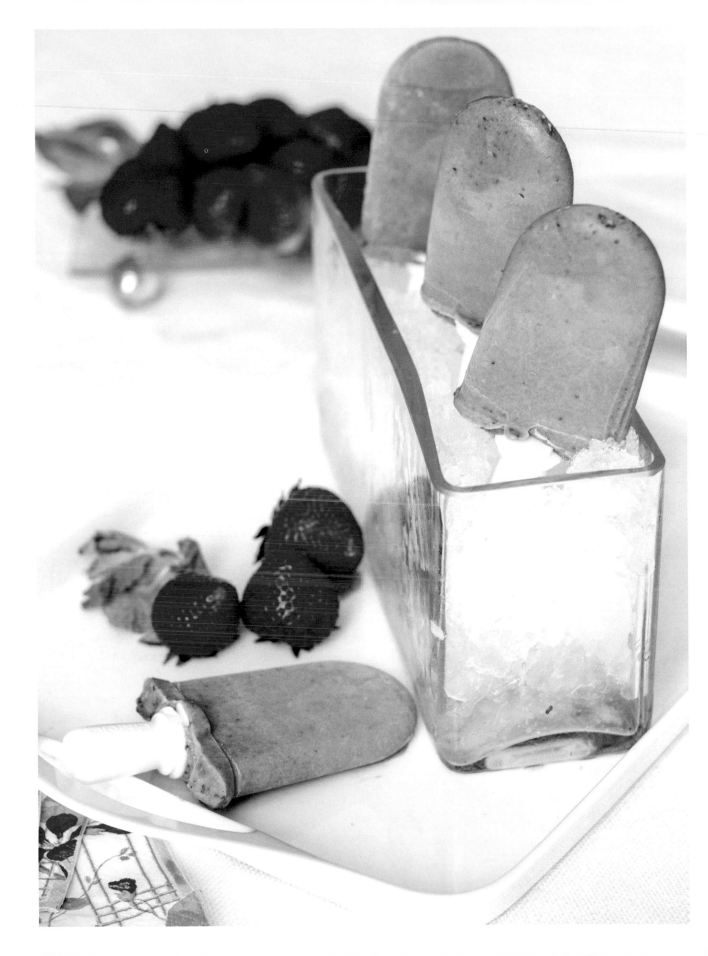

spinach & artichoke dip

MAKES about 1½ cups   PREP TIME: 20 minutes   COOK TIME: 50 minutes

Whether we are staying in for Sunday night football or having friends over for dinner, this dip is frequently on the menu. And leftovers never go to waste! This is an incredibly versatile dip. I mix it with scrambled eggs for a quick breakfast or spread it on sprouted whole-grain bread and top it with sliced jarred roasted red peppers and anchovies for a tasty open-faced sandwich. For super-easy Meatless Monday dinners, I'll serve baked potatoes stuffed with this dip and a side green salad. And of course, you can never go wrong with dip and whole-grain crackers or crudités for an afternoon snack.

2 (9-ounce) packages frozen artichoke hearts

2 tablespoons extra-virgin olive oil, divided

¾ teaspoon Himalayan pink salt, divided

½ cup chopped shallots

3 cups chopped spinach

2 teaspoons minced garlic

½ cup pine nuts (see Note)

½ cup water

2 tablespoons fresh lemon juice

¼ teaspoon ground white pepper

2 pinches of ground nutmeg

1. Preheat the oven to 400°F.

2. Place the frozen artichoke hearts on a rimmed baking sheet, drizzle with 1 tablespoon of the oil, and sprinkle with ¼ teaspoon of the salt. Roast for 40 minutes, until softened. Remove the artichokes from the oven and set aside to cool. Lower the oven temperature to 350°F.

3. Heat the remaining tablespoon of oil in a large skillet over medium heat. Add the shallots and sauté for 3 to 4 minutes, until they start to soften. Add the spinach and garlic and cook until the spinach has completely wilted, about 3 minutes. Stir in ¼ teaspoon of the salt. Slide the pan off the heat and set aside.

4. Place the pine nuts, water, lemon juice, white pepper, nutmeg, and remaining ¼ teaspoon of salt in a blender. Process on high speed until the mixture is smooth and creamy.

5. Place the pine nut cream and roasted artichoke hearts in a food processor and process until the artichoke hearts are coarsely chopped and the ingredients are just blended. Do not overblend; the mixture should still have some texture to it.

6. Transfer the artichoke–pine nut mixture to the skillet with the spinach. Use a wooden spoon to mix the ingredients together. Spoon the spinach mixture into an ovenproof 1-quart casserole dish and bake for 10 minutes.

STORAGE INFORMATION _____
This dip will keep in an airtight container in the refrigerator for up to 3 days.

NOTE _____
If you are using a conventional blender instead of a high-powered one, soak the pine nuts in water for 30 minutes, then rinse and drain them, before using them in this recipe.

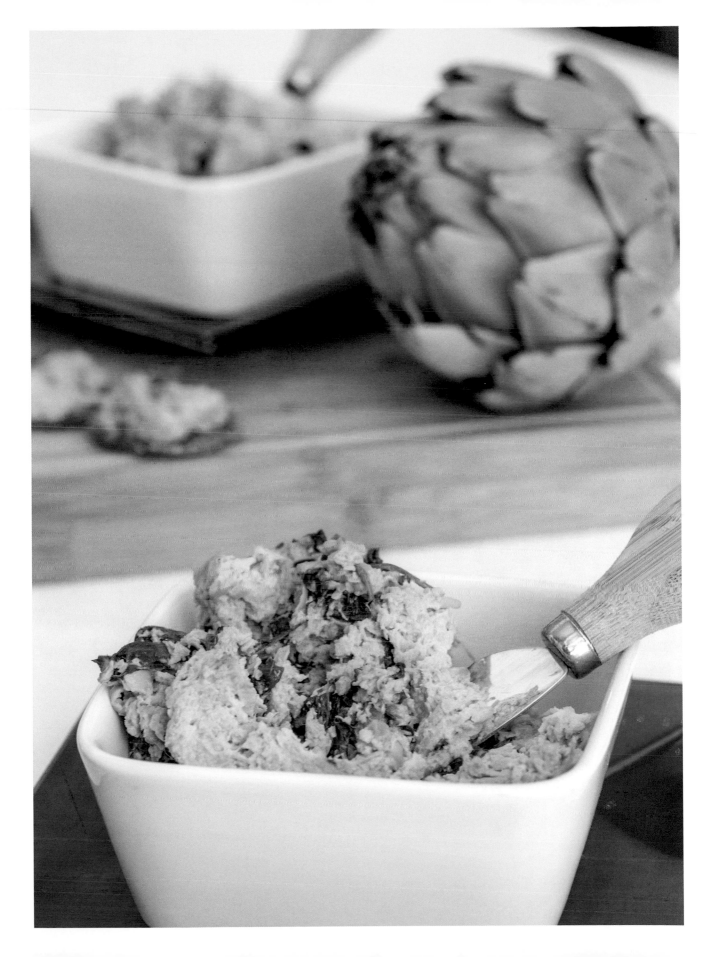

chocolate popcorn

MAKES 10 cups   PREP TIME: 5 minutes, plus time to chill   COOK TIME: 5 minutes

I've been making a version of this popcorn ever since my son, Blake, was in elementary school. Whenever his friends came over, this was the treat they all would ask for. I think his friend Naaman ate practically all of it in one sitting the first time I made it for him! The boys were about six or seven years old at the time, and I'll never forget what Naaman said to Blake after polishing off that huge bowl: "It's funny how I can always eat so much of your mom's junk food and never get sick like I do when I eat junk food at other places."

---

10 cups popped popcorn (see Note)

¼ cup plus 3 tablespoons extra-virgin coconut oil

2 tablespoons full-fat coconut milk

½ cup cacao powder

¼ cup pure maple syrup

2 tablespoons acai powder (optional)

1 teaspoon pure vanilla extract

¼ teaspoon Himalayan pink salt

2 tablespoons coconut sugar

1. Place the popcorn in a large mixing bowl and set aside.

2. Put the coconut oil and coconut milk in a small saucepan over low heat and stir together for about 1 minute, until the oil is melted. Slowly stir in the cacao powder, maple syrup, acai powder (if using), and vanilla extract. Use a whisk to mix the ingredients thoroughly until the mixture is smooth and lump-free. Stir in the salt.

3. Carefully pour the chocolate mixture over the popcorn, using a spoon to mix and toss the popcorn to evenly coat. Sprinkle with the coconut sugar. Refrigerate for about 15 minutes to harden the chocolate before serving.

NOTE _____

To get 10 cups popped popcorn, you will need ⅓ cup unpopped popcorn.

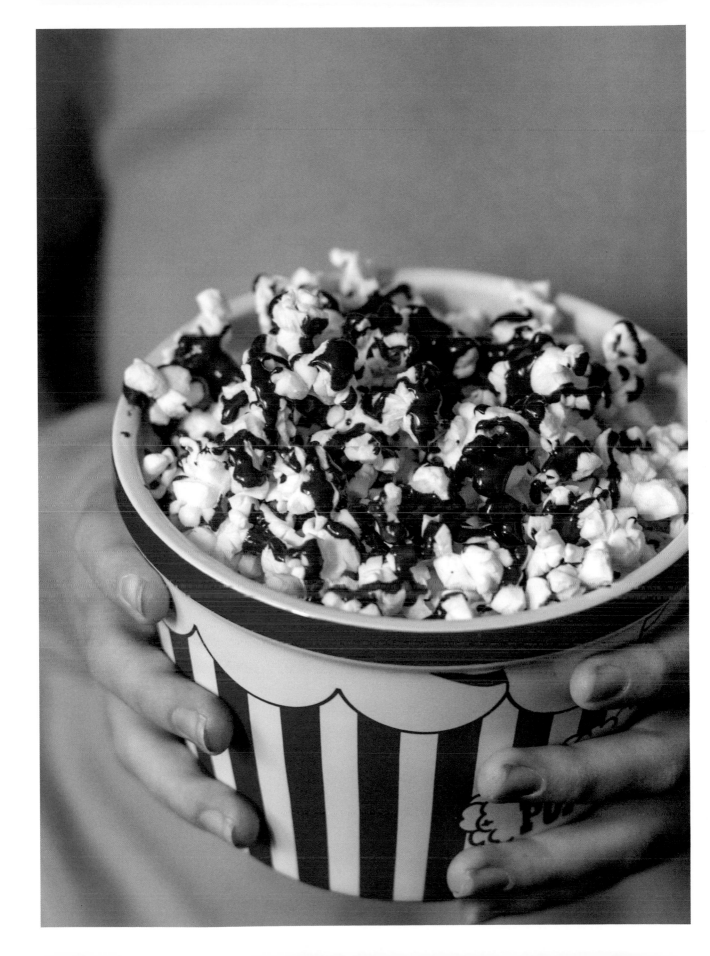

carrot hummus

MAKES about ¾ cup   PREP TIME: 10 minutes   COOK TIME: 5 minutes

As long as it is not made with refined vegetable oil, I have nothing against store-bought hummus. However, this hummus is a super-tasty way to work yet another vegetable serving into your day. And the color is so vibrant and beautiful! I first made this hummus for a dinner party and served it with olives, grapes, Sweet & Savory Party Nuts (page 132), dried fruit, crackers, and homemade beet chips. What a hit it was! But this hummus is not just for entertaining. It's so easy to make that it's a great everyday snack food, especially in the summer because, over time, the beta-carotene and phytonutrients in the carrots help protect against sunburn. Serve with beet chips (see below) or gluten-free crackers.

---

3 large carrots, peeled and cut into bite-sized pieces

3 cloves garlic, peeled

¼ cup fresh lemon juice

¼ cup tahini

3 tablespoons extra-virgin olive oil

½ teaspoon Himalayan pink salt

¼ teaspoon ground black pepper

⅛ teaspoon turmeric powder

Sprig of rosemary, for garnish (optional)

1. Place a steamer basket in a saucepan filled with about 2 inches of water. Bring the water to a boil, add the carrots to the steamer basket, cover, and steam until fork-tender, about 5 minutes. Allow the carrots to cool until they can be handled but are still warm. (Note: If you've steamed the carrots in advance, warm them in the microwave on high for about 1 minute.)

2. Place all of the ingredients in a food processor. Process for 1 full minute, until the mixture is smooth and creamy. Adjust the seasoning to taste and serve at room temperature, garnished with a sprig of rosemary, if desired.

STORAGE INFORMATION

Carrot hummus can be stored in an airtight container in the refrigerator for up to 2 days. Once refrigerated, bring to room temperature for at least an hour before serving. This recipe can easily be doubled if you're serving a crowd.

HOW TO MAKE BEET CHIPS

Beet chips are easy to make: simply slice peeled beets super thin with a mandoline, toss the slices with some extra-virgin olive oil and salt, then roast them on a rimmed baking sheet in a preheated 375°F oven for 15 to 20 minutes, until crispy, flipping them halfway through. But if you are pressed for time, Naked Beet Chips from Rhythm Superfoods are a clean store-bought option, and they are delicious!

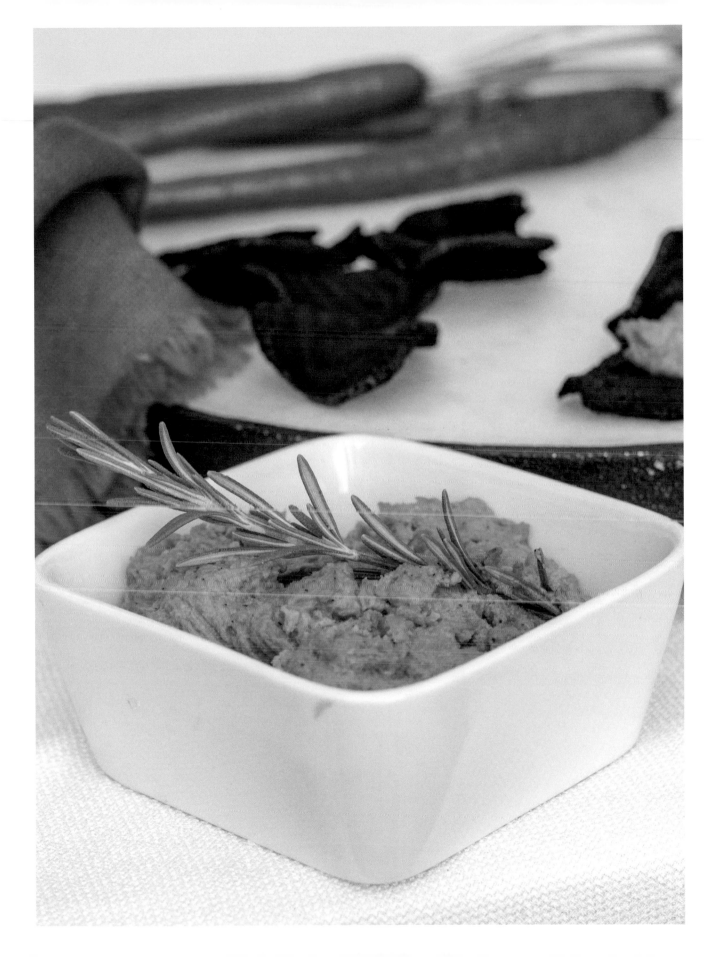

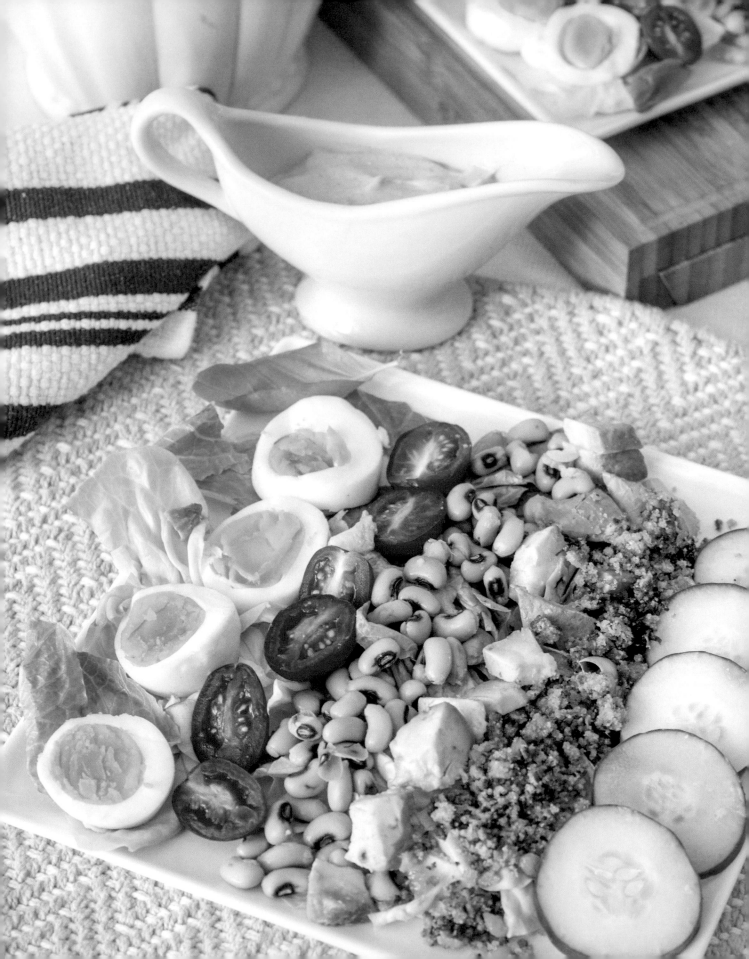

CHAPTER 10

soups and salads

cream (or no cream) of tomato soup

SERVES 6   PREP TIME: 25 minutes   COOK TIME: 25 minutes

This soup is delicious served hot, but living in South Florida, where we are lucky to have warm weather almost year-round, I frequently serve it chilled. If I want a lighter (non-creamy) soup, I simply omit the cashews. But no matter how you decide to serve it—chilled, hot, creamy or not—you will most definitely not be disappointed!

⅓ cup raw cashews, preferably soaked in water for 1 to 2 hours, then rinsed and drained (optional; see Note)

4 cups vegetable broth

5 large tomatoes

1 tablespoon plus 1 teaspoon extra-virgin olive oil

1 large onion, chopped

3 stalks celery, chopped

5 cloves garlic, smashed with the side of a knife

2 medium carrots, peeled and chopped

1 red bell pepper, chopped

¼ teaspoon Himalayan pink salt

Juice of 1 lime

2 teaspoons raw honey

½ teaspoon curry powder

For garnish (optional):

1 cup Garlic Herbed Croutons (page 358)

Coarsely chopped fresh parsley

1. If you're not using cashews, skip to step 2. In a blender, process the cashews and vegetable broth until smooth and creamy. Set the creamy broth aside.

2. Bring a large pot of salted water to a boil and fill a large bowl with ice and water and set it next to the stove. Score an X on the bottoms of the tomatoes with a paring knife, then add the tomatoes to the boiling water. When the skins of the tomatoes start to wrinkle and split, after about 1 minute, scoop them out with a slotted spoon and transfer them to the ice water bath. Once the tomatoes are cool enough to handle, carefully slip off the skins and discard. Chop the tomatoes and set aside.

3. Heat the oil in a large saucepan over medium-high heat, then add the onion and celery and sauté for about 3 minutes. Add the garlic, carrots, and bell pepper and sauté for 3 to 4 minutes, until the vegetables are soft. Add the salt. Stir in the chopped tomatoes.

4. If you completed step 1 to make the creamy broth, add that now; if you skipped step 1, add just the 4 cups of vegetable broth. Then add the lime juice, honey, and curry powder and simmer for 15 minutes, until the tomatoes are soft.

5. Use a handheld stick blender to blend the soup until it's smooth, or blend it in small batches in a jar blender. Garnish with croutons and chopped parsley if desired. Serve hot or cold.

NOTE

If you're using a high-powered blender, soaking the cashews is optional, though it creates an even smoother, creamier soup. If you are using a conventional blender, soaking the nuts first is necessary to get the right texture.

MAKE IT NUT-FREE

Omit the cashews.

MAKE IT VEGAN

Omit the honey.

MAKE IT GRAIN-FREE AND PALEO-FRIENDLY

Omit the croutons.

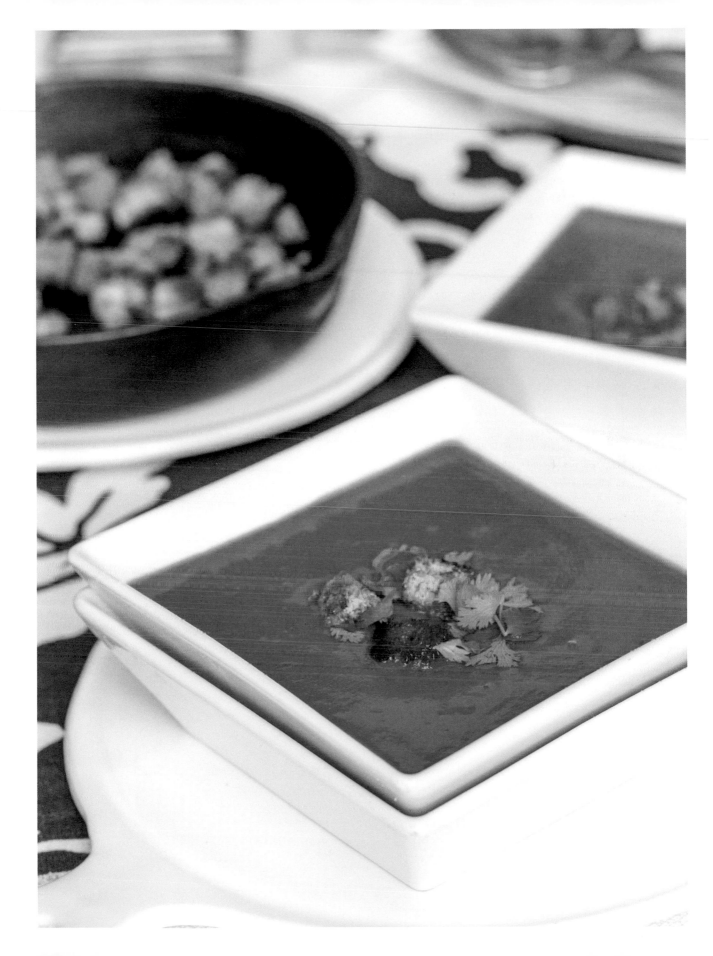

cream of mushroom soup

SERVES 4   PREP TIME: 15 minutes   COOK TIME: 30 minutes

Nobody will ever guess this rich and luscious soup is dairy-free. Savory, earthy, and mellow, it's a soup for all seasons. I actually serve it chilled in the summertime, and it's absolutely delicious! I like to use probiotic-rich chickpea miso mixed with warm water for the broth, but you can substitute vegetable broth if you prefer. By the way, chickpea miso doesn't taste at all like conventional soy-based miso; it has a mild, nutty flavor.

½ cup chickpea miso plus 5 cups warm water, or 5 cups vegetable broth

½ cup raw cashews, preferably soaked in water for 1 to 2 hours, then rinsed and drained (see Note)

¼ cup extra-virgin olive oil

¾ cup chopped onions

10 ounces shiitake mushrooms, stemmed and chopped

2 teaspoons fresh thyme

½ teaspoon Himalayan pink salt

2 tablespoons cassava flour (or sprouted spelt flour if not gluten- or grain-free)

4 thyme sprigs, for garnish (optional)

1. Put the chickpea miso and warm water (or just the vegetable broth) in a blender. Add the nuts and blend the ingredients together until smooth. Set aside.

2. Heat the oil in a stockpot over medium heat. Add the onions and cook until softened, about 8 minutes.

3. Add the mushrooms, thyme, and salt to the pot and stir to combine with the onions. Cook until the mushrooms begin to release their liquid, 5 to 6 minutes. Reduce the heat to medium-low and add the flour. Cook, stirring continuously, for about 2 minutes, until the flour, onions, and mushrooms are well combined.

4. Add the blended broth mixture to the pot and increase the heat to medium-high. Once the soup begins to boil, turn the heat down to low and simmer for 10 minutes, until the mushrooms are very soft.

5. Use a handheld stick blender to process the soup until creamy and well blended, or blend it in small batches in a jar blender. Divide evenly among 4 bowls and garnish each with a thyme sprig, if desired. Serve hot or cold.

NOTE

If you're using a high-powered blender, soaking the nuts is optional, though it creates an even smoother, creamier soup. If you are using a conventional blender, soaking the nuts first is necessary to get the right texture.

MAKE IT BEAN-FREE AND PALEO-FRIENDLY

Substitute vegetable broth for the chickpea miso broth.

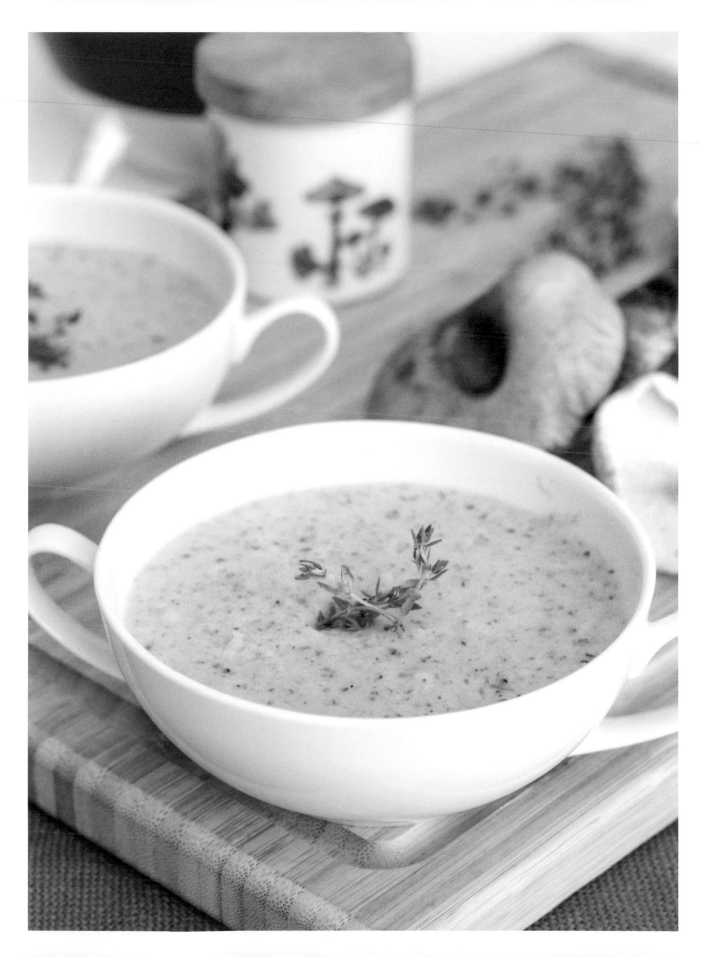

japanese restaurant–style salad with ginger dressing

SERVES 4   PREP TIME: 10 minutes

I have always loved the vibrant orange ginger dressing you get at Japanese restaurants—so much so that sometimes I would go out for Japanese food just to have the salad! The dressing always elevated the simple greens into something very special. The first time I made this dressing recipe was when we had one of my dearest friends, Gisela Tanner, and her family over to dinner. Everybody poured the dressing on top of their wild salmon before we even got to the salad. I was especially pleased that all of the kids loved it, too! All those years, I had no idea that classic Japanese dressing is so easy to make.

For the dressing:

3 small carrots, peeled and coarsely chopped

2 shallots, coarsely chopped

2 cloves garlic, peeled

½ cup unrefined macadamia nut oil

¼ cup grated fresh ginger

¼ cup unseasoned rice vinegar

¼ cup water

2 tablespoons chickpea miso

2 tablespoons fresh lime juice

2 tablespoons manuka honey or other raw honey

2 tablespoons unrefined toasted sesame oil

1 tablespoon plus 1 teaspoon gluten-free tamari (or unpasteurized soy sauce, if not gluten-free)

7 cups chopped butter lettuce

Place all of the ingredients for the dressing in a large food processor. Process until smooth and creamy. Refrigerate until chilled. Serve the chilled dressing over the butter lettuce.

STORAGE INFORMATION

The dressing will keep in a mason jar in the refrigerator for up to 4 days.

NOTE

If you want to make a more elaborate or filling salad, try topping the salad greens with avocado slices, orange slices, sliced scallions, and sliced or quartered hard-boiled eggs.

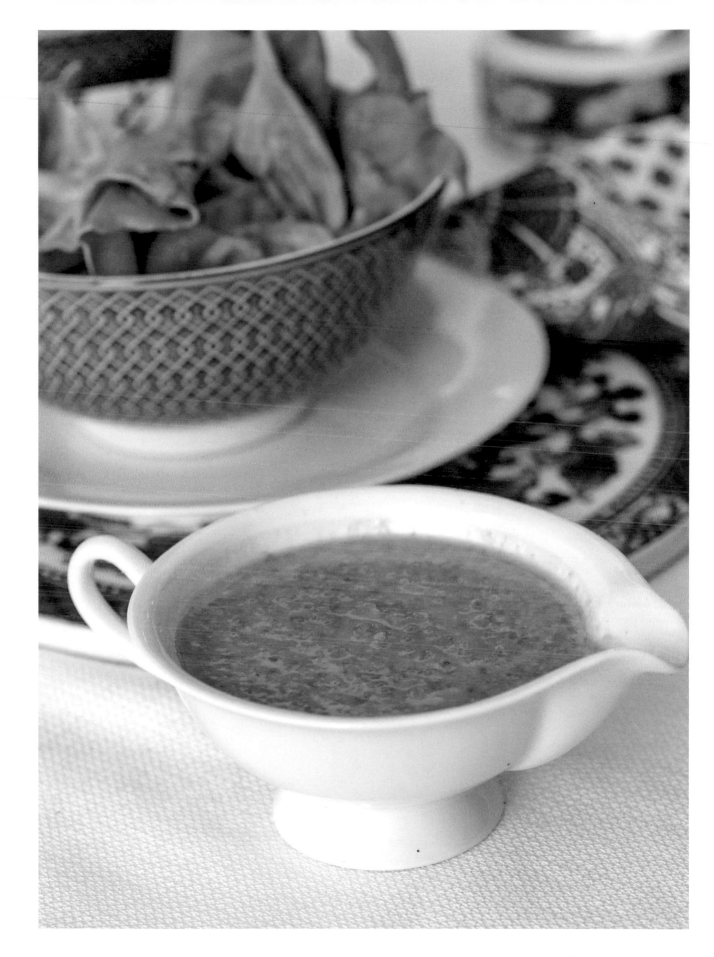

red curry butternut squash soup

SERVES 6   PREP TIME: 25 minutes   COOK TIME: 1 hour 30 minutes

I have a weakness for all things curry, so much so that my cooking notebook is filled with hand-scribbled curry recipes of all kinds. Some are admittedly a bit complicated, while others are incredibly basic and unfussy—like this one, which I am particularly fond of. It's perfect for a light lunch or supper, but it can also easily be made heartier with simple stir-ins. When I am trying to beef the recipe up a bit, I often add cooked black rice or shrimp (or both!). Tofu is also a delicious addition for Meatless Mondays.

For the squash:

1 medium butternut squash (2½ to 3 pounds)

Melted extra-virgin coconut oil

Himalayan pink salt

1 tablespoon extra-virgin coconut oil

1 medium onion, chopped

¼ teaspoon Himalayan pink salt

6 cloves garlic, minced

1 tablespoon grated fresh ginger

1 (14.5-ounce) can diced tomatoes, drained

1 tablespoon red curry paste

4 cups vegetable broth

1 cup full-fat coconut milk

2 tablespoons gluten-free tamari (or unpasteurized soy sauce, if not gluten-free)

5 cups baby spinach

2 tablespoons fresh lime juice

1. To roast the squash, preheat the oven to 400°F. Slice the butternut squash in half lengthwise and scoop out the seeds. Lightly brush the inside flesh with coconut oil and season lightly with salt. Put the squash halves on a rimmed baking sheet, cut side up, and roast for 50 to 60 minutes, until the flesh is fork-tender. Once the butternut squash is cool enough to handle, peel and cut into bite-sized cubes; set aside.

2. Heat the oil in a large pot over medium heat. When the oil is hot, add the onion and salt and sauté for 5 to 6 minutes, until the onion softens. Add the garlic and ginger and sauté for 1 to 2 minutes.

3. Add the tomatoes, red curry paste, and butternut squash and cook for 5 minutes, until warm. Add the vegetable broth, coconut milk, and tamari, bring to a rapid simmer, and cook for 10 minutes, until fragrant. Lower the temperature to a gentle simmer and continue to cook for an additional 5 minutes to deepen the flavor.

4. Transfer half of the soup to a large bowl. Use a handheld stick blender to puree the soup remaining in the pot until smooth. (Alternatively, transfer half of the soup to a jar blender, allow it to cool to room temperature, and then process until smooth.) Return the pureed soup to the pot.

5. Turn the heat up to medium and add the spinach and lime juice; cook for 1 to 2 minutes, until the spinach wilts. Serve warm.

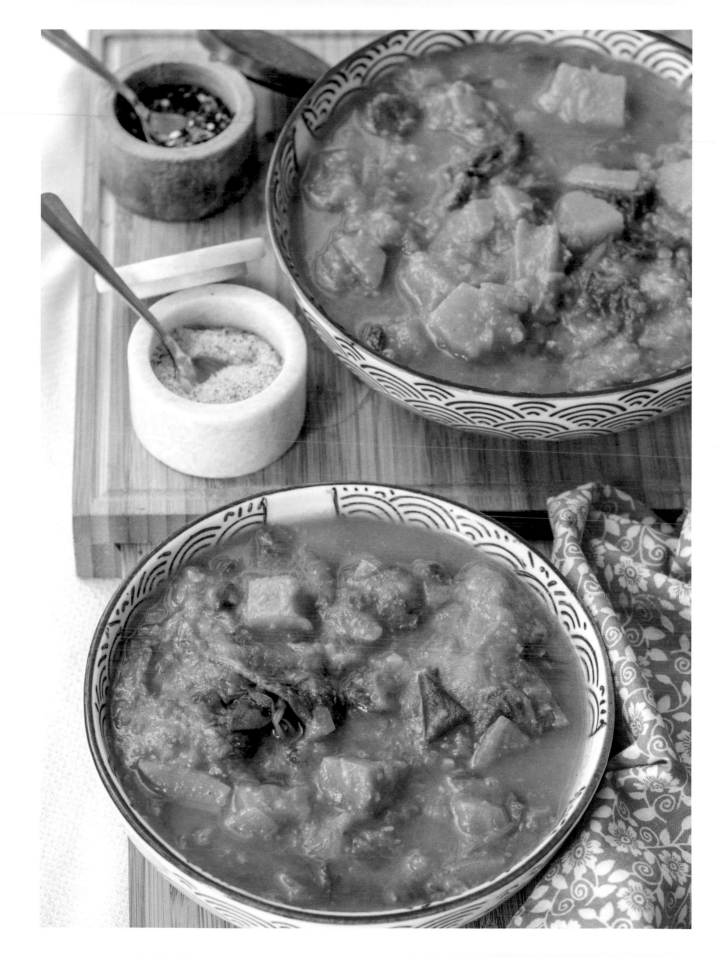

salmon niçoise salad
with lemon tarragon dressing

SERVES 4   PREP TIME: 20 minutes   COOK TIME: 35 minutes

For years, niçoise salad has been a restaurant favorite of mine. But it wasn't until I started writing this cookbook that I made it at home. I should have been doing this years ago! A true classic, it's the perfect meal-in-one salad for a weeknight dinner, but it's also great for easy entertaining. Although a niçoise salad is traditionally made with tuna, I prefer to use wild salmon because tuna is high in mercury. And of course, I couldn't help but sneak in some extra vegetables!

For the dressing:

½ cup extra-virgin olive oil

3 tablespoons fresh lemon juice

2 tablespoons chopped fresh tarragon

2 cloves garlic, peeled

1 teaspoon Dijon mustard

½ teaspoon manuka honey or other raw honey

¼ teaspoon Himalayan pink salt

For the salad:

8 new potatoes or small Yukon Gold potatoes (leave peel on)

3 cups haricots verts or regular green beans, ends trimmed

2 large carrots, peeled and cut into thin 4-inch-long strips

4 (4-ounce) wild salmon fillets

Extra-virgin olive oil

Himalayan pink salt

2 heads butter lettuce, roughly torn

4 cups mâche (corn salad) or other soft green lettuce

2 jarred roasted red peppers, patted dry and cut into thin strips

1 pint grape tomatoes, halved

½ cup niçoise olives, pitted

1 dozen olive oil–packed anchovies (optional)

4 hard-boiled eggs, halved lengthwise

TO MAKE THE DRESSING: Place all the ingredients in a blender or mini food processor and process until smooth and creamy. Taste and add more salt if desired. (Note: The dressing can be made up to 3 days in advance and stored in a covered container in the refrigerator.)

TO MAKE THE SALAD:

1. Place a steamer basket in a saucepan filled with about 2 inches of water. Bring the water to a boil, place the potatoes in the steamer basket, cover, and steam until cooked through, about 20 minutes. Remove the potatoes and set aside. Add more water if necessary and place the haricots verts and carrots in the steamer basket. Return the water to a boil, cover, and steam until fork-tender, about 7 minutes. Let the vegetables cool, then quarter the potatoes.

2. Lightly brush the salmon with oil and season lightly with salt. Oil a large heavy-bottomed skillet and heat over medium-high heat. When the skillet is hot, add the salmon and sear for about 3 minutes per side, until medium-rare. Transfer the salmon to a platter and set aside.

3. Divide the butter lettuce and mâche among 4 plates. Lay the haricots verts, carrots, peppers, tomatoes, olives, and anchovies (if using) on top of the lettuce. Arrange the potatoes and eggs around the edges. Lay the seared salmon fillets on top. Drizzle with the dressing. Serve at room temperature.

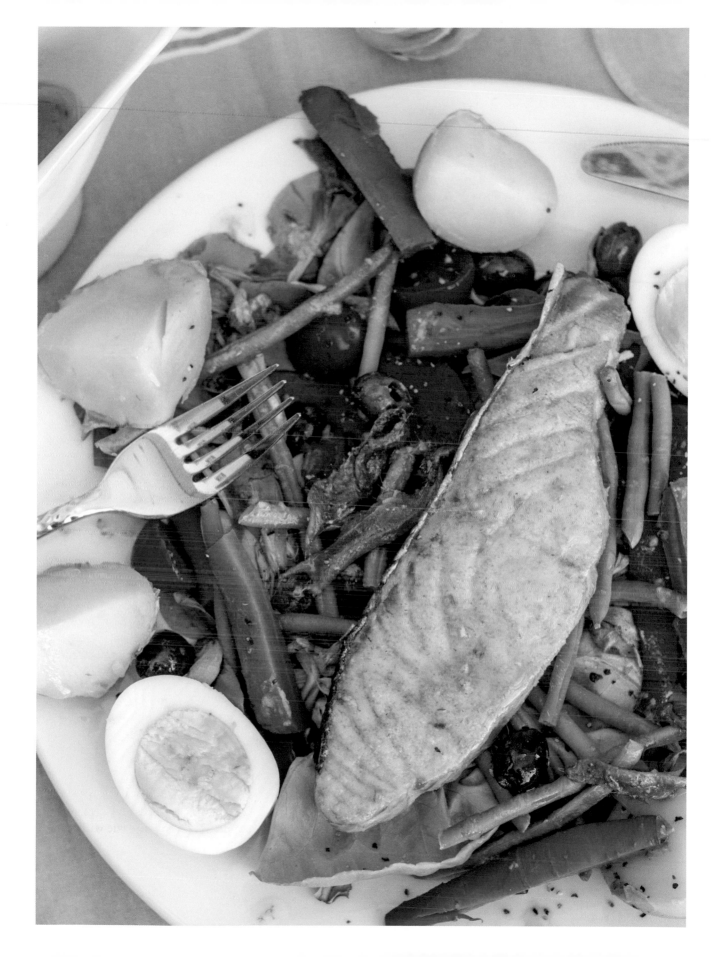

classic-style caesar salad

SERVES 6   PREP TIME: 15 minutes

If you are entertaining guests, you can't go wrong with this dish. Not only does almost everybody love Caesar salad, but this version can be made to suit just about any dietary need, yet it still tastes just like a classic Caesar salad. I first made this recipe when I was teaching an after-hours cooking class at Williams Sonoma, and I later made it at the Palm Beach Fresh Fest for a large audience. It has been tested on hundreds of people, and everyone always goes crazy over it. It never lets me down! Of course, you can always add grilled shrimp, chicken, or salmon to make a quick and easy weeknight dinner, too.

For the dressing:

¼ cup plus 1 tablespoon extra-virgin olive oil

¼ cup plus 1 tablespoon fresh lemon juice

¼ cup hemp seeds

3 cloves garlic, peeled

1 teaspoon gluten-free Worcestershire sauce

¾ teaspoon Dijon mustard

½ teaspoon anchovy paste (optional)

⅛ teaspoon ground black pepper

⅛ teaspoon Himalayan pink salt

For the salad:

10 cups coarsely chopped romaine lettuce

5 cups Garlic Herbed Croutons (page 358) (optional)

6 olive oil–packed anchovies (optional)

1. To make the dressing, put all the dressing ingredients in a blender and process on high speed until smooth and creamy. (Note: The dressing can be made 4 to 5 days in advance and stored in a covered container in the refrigerator.)

2. To make the salad, put the lettuce in a large bowl. Drizzle the dressing on top and use wooden spoons to gently toss to coat the lettuce. Divide the salad among 6 bowls, add the croutons (if using), and top each salad with one anchovy (if using). Serve the salads at room temperature.

MAKE IT VEGAN AND VEGETARIAN _____
Omit the anchovies and anchovy paste and use a vegan Worcestershire sauce.

MAKE IT GRAIN-FREE AND PALEO-FRIENDLY _____
Omit the croutons.

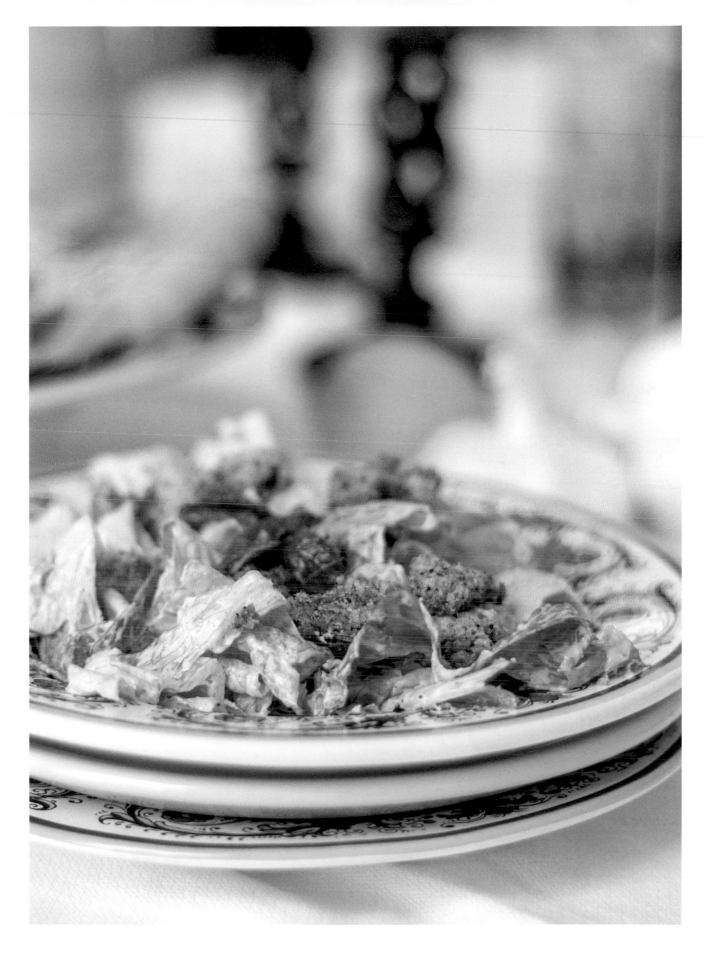

manhattan clam chowder

SERVES 8 to 10   PREP TIME: 25 minutes   COOK TIME: 45 minutes

I became fond of Manhattan clam chowder while living in New York in 2001. I was nursing our son, Blake, at the time and was always starving, and one of the things that totally hit the spot was the Manhattan clam chowder at Dock's Oyster Bar & Seafood Grill, located in Midtown East. Everything there was fresh and delicious, but I just couldn't get enough of their chowder. I ate it so much while I was nursing, I often wonder if Blake developed a taste for it (and for seafood in general) through osmosis. I re-created the recipe at home—and of course I couldn't help but beef up the vegetables—and to this day Blake still loves this recipe. One of the secrets to this recipe is to finely chop the vegetables so that they are not much bigger than the clams. Also, I use anchovy paste instead of bacon or sausage. Even if you don't like anchovy paste, use it for this recipe—it gives incredible depth of flavor, and I promise it doesn't make the chowder taste one bit anchovy-ish.

¼ cup extra-virgin olive oil

1 tablespoon plus 2 teaspoons anchovy paste

1 cup finely chopped onions

5 cloves garlic, minced

2 stalks celery, finely chopped

2 medium carrots, peeled and finely chopped

1 red bell pepper, finely chopped

2 large Yukon Gold potatoes, cubed (leave skins on)

1 teaspoon ground black pepper

1 teaspoon Himalayan pink salt

½ teaspoon crushed red pepper

1 (28-ounce) can whole peeled tomatoes, with juices, gently crushed with a potato masher

1 cup clam broth (see Note)

3 sprigs fresh thyme

3 (6.5-ounce) cans chopped clams, drained (see Note)

Chopped chives, scallions, or parsley, for garnish (optional)

1. Place the oil and anchovy paste in a large saucepan and heat over medium heat. Once the oil is hot, add the onions, garlic, celery, carrots, and bell pepper. Sauté the vegetables, stirring occasionally, for about 10 minutes, until very soft.

2. Stir in the potatoes and add the black pepper, salt, and crushed red pepper. Cook for about 7 minutes.

3. Add the tomatoes, clam broth, and thyme sprigs. Partly cover the pot, turn the heat down to low, and simmer until the potatoes are tender, 10 to 15 minutes. Smash the potatoes gently with a potato masher.

4. Add the clams and simmer, uncovered, for 10 minutes. Slide the pan off the heat and let the chowder sit to allow the flavors to develop for at least 10 minutes before serving. Taste and add additional salt if desired. Garnish with chives, scallions, or parsley, if desired, and serve warm.

NOTE

It is super important to buy the highest-quality clams and clam broth you can find for this recipe. I really love Bar Harbor brand for both; it doesn't have any funky, "non-clean" ingredients.

STORAGE INFORMATION

Manhattan clam chowder can be stored in an airtight container in the refrigerator for up to 3 days or in the freezer for up to 2 weeks.

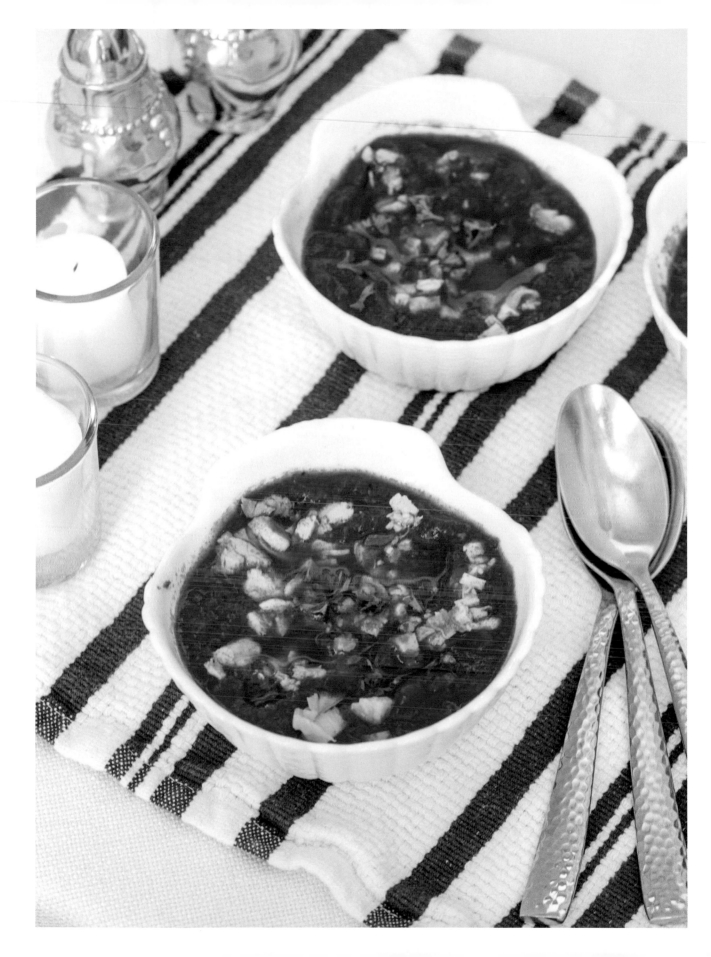

vegetable chowder

A spin-off of classic corn chowder and a great alternative to the vegetable soup on page 174, this rich and creamy chowder recipe offers yet another way to eat your vegetables! Thanks to the roux, it has a satisfyingly thick texture, and just like Hidden Veggie Marinara (page 378), this recipe works in a surprising number of vegetables. It's the perfect soup for those with picky palates who say they don't like vegetables.

4 cups vegetable broth

¾ cup raw cashews, preferably soaked in water for 1 to 2 hours, then rinsed and drained (see Note)

3 tablespoons extra-virgin olive oil or unrefined avocado oil

2 tablespoons cassava flour (or sprouted spelt flour if not gluten- or grain-free)

½ cup finely chopped onions

3 medium carrots, peeled and finely chopped

1 leek, finely chopped, thoroughly washed, and dried (see page 219)

3 stalks celery, finely chopped

3 cups frozen corn

1 teaspoon dried thyme leaves

½ teaspoon Himalayan pink salt

3 tablespoons fresh lemon juice

1. Put the broth and cashews in a blender and process until smooth and creamy. Set aside.

2. To make a roux, heat the oil in a large saucepan over medium heat. Whisk in the flour and keep whisking until the mixture darkens but does not burn, about 4 minutes.

3. To the saucepan with the roux, add the onions, carrots, leek, and celery and cook, stirring occasionally, until the vegetables begin to soften, 5 to 6 minutes. Add the corn, thyme, and salt and cook for 2 to 3 minutes, until the corn is completely thawed.

4. Pour in the reserved cashew mixture and bring to a boil. Turn the heat down to low and simmer for 10 minutes, until thickened. Add the lemon juice and turn the heat off.

5. Use a handheld stick blender to blend the chowder until mostly smooth (it should still have a slightly chunky texture), or blend it in small batches in a jar blender. Taste for seasoning and add more salt, if desired. Serve warm.

NOTE

If you're using a high-powered blender, soaking the cashews is optional, though it creates a creamier texture. If you are using a conventional blender, soaking the nuts first is necessary to get the right texture.

STORAGE INFORMATION

Store vegetable chowder in an airtight container in the refrigerator for up to 3 days or in the freezer for up to 2 weeks.

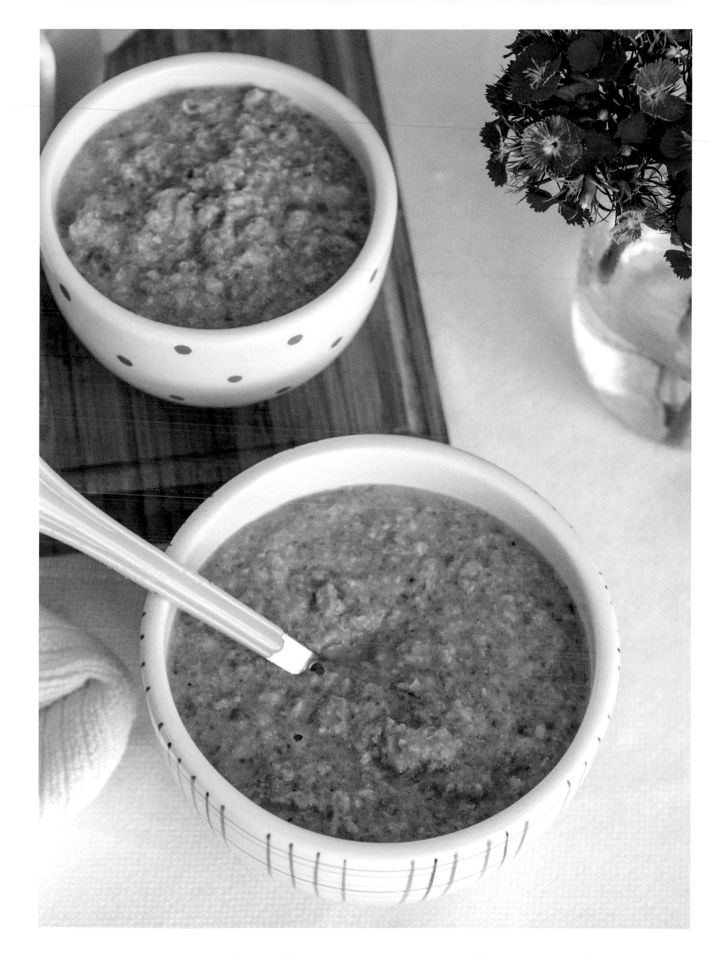

seven-layer salad

SERVES 8   PREP TIME: 10 minutes, plus time to chill   COOK TIME: 30 minutes

A seven-layer salad is always a party favorite, and if you happen to have a family of football fans (as we do), then you need touchdown-worthy football food. This dish is sure to bowl the whole gang over! Traditionally, seven-layer salad is served in a large clear bowl, but I like to serve it in individual mason jars, so we can eat it straight from the jar with a spoon. If you serve it in a large bowl, you'll want to have some healthy chips to dip in it. I make my own whole-grain baked tortilla chips (the recipe is on our blog). Thin brown-rice cakes also make great dippers.

---

2 cups cherry tomatoes

2 teaspoons extra-virgin olive oil

½ teaspoon Himalayan pink salt, divided

2 Hass avocados, peeled, halved, and pitted

Juice of 1 lime

2 cups Karen's Easy Refried Beans (page 272), room temperature

2 cups shredded butter lettuce

¾ cup canned sliced black olives

¾ cup Clean Cuisine Sour Cream (page 372)

1 cup chopped scallions

1. Preheat the oven to 400°F.

2. Arrange the tomatoes on a rimmed baking sheet and drizzle with the olive oil. Sprinkle with ¼ teaspoon of the salt. Roast the tomatoes for 30 minutes, or until soft. Remove the tomatoes from the oven and use a potato masher to lightly mash. Set aside to cool to room temperature.

3. In a medium-sized mixing bowl, mash the avocados with the lime juice and remaining ¼ teaspoon of salt. Set aside.

4. Divide the refried beans evenly among eight 8-ounce mason jars (or spread it on the bottom of a large glass bowl, if you prefer). Spread the mashed avocado on top. Spread the mashed tomatoes on top of the avocado. Scatter the lettuce on top, then the olives. Spread the sour cream on top of the olives and finish with the scallions.

5. Cover and refrigerate for at least 2 hours or overnight. Allow to come to room temperature before serving.

STORAGE INFORMATION _____
Store seven-layer salad in an airtight container in the refrigerator for up to 1 day.

MAKE IT VEGAN _____
Omit the honey in the sour cream.

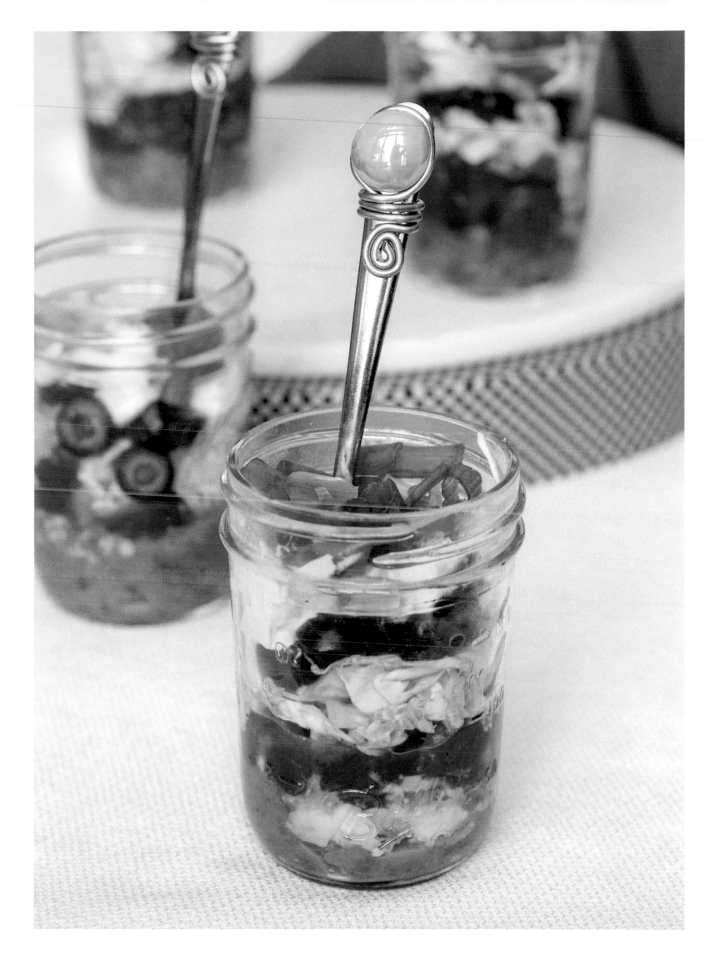

cream of broccoli soup

SERVES 6   PREP TIME: 15 minutes   COOK TIME: 35 minutes

The first time I made this soup, my son suggested I serve broccoli only this way from then on. I think it must be among the tastiest ways to eat broccoli. Okay, so broccoli cheddar soup might be even better, but for being clean and dairy-free, this one can't be beat! If I'm out running errands all day, I often pack it in a thermos and take it as a snack. (I don't even use a spoon; I just sip it straight from the thermos.) It's great for packing in school lunches, too.

2 cups water

¾ cup raw cashews or pine nuts, preferably soaked in water, then rinsed and drained (see Note)

2 tablespoons extra-virgin olive oil

1 cup finely chopped onions

½ cup finely chopped celery

1 leek, sliced, thoroughly washed, and dried (see page 219)

3 cloves garlic, chopped

¼ teaspoon Himalayan pink salt

¼ teaspoon ground white pepper

1 head broccoli, coarsely chopped (both florets and stems)

6 cups vegetable broth

Clean Cuisine Sour Cream (page 372), for garnish (optional)

1. Put the water and cashews in a blender and process until smooth and creamy. Set the nut milk aside.

2. Heat the oil over low heat in a large saucepan. Add the onions, celery, leek, and garlic to the saucepan and cook for 10 minutes, or until the vegetables are very soft. Add the salt and pepper, then add the chopped broccoli and vegetable broth. Bring to a boil, then turn the heat down to low, cover, and simmer for 10 minutes, or until thickened. Add the nut milk and simmer for an additional 10 minutes to allow the flavors to deepen.

3. Using a handheld stick blender, puree the soup until smooth and creamy, or blend it in small batches in a jar blender. Divide evenly among 6 bowls and drizzle a little sour cream on top, if desired. Serve warm.

NOTE

If you're using a high-powered blender, soaking the nuts is optional, though it creates an even smoother, creamier soup. If you are using a conventional blender, soaking the nuts first is necessary to get the right texture. Pine nuts should be soaked for 30 minutes, cashews for 1 to 2 hours.

MAKE IT VEGAN

Omit the honey in the sour cream.

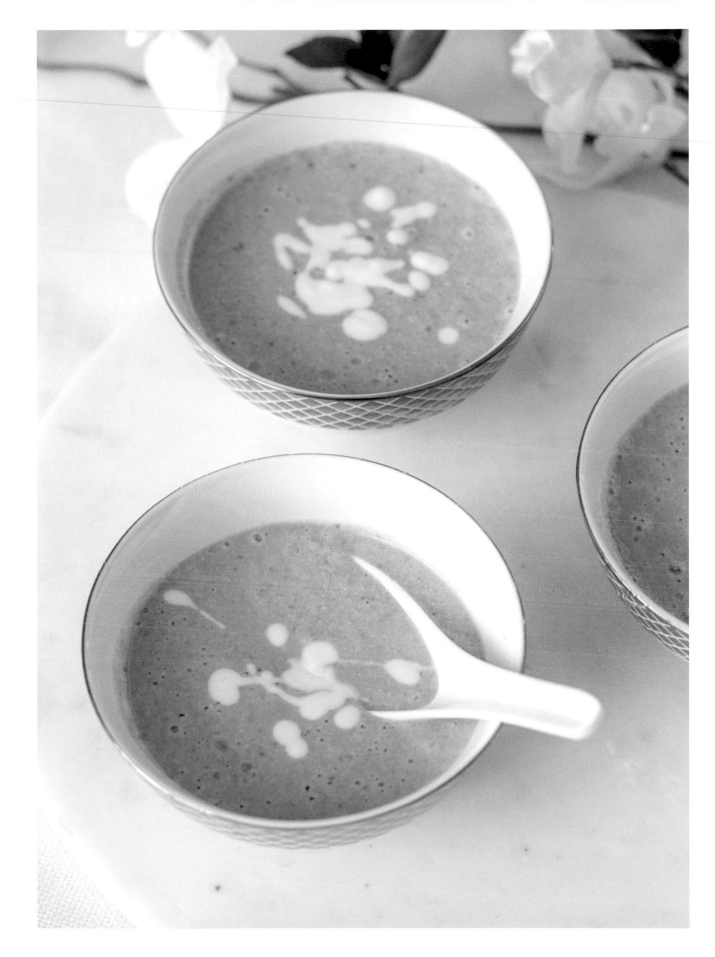

waldorf salad

SERVES 4   PREP TIME: 15 minutes

When it was created at New York's Waldorf Astoria Hotel in 1896 by a maître d', Oscar Tschirky, the Waldorf salad was an instant success. It's the perfect brunch or lunch, and my son has always loved it as an after-school snack. The original version contained only apples, celery, and mayonnaise, though variations abound. I have added grapes, pineapple, and walnuts, and I use my egg-free mayonnaise (page 392) as a base. If you don't have time to make homemade mayonnaise (totally understandable!), see page 401 for good-quality store-bought brands (they do contain eggs, however).

4 to 6 tablespoons mayonnaise, homemade (page 392) or store-bought

1 tablespoon fresh lemon juice

Pinch of ground black pepper

2 sweet apples, cored and chopped

1 cup chopped fresh pineapple or thawed frozen pineapple

1 cup red or green seedless grapes (or a combination), halved

1 cup thinly sliced celery

½ cup chopped raw walnuts

⅓ cup raisins

1 head butter lettuce, torn into bite-sized pieces

In a medium-sized bowl, whisk together the mayonnaise, lemon juice, and pepper. Stir in the apples, pineapple, grapes, celery, walnuts, and raisins. Serve on a bed of fresh lettuce.

MAKE IT EGG-FREE AND VEGAN

Use my Egg-Free Mayonnaise (page 392) rather than store-bought.

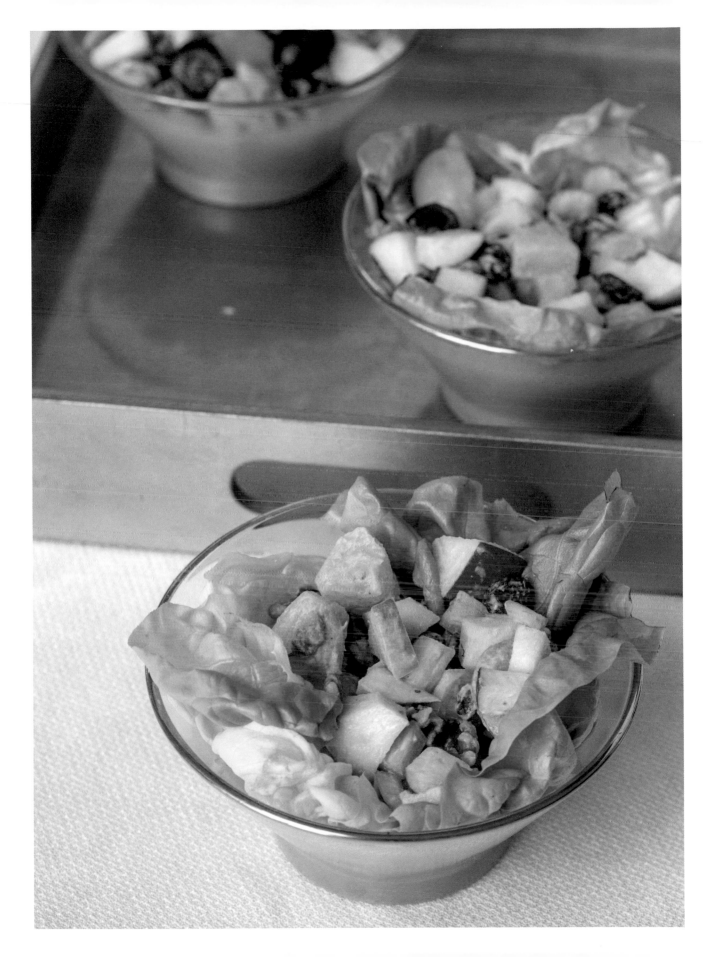

dad's chopped salad with garlic dressing

SERVES 6   PREP TIME: 20 minutes, plus time to rest

My ninety-one-year-old dad, Norman Ingram, doesn't typically cook, but the few recipes he does make are pretty amazing, and this chopped salad is one of them. It's the dish I most often ask him to make for our family dinners. When Dad initially told me the ingredients for the recipe, I thought surely he had made a mistake—twelve cloves is a lot of garlic. But that's the correct amount. The secret is to briefly cook the garlic to soften and mellow the flavor. The second secret is to chop the vegetables as uniformly as possible. With so many vegetables, chopping by hand can be a bit time-consuming; I find using a mini food processor is the easiest way to go (see note below)—but going the extra mile and chopping by hand (as shown in the photo) does make for a prettier presentation.

For the garlic dressing:

12 cloves garlic, peeled

⅓ cup unrefined avocado oil

2 tablespoons raw apple cider vinegar, plus more to taste

2½ teaspoons Italian seasoning, plus more to taste

Himalayan pink salt and ground black pepper

1 cup frozen corn, thawed

½ cup finely chopped cauliflower

½ cup finely chopped celery

½ cup finely chopped green bell peppers

½ cup finely chopped red or yellow bell peppers

½ cup finely chopped red onions

½ cup peeled and finely chopped carrots

¼ cup finely chopped or thinly sliced radishes

2 cups coarsely chopped butter lettuce, plus 6 leaves for serving if desired

1 cup dark salad greens (such as arugula or spinach)

Himalayan pink salt and ground black pepper

1. To make the dressing, put the garlic and avocado oil in a small microwave-safe bowl and microwave for about 1 minute, until the garlic is soft. Remove the bowl from the microwave and set aside to cool. Once cooled, put the garlic and oil, along with the vinegar and Italian seasoning, in a mini food processor and process to emulsify the dressing. Season with salt and pepper to taste. Set the dressing aside.

2. Put the corn, cauliflower, celery, green bell peppers, red bell peppers, onions, carrots, and radishes in a large bowl. Gently toss the ingredients together. Add the butter lettuce, dark salad greens, and garlic dressing and gently toss. Season with salt and pepper to taste, adding extra vinegar or Italian seasoning if desired.

3. Allow the salad to sit at room temperature for at least 30 minutes before serving to give time for the flavors to develop. If desired, place one lettuce leaf on each plate before scooping the salad onto it and serving. (Note: The salad dressing and chopped vegetables can be prepared up to 24 hours in advance and stored in separate sealed containers in the refrigerator. Add the dressing just prior to serving.)

NOTE

Since there's just ½ cup or less of each chopped vegetable in this recipe, I find it's best to use a mini food processor for chopping: it's much faster than chopping by hand, and it gives you more control than a large food processor. For best results, chop just one vegetable at a time.

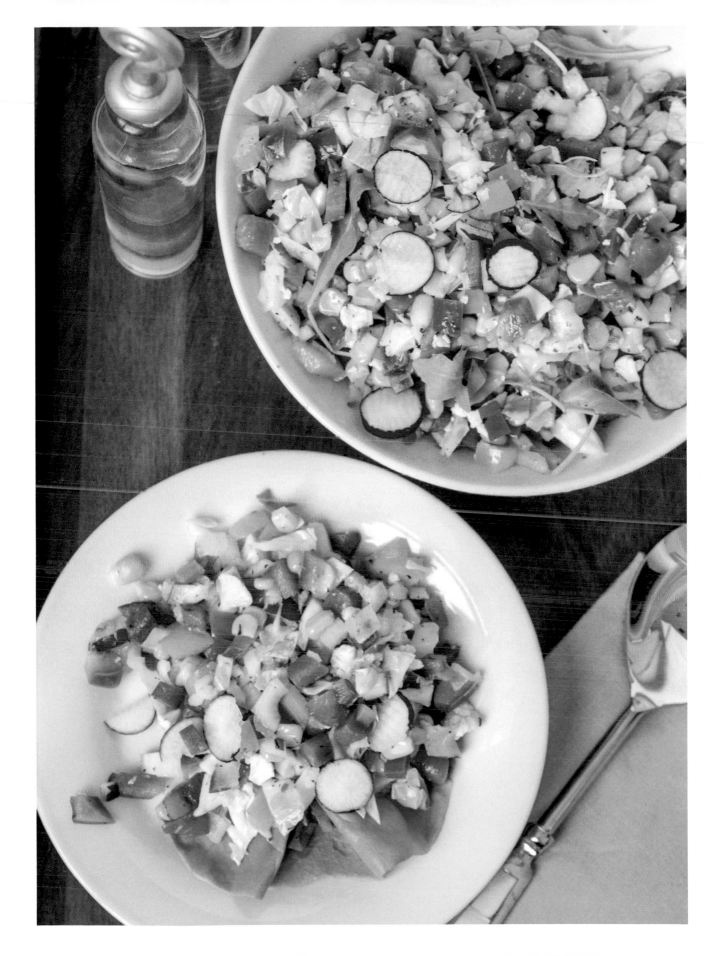

southern cobb salad

SERVES 4   PREP TIME: 15 minutes   COOK TIME: 5 minutes

I know there are variations on Cobb salad galore, but I had never heard of a southern Cobb salad until I saw it on the menu at the Regional Kitchen & Public House, where it comes topped with fried chicken and dressed with buttermilk ranch. I've swapped the chicken for black-eyed peas to keep with the southern theme and provide a vegetarian source of protein, and I've used my Green Goddess Dressing/Dip (page 394) to keep it dairy-free. I make this salad all the time for Meatless Monday, and it's one of my favorite weekend lunches. It's tasty and satisfying—you won't walk away hungry after this one!

¼ cup extra-virgin olive oil

5 Cornbread Muffins with Kale (page 124), crumbled

8 cups chopped romaine lettuce (about 2 heads)

⅓ cup Green Goddess Dressing/Dip (page 394), plus more for serving

Himalayan pink salt

8 hard-boiled eggs, halved lengthwise

1½ cups cherry tomatoes, halved

2 cups canned black-eyed peas (about 1½ [15-ounce] cans), rinsed and drained

1 just-ripe Hass avocado, diced (see Note)

2 medium cucumbers, thinly sliced

1. Heat the oil in a large skillet over medium heat. When the oil is hot, add the crumbled cornbread muffins and sauté for about 5 minutes, until the cornbread begins to brown. Slide the skillet off the heat and set the cornbread crumbs aside to cool.

2. In a large bowl, toss the lettuce with the dressing. Season the lettuce with salt to taste. Arrange the dressed greens on 4 plates.

3. On each plate, arrange 4 egg halves in a row, followed by a row each of halved cherry tomatoes, black-eyed peas, diced avocado, cornbread crumbs, and sliced cucumbers. Serve at once, with more dressing on the side.

NOTE

Just-ripe avocados that are still rather firm work best in salads because they hold their shape well.

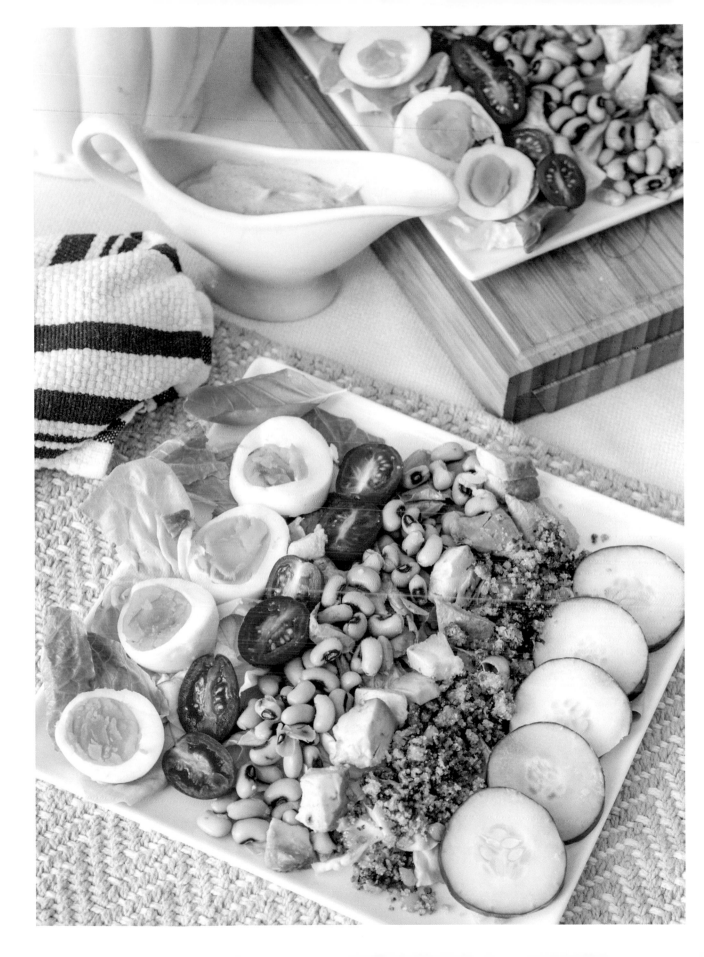

chunky (or creamy!) vegetable soup with basil pesto

SERVES 6 to 8   PREP TIME: 20 minutes   COOK TIME: 25 minutes

Eat your vegetables! How often do we hear this? I know it can be easier said than done, but the trick to eating lots of vegetables is to make sure they are ready-made and tasty, so if you have a go-to vegetable soup like this one that you can keep for three or four days in the refrigerator, I guarantee you'll eat more vegetables. It is not uncommon for me to serve a big bowl of this vegetable soup with avocado toast on a weekend morning. It's even good for a snack. For variety, you can serve this soup chunky or blend it for a creamy pureed soup.

For the soup:

2 tablespoons extra-virgin olive oil

1 teaspoon anchovy paste (optional)

2 cups chopped onions

1 leek, cut into ½-inch-thick slices, thoroughly washed, and dried (see page 219)

3 medium carrots, peeled and chopped

3 stalks celery, chopped

10 cloves garlic, sliced

¾ teaspoon dried oregano leaves

½ teaspoon Himalayan pink salt

⅛ teaspoon ground black pepper

8 cups vegetable broth

2 (14.5-ounce) cans diced tomatoes, drained

2 cups cauliflower florets

5 cups baby spinach (optional)

Juice of 1 lemon

For the pesto:

3 cloves garlic, peeled

2 lightly packed cups fresh basil leaves

3 tablespoons extra-virgin olive oil

3 tablespoons raw walnuts

3 tablespoons water, plus more if needed

2 tablespoons fresh lemon juice

2 tablespoons unfortified nutritional yeast (optional)

¼ teaspoon Himalayan pink salt

SPECIAL TOOLS _____
Mini food processor

1. To make the soup, heat the oil and anchovy paste (if using) in a stockpot over medium heat. Add the onions and leek and cook, stirring occasionally, until translucent, about 8 minutes. Add the carrots, celery, garlic, oregano, salt, and pepper. Cook, stirring occasionally, for 5 minutes, until the carrots and celery are soft.

2. Pour in the vegetable broth, cover, and bring to a boil. Add the tomatoes and cauliflower, turn the heat down to low, and simmer, uncovered, until the cauliflower softens, about 10 minutes. Meanwhile, make the pesto.

3. To make the pesto, put all the ingredients in a mini food processor and process until well blended.

4. For a thinner pesto, add up to 3 tablespoons more water, 1 tablespoon at a time. Set the pesto aside until the soup is finished. (Note: The pesto can be made up to 5 days in advance and stored in a mason jar in the refrigerator.)

5. When the cauliflower is tender, add the spinach (if using) and lemon juice to the stockpot and cook for 30 more seconds, then remove the pot from the heat. Taste and adjust the seasoning, if necessary. If you like your soup chunky, then it's ready to eat! For a smoother soup, use a handheld stick blender to puree the soup, or blend it in small batches in a jar blender.

6. To serve, ladle the soup into serving bowls and drizzle with the pesto. Serve warm.

A lot of times we eat vegetable soup as a side dish, but with some simple stir-ins it's excellent for the main event. To bulk up this vegetable soup recipe, simply stir one or two of the following ingredients into your bowl. If you are serving the soup for your family, you can even do a "soup buffet" with individual bowls of stir-ins so that each person can customize his or her soup bowl.

Frozen corn kernels, thawed

Frozen petite green peas, thawed

Cooked quinoa

Cooked brown rice, preferably sprouted short-grain brown rice

Cooked black rice

Cooked barley

Cooked millet

Canned or cooked chickpeas, rinsed and drained

Canned or cooked cannellini beans, rinsed and drained

Cooked whole-grain or garbanzo macaroni

MAKE IT VEGAN AND VEGETARIAN

Omit the anchovy paste.

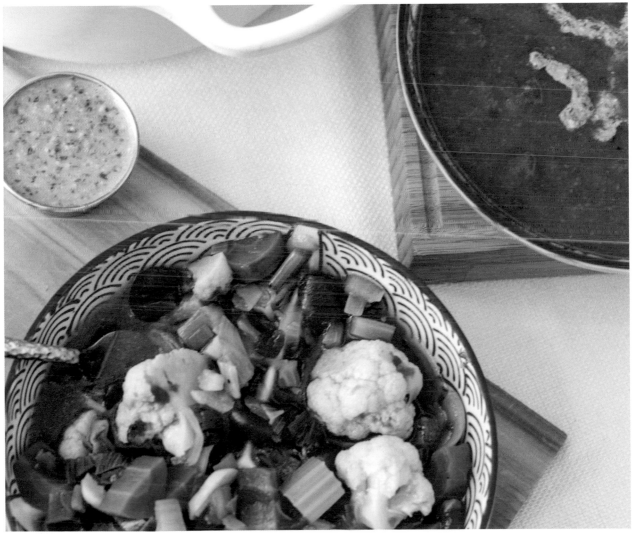

tomato-watermelon gazpacho with cilantro pesto

SERVES 4   PREP TIME: 15 minutes, plus time to chill the soup

Nothing tastes more like summer than this no-cook chilled soup! And if you are planning a day in the summer sun, this is one of the very best recipes for preventing sunburn and sun damage. Did you know the carotenoids (including lycopene) in both tomatoes and watermelon act as an edible sunscreen? These sun-protecting nutrients are best absorbed when the tomatoes and watermelon are eaten with a bit of fat, which this soup has thanks to the olive oil. A nice big bowl of this gazpacho with some crusty sprouted whole-grain bread dipped in olive oil or cilantro pesto is the perfect summer lunch.

For the pesto:

1 cup chopped fresh cilantro

¼ cup extra-virgin olive oil

¼ cup raw macadamia nuts, preferably soaked in water for 1 to 2 hours, then rinsed and drained (see Note)

¼ teaspoon Himalayan pink salt

For the gazpacho:

4 cups cherry tomatoes

4 cups seeded and coarsely chopped watermelon

2 medium cucumbers, peeled, seeded, and coarsely chopped

¼ cup extra-virgin olive oil

2 tablespoons fresh lime juice

2 teaspoons seeded and finely chopped jalapeño peppers

1 teaspoon ground cumin

½ teaspoon Himalayan pink salt

4 lime wedges, for serving (optional)

1. To make the pesto, put all the ingredients in a blender and process until smooth and creamy. Set the pesto aside until the gazpacho is ready to serve. (Note: The pesto can be made up to 3 days in advance and stored in an airtight container in the refrigerator.)

2. To make the gazpacho, put all the ingredients except the lime wedges in a food processor and pulse until just mixed. Do not overprocess; the ideal texture is ever-so-slightly chunky. Transfer the gazpacho to a large bowl and refrigerate for at least 2 hours.

3. To serve, ladle the gazpacho into 4 serving bowls and drizzle the pesto on top. Serve with lime wedges, if desired. Best served cold.

NOTE

If you're using a high-powered blender, soaking the macadamia nuts is optional, though it creates an even smoother, creamier texture. If you are using a conventional blender, soaking the nuts first is necessary to get the right texture.

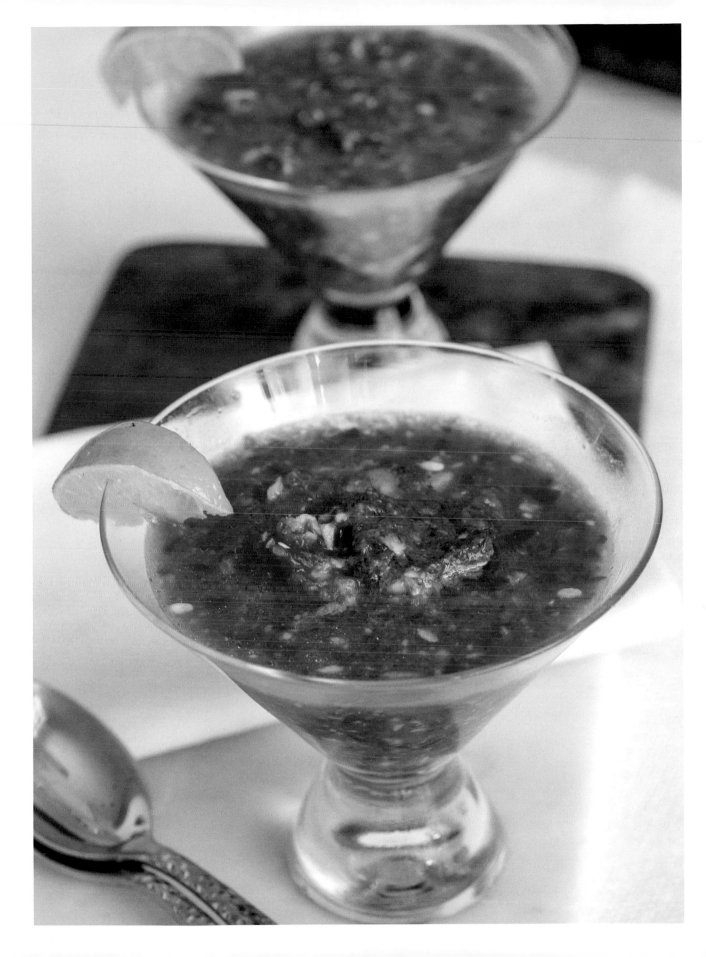

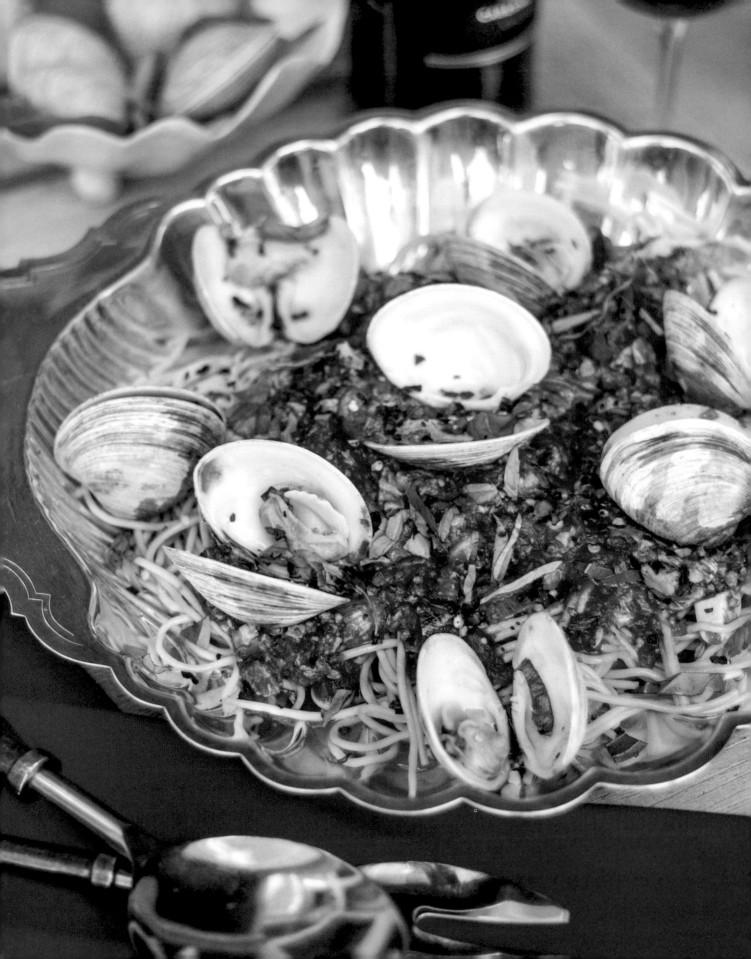

CHAPTER 11

what's for dinner?

salmon teriyaki

SERVES 4   PREP TIME: 5 minutes, plus time to marinate the salmon
COOK TIME: 7 minutes

Until I realized I could make my own clean sauce, I avoided eating salmon teriyaki for years because conventional teriyaki sauce is loaded with refined sugar. Making your own teriyaki sauce might sound a bit over the top, or at least it did to me at first. But it takes less than 10 minutes, and homemade tastes so much better than store-bought! I always serve this dish with sides of steamed frozen green peas and lemon wedges. When pineapple is in season, I sometimes add fresh pineapple chunks to the plates as well. Easy-peasy!

4 (6-ounce) wild salmon fillets, skins on

Himalayan pink salt and ground black pepper

1¼ cups Pineapple Teriyaki Sauce (page 374)

Extra-virgin coconut oil, for the pan

1. Season the salmon fillets lightly with salt and pepper and place them in a shallow 9 by 11-inch casserole dish.

2. Pour the teriyaki sauce over the fillets. Cover the dish with plastic wrap and place in the fridge to marinate for at least 20 minutes or up to 2 hours.

3. Lightly grease a large skillet with oil and place it on the stovetop over medium heat. When the oil is hot, remove the salmon from the marinade, reserving the marinade, and place it skin side down in the skillet. Cook for 2 minutes, then pour in the reserved marinade and cook for another minute or so, until the salmon fillets are opaque halfway up the sides. Turn them over and cook on the other side for 3 to 4 minutes, basting with the sauce so that the salmon is well coated. The salmon is done when it flakes easily when pierced with a fork.

4. Serve the salmon fillets on individual plates, spooning over them any teriyaki sauce left in the pan.

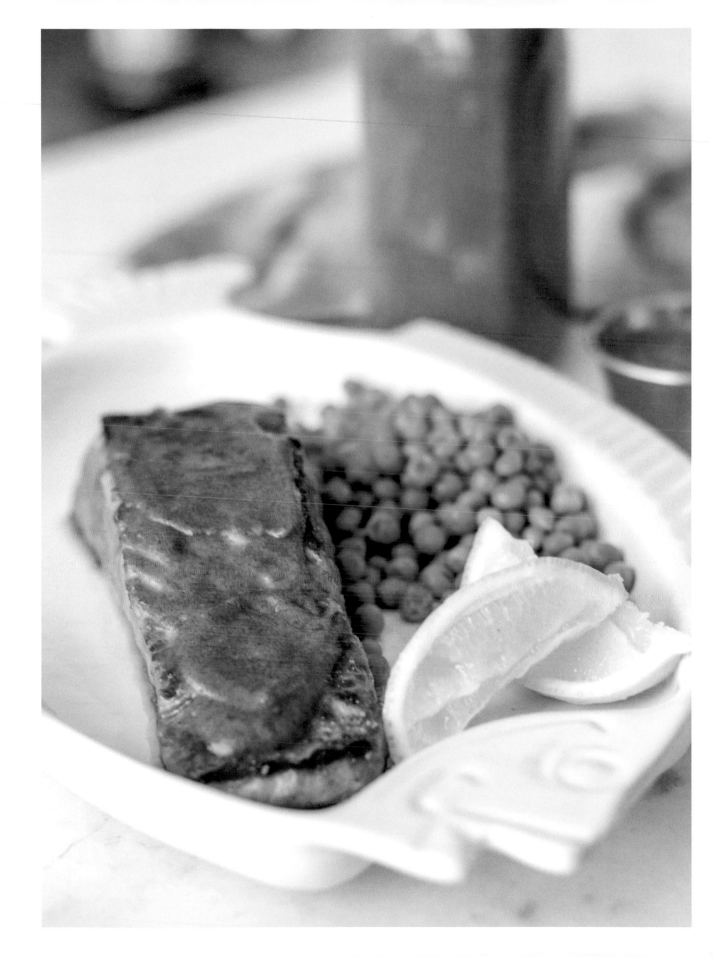

hidden veggie meatloaf

SERVES 8   PREP TIME: 20 minutes   COOK TIME: 1 hour 5 minutes

Who doesn't love a good meatloaf? It's the ultimate comfort food. I've added a lot of vegetables to this meatloaf, much more than the ¼ cup of minced onions you might see in a conventional recipe. They contribute significantly to the flavor and help keep the meatloaf moist. And if you've got kids in the house who don't like vegetables, well, nobody needs to tell them this is one very veggie-packed meatloaf!

Since I like to keep our family's red-meat consumption down, I usually make this meatloaf with turkey. But I also frequently make it with lamb, which is high in anti-inflammatory omega-3 fats. One important note on the meat: If you are using ground turkey, don't use extra-lean meat; it will be too dry.

2½ cups peeled and coarsely chopped carrots

1 medium onion, coarsely chopped

6 cloves garlic, peeled

¼ cup fresh thyme leaves

1 cup shiitake mushrooms, stemmed

2 tablespoons extra-virgin olive oil

2½ teaspoons Himalayan pink salt, divided

½ cup plus 3 tablespoons ketchup, homemade (page 390) or store-bought, divided, plus more for serving

½ cup gluten-free old-fashioned rolled oats

½ cup unsweetened, plain hemp milk or almond milk, homemade (page 368) or store-bought

2 tablespoons gluten-free Worcestershire sauce

2 teaspoons Dijon mustard

1 large egg, whisked

2 pounds ground turkey or lamb

Chopped fresh parsley, for garnish (optional)

1. Preheat the oven to 375°F and set a large pan of water on the bottom oven rack (the steam it creates will help to keep the meatloaf moist). Line a rimmed baking sheet with parchment paper.

2. Put the carrots, onion, garlic, and thyme in a food processor. Process until minced, but be sure to stop before the mixture turns into a paste. Transfer the onion-carrot mixture to a bowl.

3. Place the shiitake mushrooms in the food processor. Process until just minced, then set aside.

4. Heat the oil in a large skillet over medium heat. Add the onion-carrot mixture and cook for about 6 minutes, until the onion begins to soften. Add the mushrooms to the skillet, season with ½ teaspoon of the salt, and cook until both the onion and mushrooms are soft, 5 to 6 minutes. Set the cooked vegetable mixture aside to cool.

5. In a large mixing bowl, combine 3 tablespoons of the ketchup, the oats, hemp milk, Worcestershire sauce, Dijon mustard, egg, and remaining 2 teaspoons of salt. Use a wooden spoon to mix the ingredients until just combined. Add the cooked vegetables and the turkey to the bowl and mix with clean hands until the ingredients are just combined; do not overmix.

6. Place the meatloaf mixture on the prepared baking sheet and shape into a mounded rectangular loaf about 9 inches long, 5 inches wide, and 2½ inches tall. Brush the top with the remaining ½ cup of ketchup and bake for 50 to 55 minutes, until a thermometer inserted in the middle of the meatloaf reads 160°F. Remove the meatloaf from the oven and let it rest for at least 15 minutes before serving. Garnish with chopped parsley before serving, if desired.

This meatloaf will keep in an airtight container in the refrigerator for up to 3 days or in the freezer for up to 3 weeks.

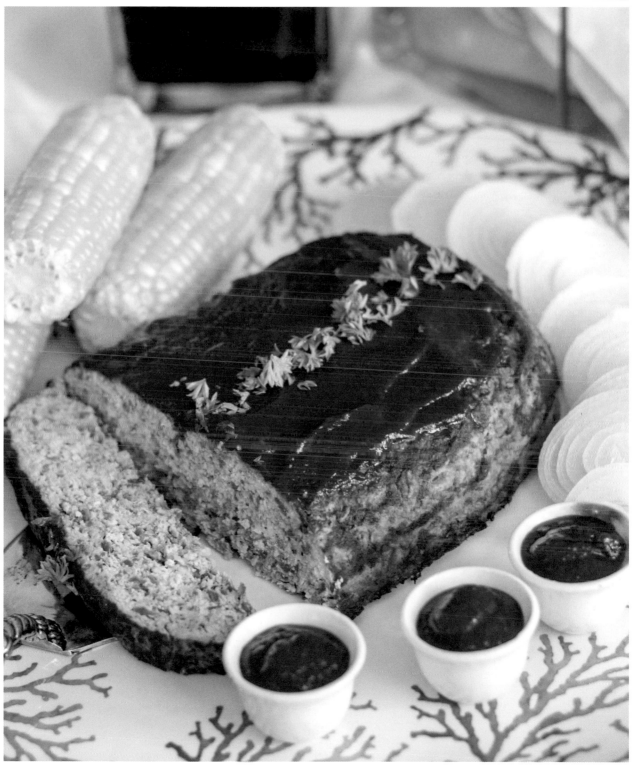

oven-style barbecue chicken

SERVES 4   PREP TIME: 15 minutes   COOK TIME: 40 minutes

I love barbecue chicken. But there are two big things I don't love about conventional barbecue chicken: (1) grilling, because it makes a huge mess, and (2) sugar—the typical serving of conventional barbecue sauce has almost the same amount of sugar as a cookie (yikes!). This oven-style barbecue chicken dinner does away with both the mess and the sugar. Not only is it healthier, but this clean version is actually considerably moister than grilled barbecue chicken. You do have to make your own barbecue sauce (page 386), but nothing could be easier—if you can use a blender, you can do it. To round out the meal, I like to serve a simple green salad, green beans, and corn on the cob.

1½ pounds boneless, skinless chicken thighs, trimmed of all visible fat (see Note)

1 tablespoon extra-virgin olive oil

1 teaspoon paprika

½ teaspoon dry mustard

Himalayan pink salt and ground black pepper

1 cup barbecue sauce, homemade (page 386) or store-bought, divided

Chopped fresh parsley, for garnish (optional)

NOTE _____

I like to use kitchen shears to trim the fat.

1. Preheat the oven to 400°F and place one oven rack in the middle and one just under the broiler. Line a rimmed baking sheet with foil for easy cleanup. If you have an ovenproof cooling rack, place it on the baking sheet on top of the foil; this will allow the excess liquid and fat to drip off the chicken thighs as they cook.

2. Put the chicken in a large bowl. Drizzle the oil on top of the chicken, then sprinkle on the paprika, dry mustard, and a generous amount of salt and pepper. Use your hands to toss the chicken to evenly coat it in the oil, spices, and salt.

3. Arrange the chicken on the cooling rack or place it directly on the foil-lined baking sheet. Place the chicken on the middle rack and bake for 20 minutes, then remove it from the oven. If you did not use a cooling rack, drain off any liquid that has accumulated in the pan.

4. Brush the chicken thighs with about ¼ cup of the barbecue sauce, then flip the chicken over and brush the other side with another ¼ cup of the sauce. Return the chicken to the oven and bake for 8 minutes. Remove the chicken from the oven, flip, and brush with another ¼ cup of the barbecue sauce. Return the chicken to the oven and bake for another 8 minutes, until the barbecue sauce has begun to thicken and caramelize.

5. Remove the chicken from the oven and brush the top with the remaining ¼ cup of sauce.

6. Turn the broiler on to high. Return the chicken to the oven and place it on the rack just under the broiler. Bake for 1 minute or so, until the sauce just begins to bubble (but be careful not to burn the sauce!). Remove the chicken from the oven, garnish with parsley, if desired, and serve warm.

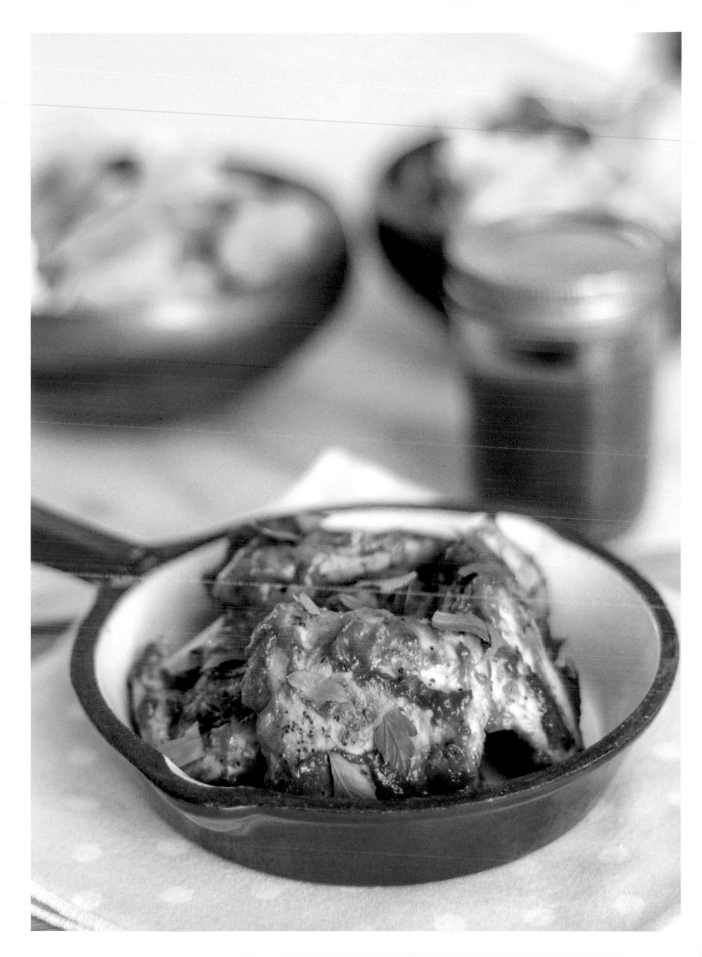

chicken cacciatore

SERVES 6 to 8   PREP TIME: 25 minutes   COOK TIME: 1 hour

If you love Italian food, then chicken cacciatore is a must-make! This is family-style rustic food, the kind of dish you can vividly imagine a big Italian family happily digging into. As with most classic Italian dishes, there must be a hundred variations of chicken cacciatore. My version, of course, has lots of vegetables! Including one that may seem more suited to a Japanese recipe than an Italian one: I use healing superfood shiitake mushrooms instead of the cultivated white button mushrooms. They contribute a subtle earthy flavor and meaty texture to the dish.

---

3 pounds boneless, skinless chicken thighs, cut into 1-inch pieces and trimmed of all visible fat (see Note, page 184)

1 teaspoon paprika

1 teaspoon Himalayan pink salt, divided

1 teaspoon ground black pepper, divided

½ cup cassava flour (or sprouted spelt flour if not gluten- or grain-free)

4 tablespoons extra-virgin olive oil, divided

2 red bell peppers, chopped

2 cups chopped onions

5 cloves garlic, minced

2½ cups stemmed and finely chopped shiitake mushrooms

¾ cup dry red wine

1 (28-ounce) can crushed tomatoes, with juices

1 (14.5-ounce) can petite diced tomatoes, with juices

½ cup chicken broth

2 teaspoons garlic powder

½ teaspoon crushed red pepper

1 teaspoon dried oregano leaves

½ cup coarsely chopped fresh parsley, for garnish

1. Sprinkle the chicken pieces with the paprika and ½ teaspoon each of the salt and pepper. Place the flour in a bowl, add the chicken pieces, and toss to coat lightly.

2. In a large sauté pan, heat 2 tablespoons of the oil over medium-high heat. Add the chicken pieces to the pan and sauté until just brown, about 3 to 4 minutes per side. (Note: If all the chicken does not fit in the pan without overcrowding it, sauté it in two batches.) Transfer the chicken to a plate and set aside. Do not clean the pan.

3. Pour the remaining 2 tablespoons of oil into the same pan used to cook the chicken. Add the bell peppers, onions, and garlic and sauté over medium heat until the onions are tender, about 5 minutes. Season with ¼ teaspoon each of the salt and pepper. Add the mushrooms and sauté for 3 to 4 minutes, until the mushrooms are soft. Add the wine, turn the heat down to medium-low, and simmer until almost no liquid remains, 8 to 10 minutes.

4. Add the crushed tomatoes and diced tomatoes, broth, garlic powder, crushed red pepper, oregano, and remaining ¼ teaspoon each of salt and pepper. Return the chicken pieces to the pan and turn them to coat in the sauce. Continue simmering until the chicken is just cooked through, about 30 minutes. Sprinkle the chicken with parsley and serve.

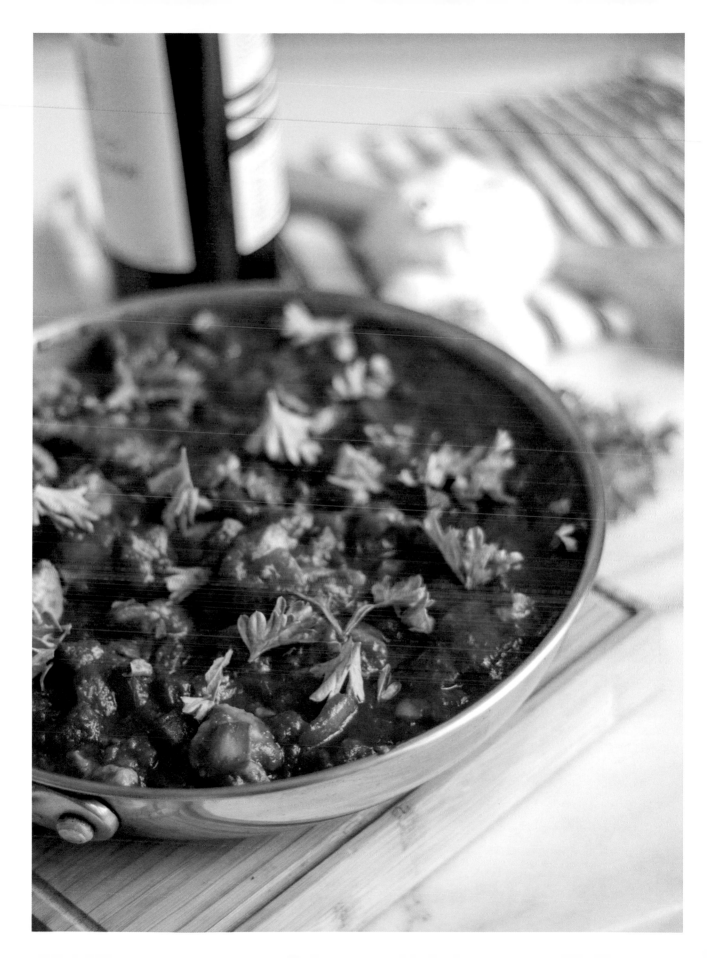

the blake burger

MAKES 8 burgers   PREP TIME: 20 minutes, plus time to chill the patties
COOK TIME: 20 minutes

If you happen to have a teenage son or growing young boy to feed, you are going to need a foolproof, super-good burger recipe. Named after our son, the Blake Burger is just that! This is one super-juicy, ultra-flavorful burger. The 1:1 ratio of ground meat to vegetables and herbs (mushrooms, onions, and parsley) might seem like it won't produce a meaty burger, but just trust me on this one. My son eats two at a time, so you may want to double the recipe (they freeze well!). And if you are looking for a fun and casual way to entertain guests and adults, be sure to check out the post "How to Set Up a Clean Burger Buffet" on our blog!

½ cup coarsely chopped onions

2 cups stemmed and coarsely chopped shiitake mushrooms

½ cup coarsely chopped fresh parsley

1½ pounds ground beef, lamb, bison, or dark-meat turkey

1 large egg, whisked

2 teaspoons anchovy paste

3 cloves garlic, crushed to a paste

1½ teaspoons Dijon mustard

1 teaspoon gluten-free Worcestershire sauce

1 teaspoon Himalayan pink salt

2 tablespoons extra-virgin olive oil, divided, for the pan

STORAGE INFORMATION _____
These burgers will keep in an airtight container in the refrigerator for 1 day or in the freezer for up to 2 weeks.

1. Preheat the oven to 425°F. Line a rimmed baking sheet with parchment paper.

2. Put the onions in a food processor and process until minced; be careful not to overprocess or they will be mushy. Transfer the onions to a medium-sized mixing bowl. Put the shiitake mushrooms in the food processor and process until just minced. Add the mushrooms to the mixing bowl with the onions. Put the parsley in the food processor and process until just minced. Add the parsley to the bowl with the onions and mushrooms.

3. To the mixing bowl with the minced vegetables, add the ground meat, egg, anchovy paste, garlic, Dijon mustard, Worcestershire sauce, and salt. Use your hands to mix until the ingredients are just blended; do not overmix. Form into 8 patties about ½ inch thick. Place them on a large plate or lightly oiled rimmed baking sheet and refrigerate for 30 minutes.

4. Heat a large, heavy-bottomed skillet over medium-high heat, then pour 1 tablespoon of the oil into the skillet and tilt to coat the bottom. When the oil is hot, put half of the patties in the pan and cook until partially cooked, 3 to 4 minutes on each side. (The burgers will finish cooking in the oven.) Transfer the burgers to the parchment-lined baking sheet. Repeat with the remaining tablespoon of oil and the rest of the patties.

5. Place the burgers in the oven and cook for about 5 minutes for medium-done burgers. (Note: If you're making turkey burgers, cook the burgers until the center of each burger reads 165°F on a meat thermometer and there is no visible pink remaining in the center of the burgers.) Remove from the oven and let sit for a couple of minutes before serving.

Sweet Potato Chili Fries (page 274)

Ketchup, homemade (page 390) or store-bought

Mayonnaise, homemade (page 392) or store-bought

Mustard

Sriracha sauce

Avocado, mashed or sliced

Lettuce or other tender greens

Naturally fermented pickles

Onion slices, sautéed, broiled, or wrapped in foil and grilled

Sliced tomato

Large lettuce leaves for the "buns" (or whole-grain buns, if not gluten free; see Resources, page 399)

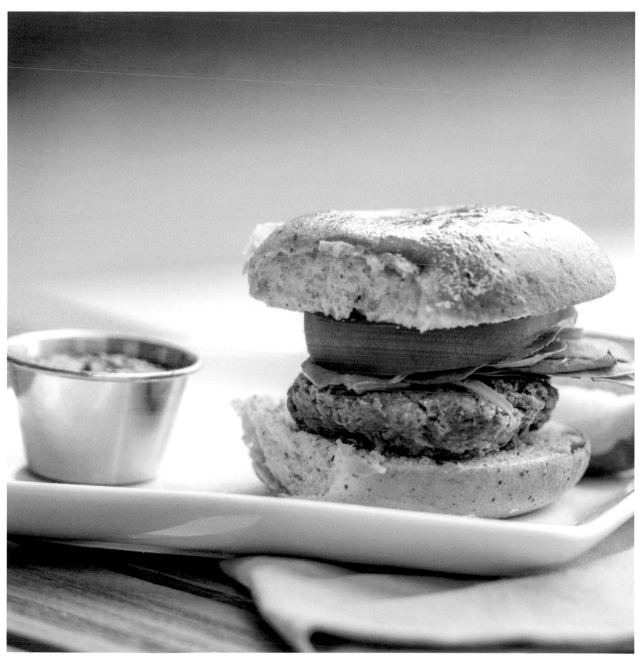

better-than-takeout cashew chicken

SERVES 6   PREP TIME: 20 minutes, plus time to soak the nuts and
marinate the chicken   COOK TIME: 20 minutes

When I was in high school, Chinese takeout was a weekly thing at our house, and cashew chicken was one of my favorites. Back then I didn't know (or care!) that my tasty takeout was stir-fried in pro-inflammatory and highly refined vegetable oil. And I had no idea that it was also surely laced with MSG, sugar, and cornstarch. So I was thrilled to figure out a clean version that tastes better than takeout! Best of all, you can get it on the table in just about the same amount of time it would take to dial out. It's delicious as is, but if you have a hungry bunch to feed, you can always add brown rice (I like to use sprouted short-grain brown rice).

¾ cup raw cashews

5 tablespoons gluten-free tamari (or unpasteurized soy sauce, if not gluten-free), divided

2 tablespoons unrefined toasted sesame oil, divided

2 tablespoons unseasoned rice wine vinegar

1 tablespoon raw honey

1 pound boneless, skinless chicken thighs, cut into bite-sized pieces

4 cloves garlic, smashed with the side of a knife

1 large onion, sliced

1 tablespoon grated fresh ginger

4 large carrots, peeled, halved crosswise, and cut into ¼-inch-thick strips

2 red bell peppers, cut into ¼-inch-thick strips

1 (8-ounce) can sliced water chestnuts, drained

1 tablespoon arrowroot

½ cup sliced scallions

½ teaspoon crushed red pepper

1. Place the cashews in a medium-sized bowl and cover with water. Soak for 30 minutes to 1 hour, then drain and set aside.

2. In a large bowl, whisk 2 tablespoons of the tamari, 1 tablespoon of the sesame oil, the vinegar, and the honey. Add the chicken to the bowl and toss to coat in the marinade. Cover, place in the fridge, and marinate for at least 20 minutes or up to 6 hours.

3. Heat the remaining tablespoon of oil in a large skillet over medium-high heat. Add the garlic, onion, and ginger and sauté for 3 to 4 minutes, until the onion starts to soften. Add the carrots and sauté for 3 to 4 minutes, until fork-tender.

4. Use tongs to remove the chicken pieces from the marinade and place them in the pan, reserving the marinade. Sauté the chicken pieces until just cooked through, about 5 minutes. Add the bell peppers and water chestnuts and sauté for 1 minute, until the ingredients are heated through. Turn off the heat and stir in the cashews.

5. Use a slotted spoon to transfer the chicken and vegetables to a large serving bowl, leaving the juices in the skillet.

6. In a small bowl, mix the reserved chicken marinade with the arrowroot and remaining 3 tablespoons of tamari. Turn the heat back on to medium, pour the mixture into the skillet, and simmer for 5 minutes. Pour the sauce over the chicken and vegetables. Scatter the scallions and crushed red pepper on top. Serve warm.

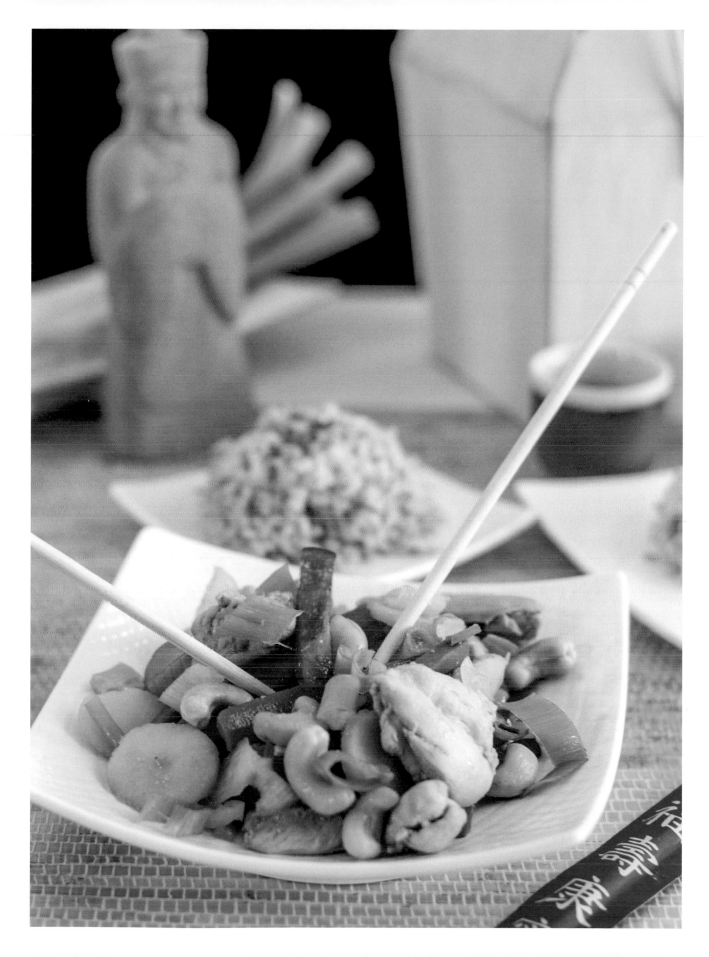

blake's bouillabaisse

SERVES 6 to 8   PREP TIME: 30 minutes   COOK TIME: 45 minutes

Bouillabaisse is a seafood stew from the South of France, and it has to be one of my favorite seafood dishes of all time. The first time our family had it was when our son, Blake, made it for my dad's eighty-ninth birthday dinner. Blake was only fifteen years old at the time, so just know that although the recipe might sound complicated, it is incredibly easy to make. These are the two most important things to keep in mind when making bouillabaisse: (1) make sure the seafood you buy is super fresh, and (2) do as professional chefs do and set up your mise-en-place—have all your ingredients measured, chopped, and set out before you begin. You want every single thing needed to make the stew prepped and ready to go before you turn on the stove.

Now, if you want your bouillabaisse to be out-of-this-world delicious and over-the-top nutritious, then the third thing you'll want to do is make your own fish broth, which is much easier than it sounds (you can easily find a recipe for fish broth online). But if you don't want to make your own fish broth, no worries. I have made bouillabaisse with ready-made fish broth and it is still incredibly delicious.

¼ cup extra-virgin olive oil

3 medium carrots, diced

2 medium onions, diced

2½ cups diced fennel (about 3 bulbs)

2 cups diced red potatoes, with skin on

1 teaspoon dried thyme leaves

¾ teaspoon Himalayan pink salt

½ teaspoon ground black pepper

2 cups crisp white wine, such as Sauvignon Blanc

1 (28-ounce) can whole peeled San Marzano tomatoes, with juices

6 cups fish broth (see Note)

6 cloves garlic, minced

1 heaping teaspoon saffron threads

2 bay leaves

1 pound large shrimp, shelled and deveined

2 dozen littleneck clams, cleaned

2 dozen mussels, cleaned

1 pound halibut fillets, cut into large chunks

1 pound monkfish fillets, cut into large chunks

1 teaspoon grated lemon zest

1 cup chopped fresh parsley, for garnish

1. Heat the oil over medium heat in a Dutch oven or stockpot. Add the carrots, onions, fennel, potatoes, thyme, salt, and pepper, then turn the heat down to medium-low and cook for 15 minutes, or until the onions begin to brown.

2. Pour in the wine and, using a wooden spoon, scrape up any brown bits from the bottom of the pot. Bring the mixture to a boil, then turn the heat down to low and simmer the vegetables in the wine for 5 minutes.

3. Add the tomatoes with their juices, fish broth, garlic, saffron, and bay leaves to the pot and simmer for 15 minutes, or until the potatoes are tender. Discard the bay leaves.

NOTE _____

Homemade fish broth is definitely best for both flavor and health, but if you don't have the time or inclination to make it, store-bought works, too. But rather than using just store-bought fish broth, I've gotten the best results by using 2½ (15-ounce) cans of Bar Harbor brand fish stock and 1 (8-ounce) bottle of Bar Harbor brand clam juice.

4. To the pot, add the shrimp, clams, mussels, and fish. (Note: If any of the mussels or clams are chipped or are not tightly shut, discard them.) Bring the liquid to a boil, then turn the heat down to low, cover, and simmer for 5 minutes, or until the shrimp and fish are just cooked through (the shrimp will have turned opaque and the fish will flake with a fork) and most or all of the mussels and clams have opened. Discard any mussels or clams that did not open. Stir in the lemon zest.

5. Ladle the bouillabaisse into large bowls and garnish with the fresh parsley. Serve warm.

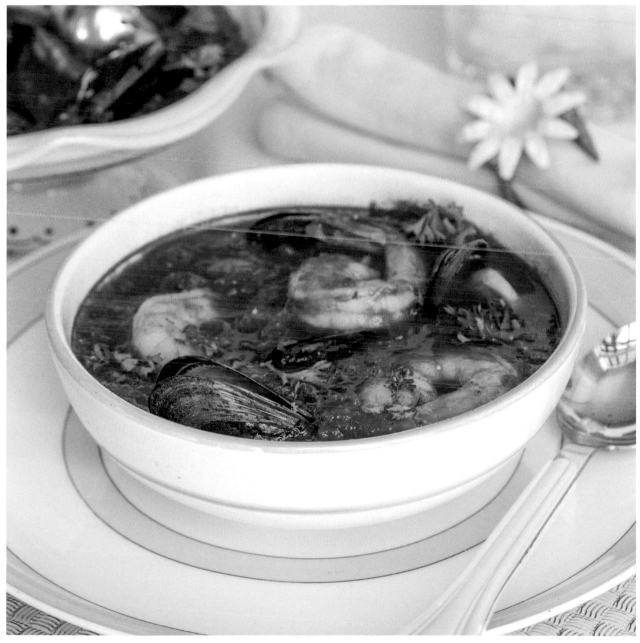

linguine with clam sauce

SERVES 4   PREP TIME: 15 minutes   COOK TIME: 25 minutes

The linguine with clam sauce that I grew up eating was made with lots of butter, heavy cream, and refined-wheat pasta. But if you love linguine with clam sauce, I promise you will fall in love with this clean and super-flavorful version. One of the things that gives it such incredible flavor is the addition of the minced and meaty shiitake mushrooms. Adding shiitakes to clam sauce might sound a bit odd, but they not only add super-healing benefits to the sauce, they really do boost the flavor and texture substantially. Best of all, you don't have to spend all day in the kitchen making this dish. You can get the whole thing on the table faster than you can call for delivery.

7 ounces shiitake mushrooms, stemmed

¼ cup plus 1 tablespoon extra-virgin olive oil, divided

1½ teaspoons anchovy paste

¾ cup finely chopped shallots

6 cloves garlic, minced

½ teaspoon Himalayan pink salt

2 (6.5-ounce) cans chopped clams, rinsed and drained

3 cups boxed chopped or canned diced tomatoes, with juices (see Note)

2 teaspoons coconut sugar

½ teaspoon crushed red pepper

8 ounces gluten-free whole-grain linguine, or 6 cups zucchini noodles (about 3 medium zucchini)

½ cup chopped fresh basil, plus more for garnish

1 pound steamed fresh clams, for serving (optional; see facing page)

1. To prepare the sauce, put the mushrooms in a food processor and pulse until finely chopped (be careful not to overprocess or the mushrooms will get mushy). Set the mushrooms aside.

2. Heat ¼ cup of the oil and the anchovy paste in a large saucepan over medium heat. Add the shallots and sauté for 3 to 4 minutes, until they soften. Add the garlic, minced mushrooms, salt, and remaining tablespoon of oil and sauté for 3 to 4 minutes, until the mushrooms are soft. Stir in the clams, tomatoes, coconut sugar, and crushed red pepper and simmer for 15 minutes.

3. While the sauce is simmering, cook the linguine according the package directions. If using zucchini noodles, set them in a steamer basket placed in a pot over an inch of boiling water and steam them for about 3 to 4 minutes, until tender.

4. After the sauce has simmered for 15 minutes, add the basil and cook for an additional minute.

5. Divide the cooked noodles among 4 serving bowls and top with the clam sauce. Garnish with basil and steamed fresh clams, if desired. Serve warm.

MAKE IT GRAIN-FREE
Use chickpea linguine or zucchini noodles.

MAKE IT PALEO-FRIENDLY
Use zucchini noodles.

NOTE
Pomi brand BPA-free boxed chopped tomatoes from Italy are particularly delicious in this dish.

Thoroughly rinse the clams to remove any traces of sand. In a stockpot, bring 1 cup canned clam juice, 2 cups water, 2 tablespoons lemon juice, and ¼ cup wine to a boil. Add the clams, cover, turn the heat down to low, and simmer until the clams just open, 2 to 3 minutes. Discard any clams that do not open on their own (never force a clam open).

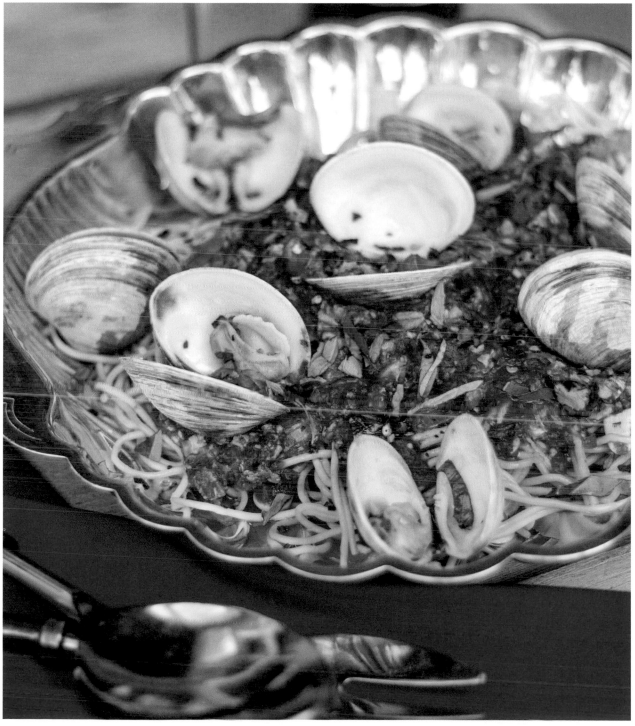

chicken tikka masala

SERVES 6   PREP TIME: 25 minutes, plus time to marinate the chicken
COOK TIME: 25 minutes

Before I moved to London to study abroad in college, I'd never had chicken tikka masala. London is very well known for having top-notch Indian eateries, and it's where I fell in love with Indian food. And if there is one dish guaranteed to be on every Indian restaurant menu, it's chicken tikka masala. Conventional recipes do not include chickpeas, which I've added here, but their mild flavor does not detract from the recipe at all, and they help give the dish more substance (along with fiber, plant protein, antioxidants, and phytonutrients!). I've also swapped cashew cream for the traditional dairy cream, but you can't tell the difference. I usually serve this dish with sprouted short-grain brown rice and sautéed spinach.

¼ cup full-fat coconut milk

1 tablespoon fresh lime juice

1½ teaspoons Himalayan pink salt, divided

5 large cloves garlic, peeled, divided

1¾ pounds boneless, skinless chicken thighs, trimmed of all visible fat and cut into bite-sized pieces (see Note, page 184)

¾ cup water

½ cup raw cashews, preferably soaked in water for 1 to 2 hours, then rinsed and drained (see Notes)

2 tablespoons paprika

1 tablespoon grated fresh ginger

½ teaspoon turmeric powder

¼ teaspoon cayenne pepper

5 tablespoons extra-virgin coconut oil, divided

1 large onion, finely chopped

2 (14.5-ounce) cans diced tomatoes, with juices

1 tablespoon garam masala (see Notes)

1 (15-ounce) can chickpeas, rinsed and drained

½ cup chopped fresh cilantro, for garnish

1. In a medium-sized bowl, mix together the coconut milk, lime juice, and ½ teaspoon of the salt. Thinly slice one of the garlic cloves and add it to the bowl. Add the chicken to the bowl and turn to evenly coat. Cover and place in the fridge to marinate for at least 20 minutes.

2. Put the water and cashews in a blender or food processor. Process on high speed until the mixture is smooth and creamy. Set the cashew cream aside.

3. Crush the remaining 4 cloves of garlic to a paste and add it to a small bowl along with the paprika, ginger, turmeric, and cayenne pepper. Mix to combine, then set the spice blend aside.

4. In a large saucepan, heat 4 tablespoons of the coconut oil over medium heat. Add the onion and sauté for 5 to 6 minutes, until soft. Turn the heat down to low and stir in the spice mixture. Cook for 1 minute, then add the tomatoes, cashew cream, and remaining teaspoon of salt. Bring the sauce to a boil, then turn the heat down to low and simmer for 5 minutes, until ever-so-slightly thickened. Stir in the garam masala and continue simmering for another 5 minutes, until fragrant.

5. Meanwhile, heat the remaining tablespoon of coconut oil in a large skillet over medium heat. Remove the chicken from the marinade (discard the marinade) and cook, stirring occasionally, for 5 to 7 minutes, until cooked through.

6. Add the chicken to the pot with the tomatoes and spices. Stir in the chickpeas and cook for another 3 to 4 minutes, until the chickpeas are heated through.

7. Divide among 6 bowls, garnish with the cilantro, and serve warm.

Omit the chickpeas.

NOTES_____

If you're using a high-powered blender, soaking the cashews is optional, though it creates an even smoother, creamier texture. If you are using a conventional blender, soaking the nuts first is necessary to get the right texture.

Garam masala is a spice blend that's essential to Indian cooking. Typical ingredients include black pepper, cinnamon, mace, cloves, cardamom, nutmeg, and cumin. You can certainly make your own garam masala, and there are umpteen different recipes online, but I almost always buy mine. Many good-quality brands exist, but I have good luck with the blend from The Spice Hunter, which is salt-free. As a general rule (one that certainly gets broken at times), garam masala is typically added toward the end of cooking because it tends to become bitter if cooked too long.

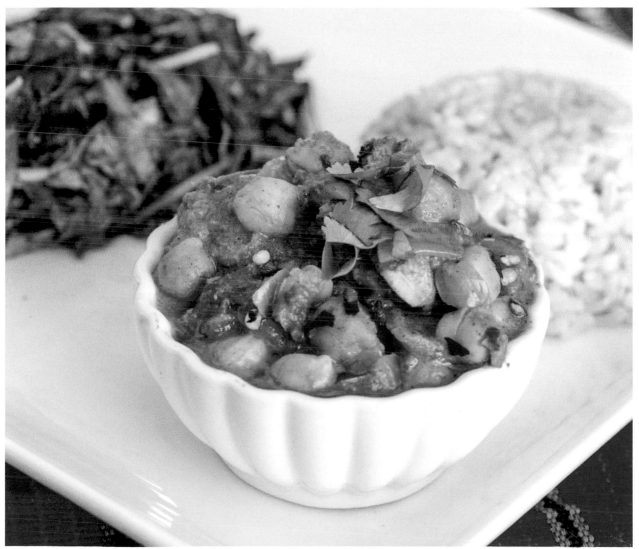

crab cakes

MAKES 8 crab cakes (4 servings)   PREP TIME: 20 minutes, plus
time to chill the crab cake mixture   COOK TIME: 10 minutes

I've put a lot of effort into trying to come up with (what I think!) is the best crab cake recipe. That's because, along with Key lime pie, crab cakes are one of Andy's absolute favorite foods. Living in South Florida, we've tried countless crab cake recipes over the years, mostly in various restaurants, and our biggest complaint is that they typically scrimp big-time on the crab and use cheap fillers instead. Rest assured, this recipe is not skimpy on the crab! I like to serve these with ketchup (page 390), egg-free mayonnaise (page 392), and lemon wedges.

---

1 pound cooked wild crab meat, large pieces broken up

3 scallions, thinly sliced

2 slices gluten-free whole-grain bread, toasted and processed into coarse breadcrumbs with a food processor

1 large egg

3 tablespoons mayonnaise, homemade (page 392) or store-bought

2 tablespoons finely chopped fresh parsley

1 tablespoon fresh thyme leaves

1 tablespoon Old Bay Seasoning (see Note)

½ teaspoon grated lemon zest

½ teaspoon hot sauce, such as Tabasco

Unrefined red palm oil, extra-virgin coconut oil, or unrefined macadamia nut oil, for the pan

1. In a large bowl, combine all of the ingredients except the oil. Mix the ingredients well with your hands. Cover with plastic wrap and let firm in the fridge for at least 25 minutes or up to 24 hours.

2. When ready to eat, form the crab cake mixture into 8 patties, each about 4 inches in diameter, then compact them a bit so everything sticks together.

3. Wipe a large skillet with oil and heat over medium-high heat. Put half of the crab cakes in the hot pan and cook until crispy on both sides, about 5 minutes total. Repeat with the remaining crab cakes. Serve warm.

NOTE

Old Bay Seasoning has been around for more than seventy-five years now, and in all that time the ingredients have not changed. Here's what's in it: celery salt (salt, celery seed), eighteen herbs and spices (including crushed red pepper and ground black pepper), and paprika. If you love seafood, this is a must-have pantry staple. It is very affordable, too. Old Bay is sold nationwide at pretty much any supermarket.

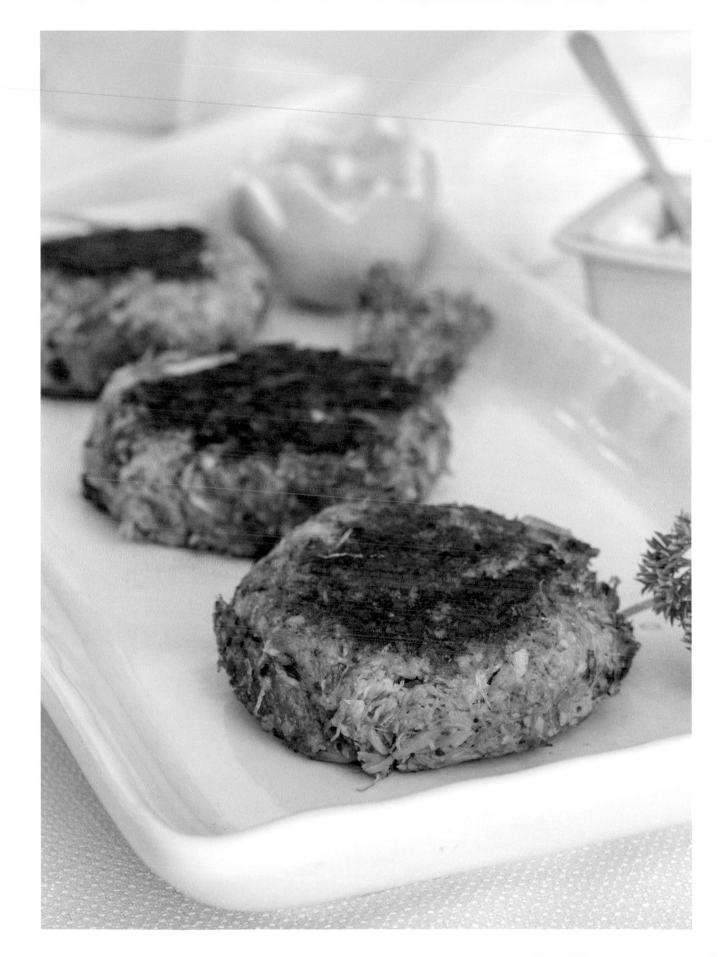

chinese takeout chicken lo mein

SERVES 6 to 8   PREP TIME: 30 minutes, plus time to rest the chicken in hot broth   COOK TIME: 1 hour

If you love chicken lo mein, this might end up being one of your favorite weeknight recipes. Conventional lo mein recipes use refined-wheat-flour egg noodles. I use gluten-free soba (buckwheat) noodles instead, which are far more nutritious and have such a mild flavor that they don't distract from the flavor of the dish at all. There are two secrets to making this recipe: (1) be sure to cut the vegetables as uniformly as possible, and (2) boil the chicken instead of pan-frying it, as in most chicken lo mein recipes (boiling the chicken will make it very tender, and the chicken broth adds incredible flavor to the dish). Serve with gluten-free tamari or unpasteurized soy sauce on the side.

For the chicken:

2 pounds boneless, skinless chicken thighs, trimmed of all visible fat (see Note, page 184)

2 cups water

½ medium onion, quartered

3 cloves garlic, peeled

1 teaspoon Himalayan pink salt

½ teaspoon ground black pepper

For the noodles:

8 ounces 100% buckwheat soba noodles

For the sauce:

½ cup gluten-free tamari (or unpasteurized soy sauce, if not gluten-free)

⅓ cup chicken broth reserved from cooking the chicken

1 teaspoon unrefined toasted sesame oil

1 tablespoon plus 1 teaspoon arrowroot

For the vegetables:

2 tablespoons extra-virgin coconut oil

1 large onion, thinly sliced

4 medium carrots, peeled, cut crosswise into thirds, then sliced lengthwise into thin strips

4 cloves garlic, crushed to a paste

1 green bell pepper, cut into thin strips

1 orange bell pepper, cut into thin strips

1 red bell pepper, thinly sliced

4 stalks celery, cut crosswise into thirds, then sliced into thin strips

6 cups shredded savoy or green cabbage

For garnish (optional):

Sliced scallions

Sesame seeds

TO MAKE THE CHICKEN:

1. Put the chicken thighs, water, onion, garlic, salt, and pepper in a medium-sized saucepan, cover, and bring to a rolling boil over high heat. As soon as the water reaches a vigorous boil, turn the heat down to low and simmer the chicken, uncovered, for 10 minutes. Then remove the pot from the heat, cover, and let it stand until the chicken is no longer pink in the center, 25 to 30 minutes. (Test for doneness by removing a thigh and cutting into it. When done, there will be no pink left in the center. The exact time will depend on the size of the thighs.)

2. When the chicken is done, remove it from the pot using tongs or a slotted spoon. Reserve ⅓ cup of the chicken broth for the sauce; save the rest for another use. Allow the chicken to cool. Shred the chicken by pulling it apart with two forks. Set the shredded chicken aside.

TO PREPARE THE NOODLES: Cook the noodles following the package directions; set aside.

TO MAKE THE SAUCE: Put the tamari, reserved chicken broth, and sesame oil in a medium-sized mixing bowl. Whisk in the arrowroot. Set the sauce aside.

TO MAKE THE VEGETABLES: Heat the oil in a large skillet over medium-high heat. Add the onion and carrots and stir-fry for 2 to 3 minutes, until slightly softened. Add the garlic, bell peppers, and celery and stir-fry for another 2 minutes, until the peppers and celery are beginning to soften. Add the cabbage and stir-fry for about 2 minutes, until softened.

TO PUT IT ALL TOGETHER: Add the sauce to the vegetables (still over medium-high heat) and cook for about 2 minutes, until everything is warm. Add the shredded chicken and noodles and continue cooking until they are heated through, about 2 minutes. Transfer to a serving dish, garnish with sliced scallions and sesame seeds, if desired, and serve at once.

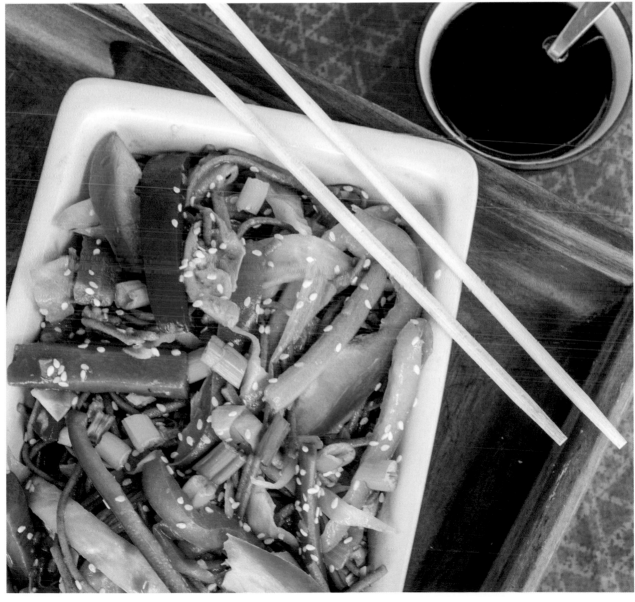

dawn's italian meatballs

MAKES about 20 meatballs (4 to 5 servings)
PREP TIME: 15 minutes   COOK TIME: 20 minutes

This is the easiest and most amazing meatball recipe ever. I wish I could say it was mine, but it came from my friend Dawn Rofrano (SpoonfulofHealth.com). An incredibly talented clean-food recipe developer, Dawn runs the Natural Medicine Clinic in Palm Beach Gardens with her husband, Dr. Tom Rofrano. When she's not at the clinic, Dawn is busy cooking up a storm! Like me, she's always looking for ways to sneak in extra vegetables, and in this meatball recipe she does a brilliant job of working in one whole zucchini (that is impossible to taste, I should add). One of our favorite ways to eat these meatballs is with our Tomato Sauce with Garlic & Italian Herbs (page 380) and gluten-free whole-grain pasta.

1 pound lean ground beef

3 tablespoons chickpea miso

1 tablespoon Italian seasoning

1 tablespoon onion flakes

2 cloves garlic, crushed to a paste

½ teaspoon Himalayan pink salt

1 medium zucchini, shredded (see Note)

Extra-virgin olive oil, for drizzling

1. Preheat the oven to 350°F. Line a rimmed baking sheet with parchment paper.

2. Put the beef, miso, Italian seasoning, onion flakes, garlic, and salt in a large bowl. With your fingers, gently mix until thoroughly combined. Gently fold in the shredded zucchini.

3. Scoop out about 2 tablespoons of the meat-zucchini mixture and use your hands to roll it into a ball. Place the meatball on the parchment-lined baking sheet. Repeat with the rest of the mixture to make about 20 meatballs. Drizzle the meatballs lightly with olive oil and bake until cooked through, about 20 minutes.

NOTE _____

For best results, shred the zucchini, with the skin on, using the largest holes of a box grater.

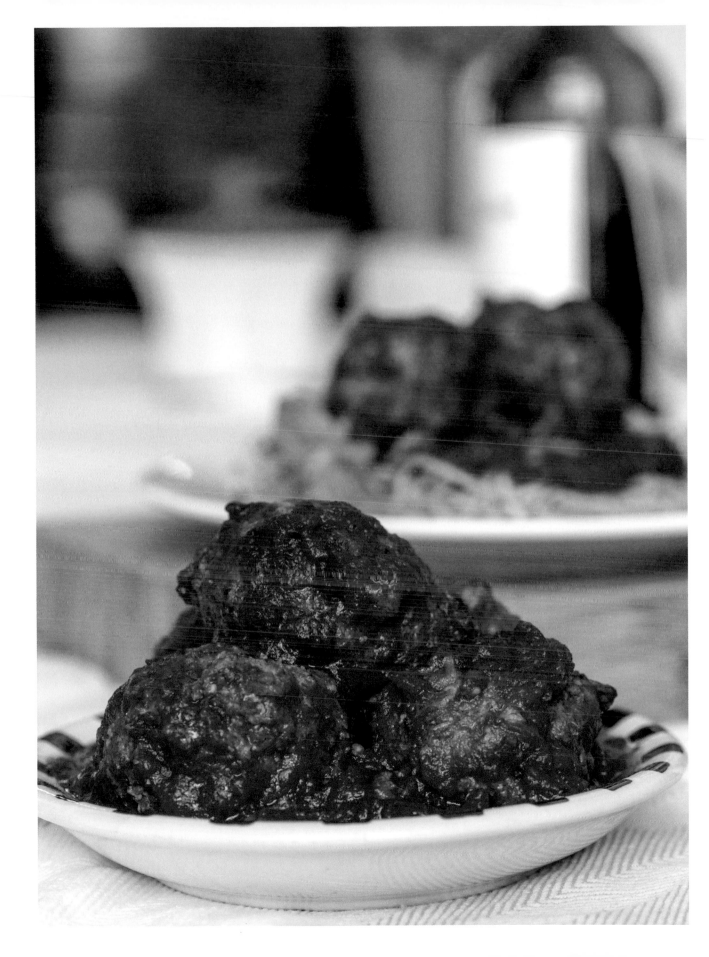

shrimp & grits

SERVES 4   PREP TIME: 25 minutes   COOK TIME: 25 minutes

As a fifth-generation Floridian, I grew up eating (and loving!) my grandma's delicious southern-style shrimp and grits recipe. But I never actually made the southern classic myself until after I turned forty. I knew that she included what she called her "fish salt," Old Bay Seasoning, but otherwise I had no idea how Grandma made her version. It turns out that since Grandma was not at all into cooking clean, her grits were always made with butter and milk, and other than collards (cooked in ham fat!), she didn't use a lot of vegetables. Grandma didn't serve her shrimp and grits with a side of green peas, like I often do, either. I am so excited that my clean version—with extra veggies and without any dairy—tastes similar enough to Grandma's to bring back many, many fond memories of eating shrimp and grits at her house.

For the shrimp:

30 large shrimp (preferably tail on), peeled and deveined

2 teaspoons extra-virgin olive oil or unrefined avocado oil

2 teaspoons Old Bay Seasoning

For the pine nut cream:

1 cup pine nuts (see Note)

1¾ cups water

For the grits:

1¼ cups pine nut cream (from above)

4 cups water, plus more if needed

1 teaspoon Himalayan pink salt

2 cups corn grits or polenta

For the vegetables:

1 tablespoon extra-virgin olive oil

1 green bell pepper, diced

1 red bell pepper, diced

1 yellow bell pepper, diced

1 cup chopped leeks, thoroughly washed and dried (see page 219)

3 cloves garlic, crushed to a paste

Himalayan pink salt

3 tablespoons dry white wine

Reserved pine nut cream (from above)

1. Rinse the peeled and deveined shrimp with cool water and pat very, very dry with paper towels. Coat the shrimp with the oil using your hands and then season with the Old Bay Seasoning. Set the seasoned shrimp aside.

2. To make the pine nut cream, put the pine nuts and 1¾ cups of water in a blender and process on high speed for 1 full minute, until the mixture is rich and creamy. Transfer 1¼ cups of the pine nut cream to a medium-sized saucepan and reserve the remaining cream for later.

3. To make the grits, pour the 4 cups of water and the salt into the saucepan with the nut cream and stir to combine. Bring the liquid to a boil over medium heat, then slowly stir in the grits. Let the liquid return to a boil, then turn the heat down to low, cover, and cook, stirring frequently, until the grits are fully cooked, smooth, and creamy, about 20 minutes. Keep your eye on the pot and add more water, 3 tablespoons at a time, if necessary. When the grits are done, remove the saucepan from the heat and cover to keep them warm.

4. While the grits are cooking, cook the vegetables and shrimp: In a large skillet, heat the oil over medium heat. Add the bell peppers, leeks, and garlic and sauté for 6 to 7 minutes, until the vegetables soften but are still firm. Season with salt to taste.

If you are using a conventional blender instead of a high-powered one, soak the pine nuts in water for 30 minutes, then rinse and drain them, before using them in this recipe.

5. Turn the heat to medium-high, push the vegetables to the sides of the skillet, and add the seasoned shrimp in the middle. Sear the shrimp briefly for about 1½ minutes per side, turning only once, until pink and cooked through. (Note: Be careful not to overcook the shrimp!)

6. To the skillet, add the wine and the reserved pine nut cream and cook for about 2 minutes, until the sauce thickens just a bit, stirring frequently to coat all of the vegetables and shrimp.

7. Serve the shrimp and vegetables alongside or on top of the grits. Eat at once.

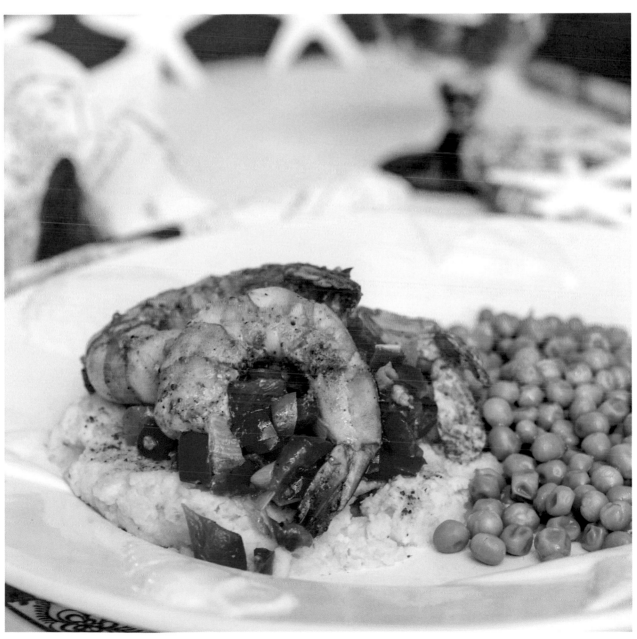

macadamia-crusted baked fish

SERVES 6   PREP TIME: 20 minutes   COOK TIME: 15 minutes

I'm not sure if nut-crusted fish is as big a deal in other parts of the country as it is here in South Florida, but if you go to a seafood restaurant in our neck of the woods, you are sure to see some variety of nut-crusted fish on the menu. Macadamia-crusted fish is one of my absolute favorite ways to prepare fish: not only is it super easy to make, but the fish always turns out just perfect. Just be sure to buy the freshest fish! (See page 86 for more on buying seafood.) I like to serve this macadamia-crusted fish with a side of steamed green beans.

6 (6-ounce) wild white-fleshed fish fillets (such as cod, halibut, or mahi) or wild salmon fillets

¼ teaspoon Himalayan pink salt

¾ cup raw macadamia nuts

2 tablespoons chopped fresh dill

1 clove garlic, coarsely chopped

1 teaspoon grated lemon zest

½ teaspoon Dijon mustard

½ teaspoon onion powder

½ teaspoon raw honey

⅓ cup mayonnaise, homemade (page 392) or store-bought

Lemon slices, for serving (optional)

1. Preheat the oven to 425°F. Lightly oil the bottom of a 9 by 13-inch baking dish.

2. Rinse the fish fillets with cold water and pat very, very dry with paper towels. Season both sides of the fillets with the salt. Arrange the fillets on the bottom of the baking dish, leaving space around each fillet.

3. Put the macadamia nuts, dill, garlic, lemon zest, Dijon mustard, onion powder, and honey in a food processor. Process until all the ingredients are thoroughly combined and finely chopped.

4. Spread the mayonnaise over the fish fillets and top with the macadamia-dill crumbs. Bake for 12 to 15 minutes, until the fish is flaky when pierced with a fork. (Note: Cooking time will vary depending on the type and thickness of the fish. But be sure to check the fish after 12 minutes so as not to overcook it. Nothing is worse than overcooked fish!) Serve with lemon slices, if desired.

MAKE IT EGG-FREE

Use my Egg-Free Mayonnaise (page 392).

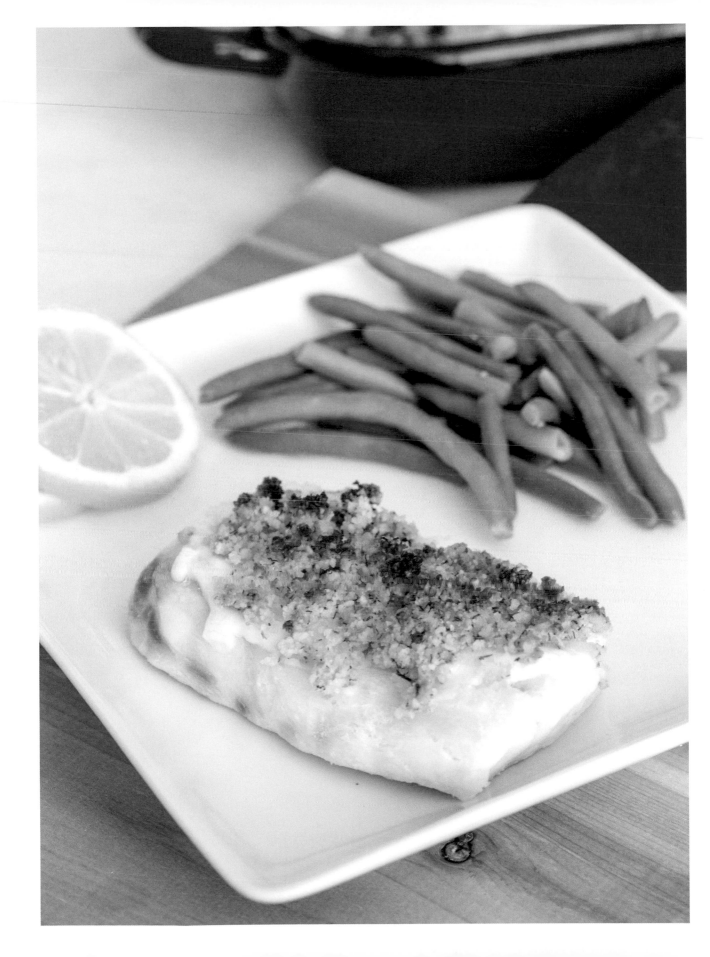

dinner party stuffed cornish hens

SERVES 4   PREP TIME: 15 minutes   COOK TIME: 1 hour

If you love the idea of hosting a dinner party but just don't have the time to spend all day in the kitchen, then you need this recipe. It's the easiest fancy-looking entrée in the world! Incredibly moist and flavorful, Cornish hens are just like little chickens. Aside from their diminutive size, their most notable trait is the tenderness of their meat. And nothing could be easier than roasting whole Cornish hens: you just rub them with oil and seasonings, stuff the cavities, and pop them in the oven. I use my Wild Rice Pilaf (page 262) for stuffing, but you can also just use steamed sprouted short-grain brown rice. Serve the stuffed hens with steamed green beans and roasted grape tomatoes and you've got a super-easy, delicious, impressive-looking, dinner party–worthy meal.

4 Cornish hens (about 1½ pounds each)

¼ cup fresh thyme leaves

Juice of 3 lemons

¼ cup extra-virgin olive oil

1 teaspoon Himalayan pink salt

½ teaspoon garlic powder

½ teaspoon ground black pepper

½ teaspoon onion powder

2 cups Wild Rice Pilaf (page 262) or steamed short-grain brown rice (preferably sprouted)

1. Preheat the oven to 375°F.

2. Rinse the hens in water and pat the insides and outsides as dry as possible with paper towels. Gently lift the skin from the breasts and put 1 tablespoon of thyme leaves under the skin of each hen. Use your hands to rub the inside and outside of each hen with the lemon juice, followed by the olive oil.

3. In a small bowl, mix together the salt, garlic powder, pepper, and onion powder. Use your hands to rub the seasoning on the inside and outside of each hen. Stuff the cavity of each bird with the rice pilaf.

4. Transfer the hens to a roasting pan and cook, uncovered, for 1 hour, or until the juices run clear when you cut between a leg and thigh and a meat thermometer inserted into each hen reads 170°F to 175°F (don't let the thermometer touch the bone). Let the hens rest for 10 to 15 minutes before serving. Serve warm.

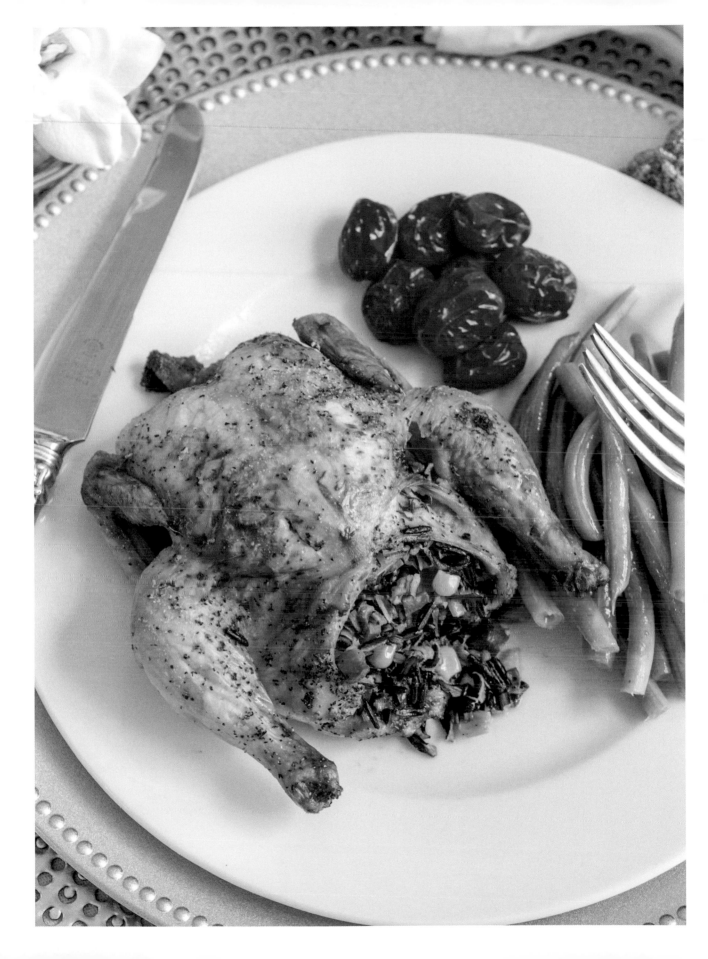

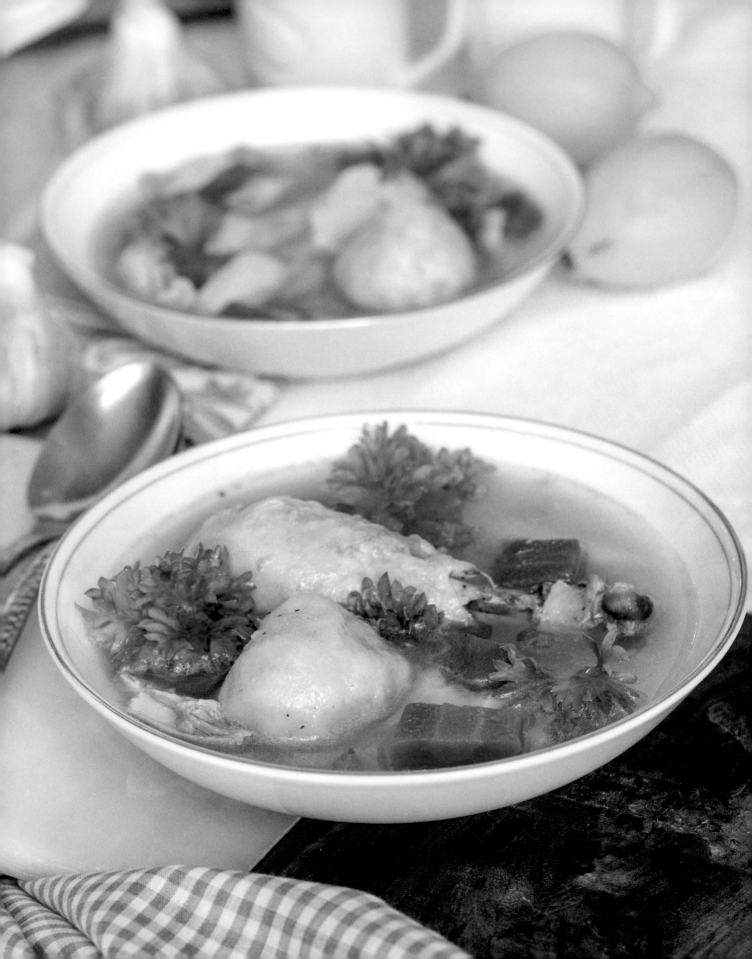

CHAPTER 12

easy one-pot meals

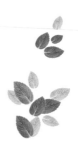

honey mustard sheet pan chicken dinner

SERVES 4   PREP TIME: 20 minutes   COOK TIME: 50 minutes

If you have Honey Mustard Sauce (page 388) already made, then this entire meal takes less than twenty minutes of hands-on prep. But even if you don't have the sauce made, it's still quick to pull together since the sauce takes less than ten minutes to whip up. That, in my book, makes it a perfect weeknight dinner!

---

2 pounds boneless, skinless chicken thighs, trimmed of all visible fat (see Note, page 184)

Himalayan pink salt and ground black pepper

¼ cup plus 3 tablespoons Honey Mustard Sauce (page 388), divided

1¼ pounds red potatoes (aka Red Bliss potatoes), quartered (4 cups)

4 cups Brussels sprouts, trimmed and halved

4 large shallots, quartered

1 tablespoon extra-virgin olive oil

5 sprigs fresh rosemary

1. Preheat the oven to 425°F. Line a rimmed baking sheet with parchment paper.

2. Generously season the chicken with salt and pepper. Rub ¼ cup of the honey mustard sauce all over the chicken. Place the chicken on the prepared baking sheet.

3. Put the potatoes, Brussels sprouts, and shallots in a large mixing bowl. Drizzle the vegetables with the olive oil and the remaining 3 tablespoons of the honey mustard sauce, then sprinkle ¼ teaspoon each of salt and pepper over them. Toss to coat the vegetables in the sauce. Spread the vegetables in an even layer around the chicken on the baking sheet. Arrange the rosemary sprigs on top of the vegetables.

4. Roast for 45 to 50 minutes, until the chicken is no longer pink in the center and the potatoes are fork-tender. Serve warm.

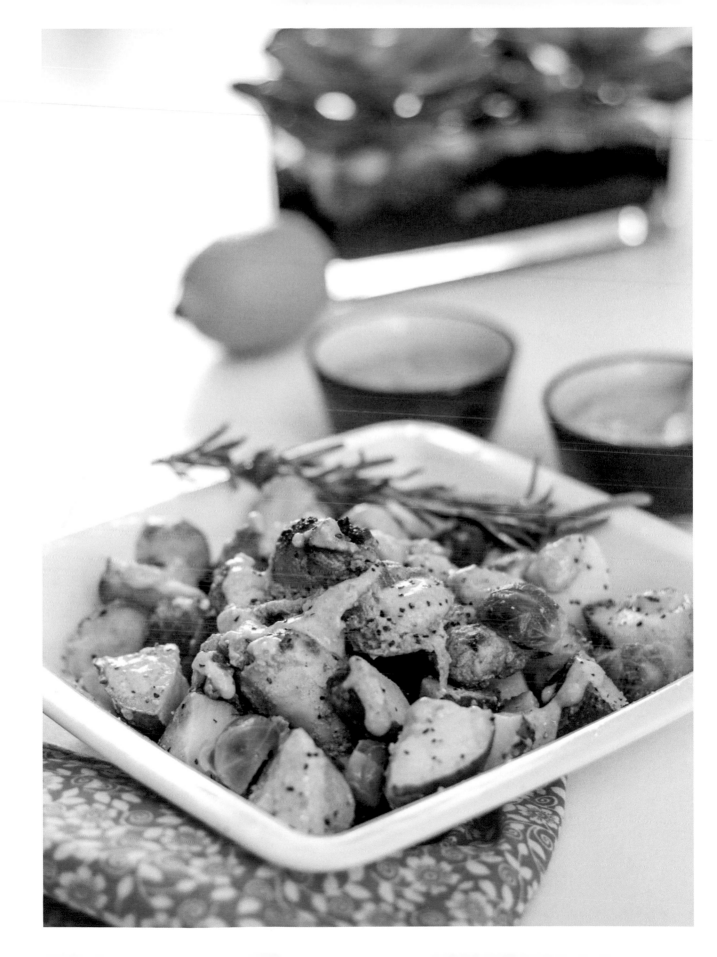

salmon noodle casserole

SERVES 6 to 8   PREP TIME: 20 minutes   COOK TIME: 30 minutes

I don't know what I would have done without this staple one-dish wonder when my son was growing up. It takes no time to make, and I almost always have all of the ingredients on hand as pantry staples. If you have kids in your family, this is a dinner recipe you'll find yourself going back to again and again! One quick note on the fish: I like to use canned wild salmon instead of tuna because it's considerably lower in mercury. But the classic choice of tuna works, too—just don't eat it often, to be on the safe side.

¾ cup raw walnuts

½ cup plus 3 tablespoons chopped fresh parsley, divided

1 cup raw cashews, preferably soaked in water for 1 to 2 hours, then rinsed and drained (see Note)

1 cup water

2 tablespoons fresh lemon juice

1 teaspoon Dijon mustard

½ teaspoon hot sauce, such as Tabasco

2 tablespoons extra-virgin olive oil, for the pan

1¼ cups finely chopped onions

3 stalks celery, finely chopped

3 medium carrots, peeled and finely chopped

1¼ cups frozen petite green peas

1 teaspoon Himalayan pink salt

1 (5-ounce) can wild salmon or tuna (packed in water), drained

10 ounces gluten-free whole-grain pasta shells, cooked according to package directions

Lemon wedges, for serving (optional)

SPECIAL TOOLS _____

Mini food processor

1. Preheat the oven to 400°F. Lightly oil the bottom and sides of an ovenproof 8-inch casserole dish.

2. Put the walnuts and 3 tablespoons of the parsley in a mini food processor. Pulse into crumb-sized pieces and set aside.

3. Put the cashews, water, lemon juice, Dijon mustard, and hot sauce in a blender and process until smooth and creamy. Set the cashew cream aside.

4. Heat the oil in a large skillet over medium heat. Add the onions, celery, and carrots and cook for 5 to 6 minutes, until the vegetables are soft. Add the peas, salt, and cashew cream and cook, stirring occasionally, for 2 to 3 minutes, until the peas are thawed. Stir in the remaining ½ cup of parsley. Add the salmon to the skillet, use a fork to break up the pieces, and cook for an additional minute.

5. Put the cooked pasta shells in the casserole dish. Spoon the vegetable-and-cashew-cream mixture over the noodles and stir to combine. Sprinkle the walnut-parsley crumbs on top.

6. Bake for 20 minutes, until no longer liquidy. Allow the casserole to cool for 10 minutes before serving. Serve warm with lemon wedges, if desired.

MAKE IT GRAIN-FREE _____
Use a chickpea (aka garbanzo bean) pasta.

NOTE _____
If you're using a high-powered blender, soaking the cashews is optional, but it does create a creamier texture. If you're using a conventional blender instead of a high-powered one, soaking the cashews is necessary to get the right texture.

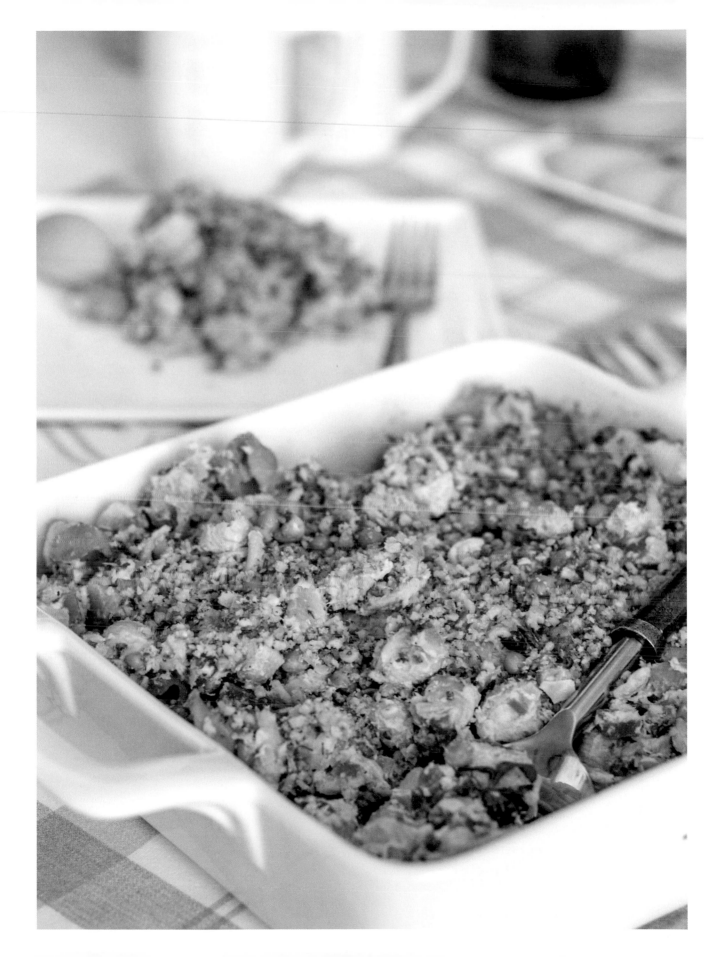

slow cooker beef stroganoff

SERVES 8   PREP TIME: 30 minutes   COOK TIME: 3 hours 20 minutes
or 5 hours 20 minutes, depending on heat level used

Until I started writing this cookbook, I always assumed beef stroganoff was a classic American dish. Turns out, it was born in Russia and has been around for several centuries. The classic version is made with lots of butter, lots of cream, and even more sour cream. It does not call for superfood shiitake mushrooms, does not include peas, and certainly doesn't use a macadamia nut–based sour cream. But don't worry! Even with all of these swaps, this version tastes just as good as the original. If you've got meat-loving family members who insist they don't want to try anything Clean Cuisine, this is the dish to make. Note: Traditionally, beef stroganoff is served over buttered egg noodles. However, since I have yet to find a clean egg-noodle brand, I usually serve it over gluten-free brown rice penne pasta. If you have a grain intolerance, you can always substitute lightly cooked zucchini noodles (see page 194).

4 tablespoons cassava flour (or sprouted spelt flour if not gluten- or grain-free), divided

2 teaspoons Himalayan pink salt, divided

1 teaspoon ground black pepper, divided

8 tablespoons extra-virgin olive oil, divided

2 pounds boneless top sirloin steak, cut crosswise into ½-inch-wide strips

1 large onion, thinly sliced

5 cloves garlic, minced

2 cups beef broth

1 cup dry red wine

4 sprigs fresh thyme

8 cups shiitake mushrooms, stemmed and sliced into thin strips

1¼ cups Clean Cuisine Sour Cream (page 372)

2 tablespoons gluten-free Worcestershire sauce

1 tablespoon sherry

2 teaspoons Dijon mustard

1 pound gluten-free whole-grain penne pasta or fettuccine, cooked according to package directions, for serving

2 cups frozen petite green peas, steamed, for serving

½ cup chopped fresh parsley, for garnish

1. In a medium-sized bowl, stir together 3 tablespoons of the cassava flour, 1 teaspoon of the salt, and ½ teaspoon of the pepper. Heat 2 tablespoons of the oil in a large skillet over medium-high heat. Working in batches, roll the steak strips in the seasoned flour, shake off the excess flour, and fry them in the hot oil, turning occasionally, until brown on all sides, about 5 minutes. Transfer the browned steak to a 5- or 6-quart slow cooker. Repeat with the remaining beef strips.

2. Turn the heat down to medium, then add 3 tablespoons of the oil and tilt the pan to coat its surface. Add the onion and sauté until tender, about 5 minutes. Add the garlic and sauté for about 30 seconds, until softened. Add ½ teaspoon of the salt and ¼ teaspoon of the pepper. Add the broth and wine and bring to a boil, stirring and scraping up the browned bits on the bottom of the pan with a wooden spoon.

3. Transfer the onion to the slow cooker. Pour the broth mixture over the steak and onion and add the thyme.

4. Wipe the pan dry with a paper towel, then pour in the remaining 3 tablespoons of oil and heat over medium heat. Add the mushrooms and sauté until they begin to brown, about 4 minutes. Season with the remaining ½ teaspoon of salt and ¼ teaspoon of pepper. Transfer the mushrooms to the slow cooker.

MAKE IT GRAIN-FREE AND PALEO-FRIENDLY _____
Swap the penne pasta for 6 cups zucchini noodles (about 3 medium zucchini), lightly cooked.

5. In a medium-sized bowl, stir together the sour cream, Worcestershire sauce, sherry, and Dijon mustard. Stirring constantly, sprinkle in the remaining 1 tablespoon of cassava flour and mix until thoroughly blended. Pour the sauce into the slow cooker on top of the beef, onion, and mushrooms.

6. Cover and cook until the steak is tender, 2 hours on high or 4 hours on low. Serve over penne pasta with steamed peas on top or on the side. Garnish with parsley.

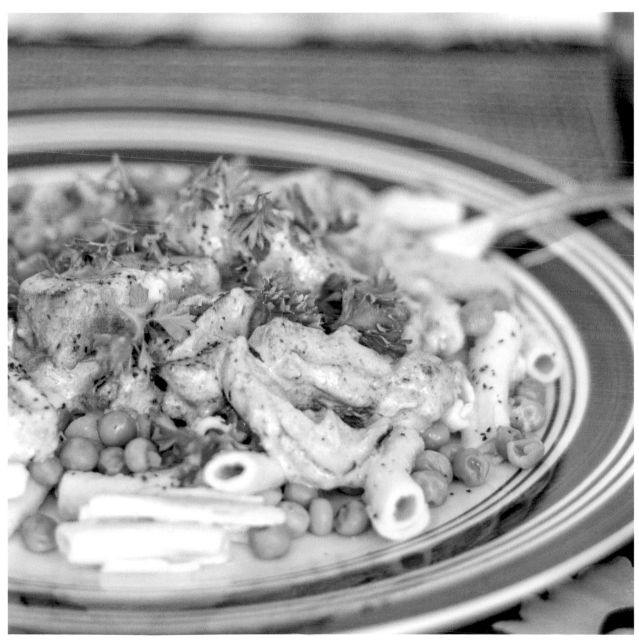

lemony chicken & dumplings

SERVES 6   PREP TIME: 30 minutes   COOK TIME: 1 hour 40 minutes

Who doesn't love chicken and dumplings? When I was growing up, my mom made it whenever anybody in our house got sick. It was my favorite thing about getting sick! Mom always added lemon juice because she figured the vitamin C would help us get better sooner. Not only does the lemon juice give an antioxidant and nutrition boost, but it really does wonders for brightening the overall flavor of the dish. I worked with my mom closely on revamping this recipe for clean eating, and the clean version has been a big hit with everyone in our family.

For the chicken:

1 whole small chicken (about 3 pounds)

Himalayan pink salt and ground black pepper

12 cups water

¼ cup fresh lemon juice

1 bay leaf

2 tablespoons extra-virgin olive oil

6 large carrots, peeled and chopped

5 cloves garlic, chopped

3 stalks celery, chopped

1 large onion, finely chopped

1 medium leek, chopped, thoroughly washed, and dried (see facing page)

½ teaspoon turmeric powder

For the dumplings:

2 cups cassava flour (or sprouted spelt flour if not gluten- or grain-free)

¼ cup brown rice flour

2 teaspoons baking powder

¾ teaspoon Himalayan pink salt

2 large eggs, beaten

1¼ cups chicken broth (from above)

1 cup plus 1 tablespoon finely chopped fresh parsley, divided, plus 6 sprigs for garnish

TO MAKE THE CHICKEN:

1. Pat the inside and outside of the chicken dry with paper towels and generously season it with salt and pepper. Put the chicken in a large pot and add the water, lemon juice, bay leaf, ½ teaspoon of salt, and ¼ teaspoon of pepper. Bring the water to a boil, then turn the heat down to low, cover, and simmer until the chicken is fully cooked and fork-tender, about 1 hour. As the chicken cooks, periodically skim off the foam and scum from the top of the water.

2. When the chicken is done, remove it from the pot and set aside to cool. Transfer 1¼ cups of the broth to a bowl and set aside; you'll use it later for the dumplings. Pour the rest of the broth into a second bowl and wipe out the pot with a paper towel.

3. Heat the oil in the pot over medium heat, then add the carrots, garlic, celery, onion, and leek. Sauté the vegetables for 6 to 7 minutes, until soft. Season with ¼ teaspoon each of salt and pepper.

4. Pour in the broth from the second bowl and turn the heat down to medium-low heat. Add the turmeric, stir to combine, and simmer, uncovered, for 10 minutes, or until fragrant.

TO MAKE THE DUMPLINGS:

1. Put the cassava flour, brown rice flour, baking powder, and salt in a medium-sized mixing bowl; whisk together until well blended. Add the beaten eggs, broth, and 1 tablespoon of the parsley and whisk until you have a dough; it will be thick and sticky.

2. Spoon out about 2 heaping tablespoons of the dumpling mixture and, using your hands, gently form the dough into a ball. Transfer the dough ball to a plate. Repeat with the rest of the dough.

3. Bring the broth and chicken back to a simmer over medium-low heat. Carefully add the dumplings to the soup one at a time. Cover and simmer until the dumplings expand in size and are no longer doughy inside, about 20 minutes. Stir in the remaining cup of parsley and serve warm, garnished with parsley sprigs.

HOW TO CLEAN A LEEK _____

Place the leek on a cutting board. If the root hairs are still attached to the root end, cut them off. Cut off the very dark green (and tough) tops, leaving just the white and pale green part of the leek. (Save the dark green tops for broth, soup, or other slow-cooking recipes.) Chop the leek as the recipe instructions dictate.

Transfer the cut-up leek to a bowl of cold water and swish it around to remove the dirt. Scoop out the leek, leaving the dirt behind in the bowl, and place in a colander to drain. If you'll be cooking the leek in oil or fat, be sure to dry it well.

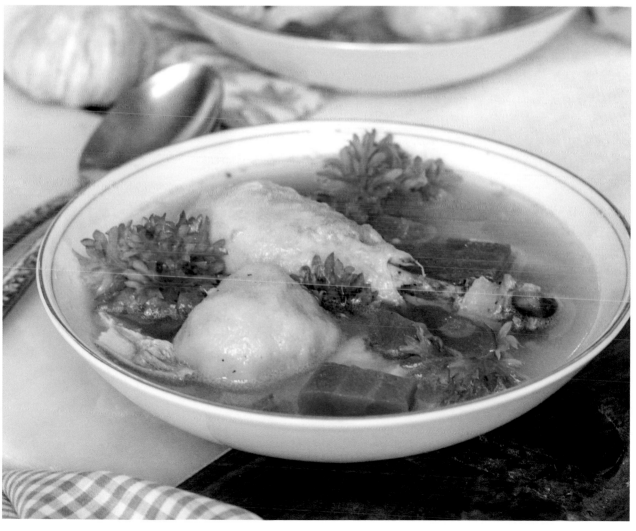

turkey shepherd's pie
with whipped sweet potatoes

SERVES 8   PREP TIME: 40 minutes   COOK TIME: 55 minutes

I grew up in a real meat-and-potatoes kind of family. My mom's shepherd's pie was a staple, so I grew up eating and loving this classic British dish. When I moved to London in college, I found myself ducking into pub after pub in search of the best shepherd's pie across the pond. Back then, the only criteria I had was that it taste good. Thanks to the sweet potatoes and the addition of a lot more vegetables to the meat mixture, this cleaned-up version actually has more flavor than the traditional versions I taste-tested back in the day. Feel free to substitute grass-fed beef or pasture-raised lamb for the turkey if you like.

For the whipped sweet potato topping:

1¼ pounds sweet potatoes, peeled and cubed (about 6 cups)

¼ cup pine nuts (see Note)

1 tablespoon fresh lemon juice

¼ teaspoon Himalayan pink salt

For the filling:

1 medium leek, sliced, thoroughly washed, and drained (see page 219)

4 medium carrots, peeled and coarsely chopped

½ medium onion, coarsely chopped

1 tablespoon extra-virgin olive oil

2 tablespoons fresh thyme leaves

Himalayan pink salt

1¼ pounds ground turkey

2 tablespoons brown rice flour

1½ cups frozen petite green peas

⅓ cup white wine

2 tablespoons tomato paste, plus more to taste

2 teaspoons gluten-free Worcestershire sauce

8 sprigs thyme, for garnish

TO MAKE THE WHIPPED SWEET POTATOES:

1. Bring a large pot of water to a boil. Add the sweet potatoes, turn the heat down to low, and simmer for 15 to 20 minutes, until the potatoes are soft.

2. Meanwhile, put the pine nuts, lemon juice, and salt in a blender and process on high speed until smooth and creamy. (Note: If you need to add more liquid, add 1 tablespoon of water at a time.)

3. Once the sweet potatoes are cooked, drain them and transfer to a large mixing bowl. Drizzle the pine nut cream over the sweet potatoes and use a handheld stick blender or mixer to whip until smooth and lump-free. Season with additional salt to taste. Set the whipped sweet potatoes aside.

TO MAKE THE FILLING:

1. Preheat the oven to 450°F.

2. Place the sliced leek in a food processor and pulse several times to finely chop. Remove the leek from the food processor and set aside. Finely chop the carrots and then the onion in the food processor in the same manner, keeping all of the vegetables separate.

3. Heat the 1 tablespoon of oil in a large skillet over medium heat. Add the finely chopped leek, carrots, and onion and sauté for 6 to 7 minutes, until the vegetables soften a bit. Stir in the fresh thyme and a few pinches of salt.

4. Add the ground turkey to the skillet and use a spatula to fully incorporate the meat into the vegetables. Cook until the meat is no longer pink, about 5 minutes, stirring occasionally to break up the meat as it cooks.

STORAGE INFORMATION ─────────
Shepherd's pie will keep in an airtight container in the refrigerator for up to 2 days.

MAKE IT PALEO-FRIENDLY AND GRAIN-FREE ─────────
Replace the brown rice flour with almond flour or cassava flour.

NOTE ─────────────
If you are using a conventional blender instead of a high-powered one, soak the pine nuts in water for 30 minutes, then rinse and drain them, before using them in this recipe.

5. Use a fork to whisk in the flour. Add a few more pinches of salt. Stir in the peas, wine, tomato paste, and Worcestershire sauce and cook for about 8 minutes, until all the ingredients are fully incorporated and all the liquid is gone. Taste and add more salt if desired.

TO ASSEMBLE THE PIE: Spread the turkey mixture on the bottom of an ovenproof 9-inch square casserole dish or on the bottoms of eight 6-ounce ramekins. Spoon the whipped sweet potatoes over the turkey mixture and smooth with the back of a spoon, then brush the sweet potatoes lightly with oil. Bake for 15 minutes, until the sweet potatoes are lightly browned. Remove from the oven and let sit 15 minutes before serving. Garnish with a sprig of thyme and serve warm.

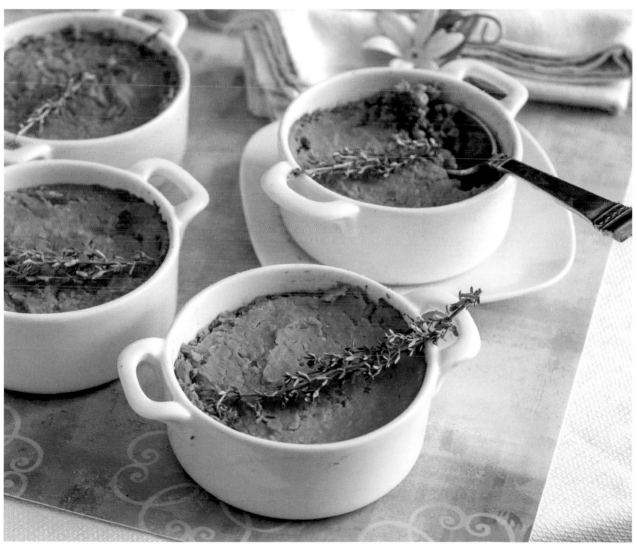

skillet meat & bean casserole with cornbread topping

SERVES 6 to 8   PREP TIME: 20 minutes   COOK TIME: 40 minutes

My grandma always made meat-and-bean casserole when I was growing up, and I've made a plant-based slow cooker version in the past. But when I saw blogger and cookbook author Robyn Stone (of AddaPinch.com) on the Food Network making her version of this dish, I immediately bought her cookbook just to get this recipe. My version here eliminates the cheese, sneaks in more vegetables, cuts down on the meat, adds tempeh, and uses a gluten-free cornbread topping that doesn't have butter. I have a hunch Robyn's version probably would win in a taste-test competition, but I think my version is pretty darn good too! And it's the perfect easy weeknight dinner.

---

1 pound ground buffalo, turkey, or beef

1 teaspoon Himalayan pink salt

2 medium carrots, peeled and chopped

2 stalks celery, chopped

½ medium onion, chopped

1 (8-ounce) package tempeh, crumbled

6 cloves garlic, minced

2 (15-ounce) cans tomato sauce

1 (15-ounce) can pinto beans, rinsed and drained

1 (4-ounce) can chopped green chiles

1 tablespoon ground cumin

2 teaspoons coconut sugar

1 recipe prepared batter for Cornbread Muffins with Kale (page 124)

1. Preheat the oven to 375°F.

2. In a large ovenproof skillet or Dutch oven set over medium heat, cook the ground meat until browned through, about 5 minutes, breaking it up with a wooden spoon as it cooks. Season the meat with the salt. Add the carrots, celery, and onion and cook for 5 minutes, until the vegetables soften. Add the tempeh and garlic and cook an additional 2 minutes, until the tempeh is warmed through.

3. Remove the skillet from the heat. Stir in the tomato sauce, beans, green chiles, cumin, and coconut sugar. Spoon the cornbread batter on top in dollops.

4. Transfer the skillet to the oven and bake for 23 to 25 minutes, until a toothpick inserted in the cornbread topping comes out clean. Serve warm.

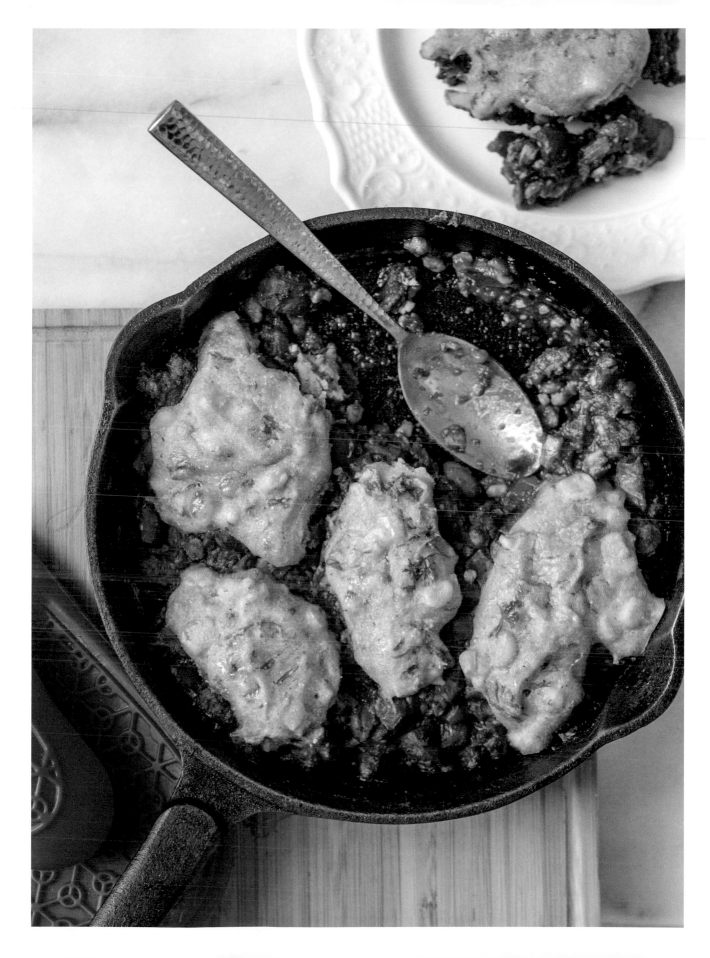

slow cooker bolognese

SERVES 8   PREP TIME: 25 minutes   COOK TIME: 2 hours 25 minutes
or 4 hours 25 minutes, depending on heat level

If spending hours in the kitchen while laboring over a hot stove is not your cup of tea, then this sauce (with hidden veggies galore!) is just for you. Traditionally, Bolognese sauce is exceptionally meat-heavy. However, I've found you can drastically reduce the meat without sacrificing richness or flavor. Secret number one is to mix in lots of meaty-textured shiitake mushrooms. Secret number two is the pine nut cream. It takes all of two minutes to make and contributes substantially to the full-bodied end result. Serve this sauce over noodles of your choice, whether that's whole-grain spaghetti noodles, zucchini noodles, or a combination of the two. (I like to mix the two types of noodles to boost my vegetable intake.)

¼ cup pine nuts (see Note)

¼ cup plus 1 tablespoon water

3 large carrots, peeled and coarsely chopped

2 cups shiitake mushrooms, stemmed

3 tablespoons extra-virgin olive oil

6 cloves garlic, minced

2 large shallots, finely chopped

1 teaspoon dried oregano leaves

½ teaspoon Himalayan pink salt, divided

½ teaspoon ground black pepper, divided

1¼ pounds ground turkey or lean beef

1 (8-ounce) package tempeh, crumbled

¼ cup red wine

1 (15-ounce) can tomato sauce

¼ cup tomato paste

STORAGE INFORMATION _____
Bolognese sauce can be stored in a covered container in the refrigerator for up to 5 days or in the freezer for up to a month.

MAKE IT PALEO-FRIENDLY _____
Omit the tempeh.

1. In a blender, process the pine nuts and water until smooth and creamy, then set aside.

2. Put the carrots in a food processor and pulse several times to finely chop; remove from the food processor and set aside. Put the mushrooms in the food processor and pulse several times to finely chop; remove from the food processor and set aside.

3. Heat the oil in a large skillet over medium heat. Add the garlic, shallots, and chopped carrots and sauté for 5 to 6 minutes, until the vegetables are soft. Add the mushrooms and sauté for 3 to 4 minutes, until the mushrooms are soft. Season with the oregano and ¼ teaspoon each of the salt and pepper. Transfer the vegetables to a 5- or 6-quart slow cooker.

4. Put the ground meat and tempeh in the same pan, season with the remaining ¼ teaspoon each of salt and pepper, and cook, stirring occasionally to break up the meat, until the meat is no longer pink, about 5 minutes. Pour the wine into the skillet and cook until the liquid evaporates, about 3 minutes or so. Stir in the pine nut cream, tomato sauce, and tomato paste and simmer for 5 minutes, until fragrant. Taste and season with additional salt and pepper if desired.

5. Transfer the meat mixture to the slow cooker. Gently stir the meat and vegetables together. Cover and cook on high for 2 hours or on low for 4 hours. Let the Bolognese sit 30 minutes for the flavors to deepen before serving. Serve warm.

NOTE _____
If you are using a conventional blender instead of a high-powered one, soak the pine nuts in water for 30 minutes, then rinse and drain them, before using.

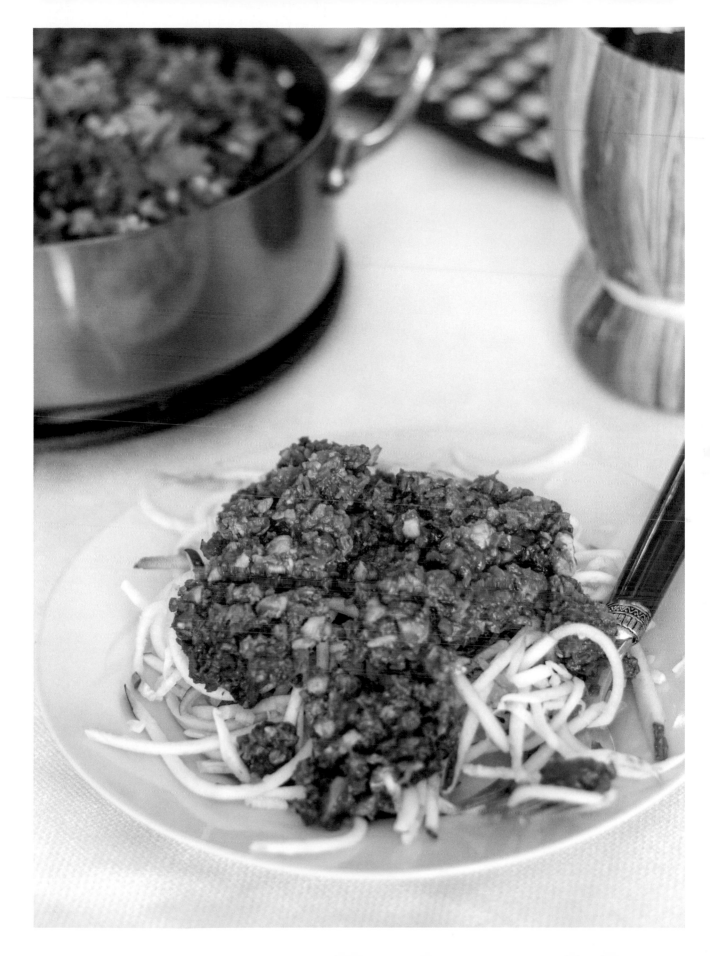

slow cooker chicken & vegetable thai curry

SERVES 4   PREP TIME: 20 minutes   COOK TIME: 2 hours 50 minutes or
6 hours 30 minutes, depending on heat level

This was the first official recipe I made in my Instant Pot, but it is every bit as tasty made in the slow cooker. (If you want the Instant Pot version, you can find it on our blog.) The flavor is pretty amazing. Even though it's unusual to put curry and beans together, adding the chickpeas at the end works surprisingly well, and they give the dish a great fiber boost.

For the sauce:

1 cup full-fat coconut milk

¼ cup chicken broth

¼ cup unsalted, unsweetened smooth peanut butter

2 tablespoons red curry paste

4 medjool dates, pitted (see Note)

1 tablespoon grated fresh ginger

2 tablespoons gluten-free tamari (or unpasteurized soy sauce, if not gluten-free)

2 tablespoons fresh lime juice

1 tablespoon fish sauce

3 cloves garlic, peeled

For the stew:

1½ pounds boneless, skinless chicken thighs, trimmed of all visible fat (see Note, page 184)

Himalayan pink salt

1 tablespoon extra-virgin coconut oil

5 medium carrots, peeled and cut into thin strips

2 red bell peppers, cut into thin strips

1 medium onion, sliced

2 (15-ounce) cans chickpeas, rinsed and drained (optional)

½ cup chopped fresh cilantro, for garnish (optional)

TO MAKE THE SAUCE: Put the ingredients in a blender in the order given in the ingredients list. Process until smooth, then set aside. (Note: The sauce can be prepared up to 3 days in advance.)

TO MAKE THE STEW:

1. Season the chicken lightly with salt on all sides. Heat the oil in a large heavy-bottomed skillet over medium-high heat. Add the chicken to the skillet and brown for about 3 minutes on each side. Remove the chicken from the skillet with a slotted spoon and transfer to a 5- or 6-quart slow cooker.

2. Add the carrots, red bell peppers, and onion to the skillet and sauté for 5 or 6 minutes, until the vegetables start to soften. Transfer the vegetables to the slow cooker.

3. Pour the sauce into the slow cooker and stir to combine with the chicken and vegetables.

4. Cover the slow cooker and cook until the chicken is cooked through and the vegetables are soft, 5 to 6 hours on low heat or about 2½ hours on high heat.

5. Stir in the chickpeas (if using) and cook until heated through, about 10 minutes on high or 20 minutes on low. Ladle the stew into individual bowls, garnish with the cilantro, if desired, and serve warm.

NOTE _____

If you're using a conventional blender rather than a high-powered one and your dates are on the dry side, soak them in water for 15 to 30 minutes to soften them before pureeing (very moist, succulent medjool dates do not require soaking).

MAKE IT BEAN-FREE

Omit the chickpeas. Substitute unsalted, unsweetened smooth raw almond butter for the peanut butter.

MAKE IT SOY-FREE

Substitute coconut aminos for the tamari.

MAKE IT PALEO-FRIENDLY

Omit the chickpeas. Substitute unsalted, unsweetened smooth raw almond butter for the peanut butter. Substitute coconut aminos for the tamari.

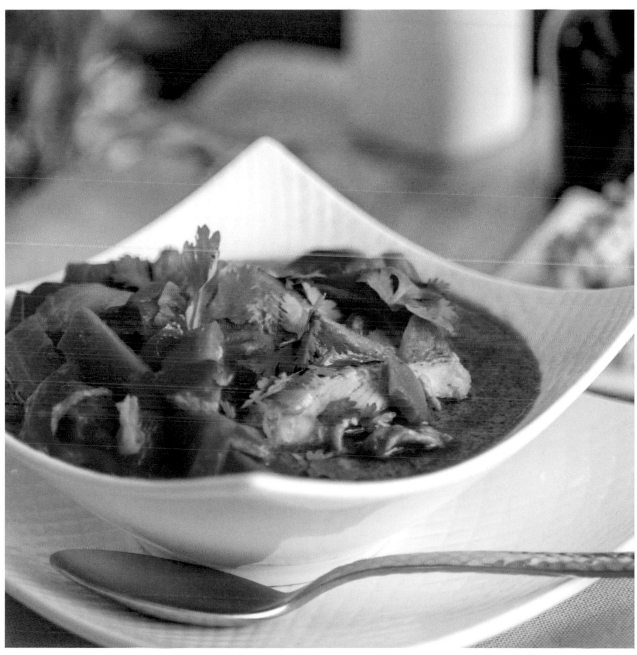

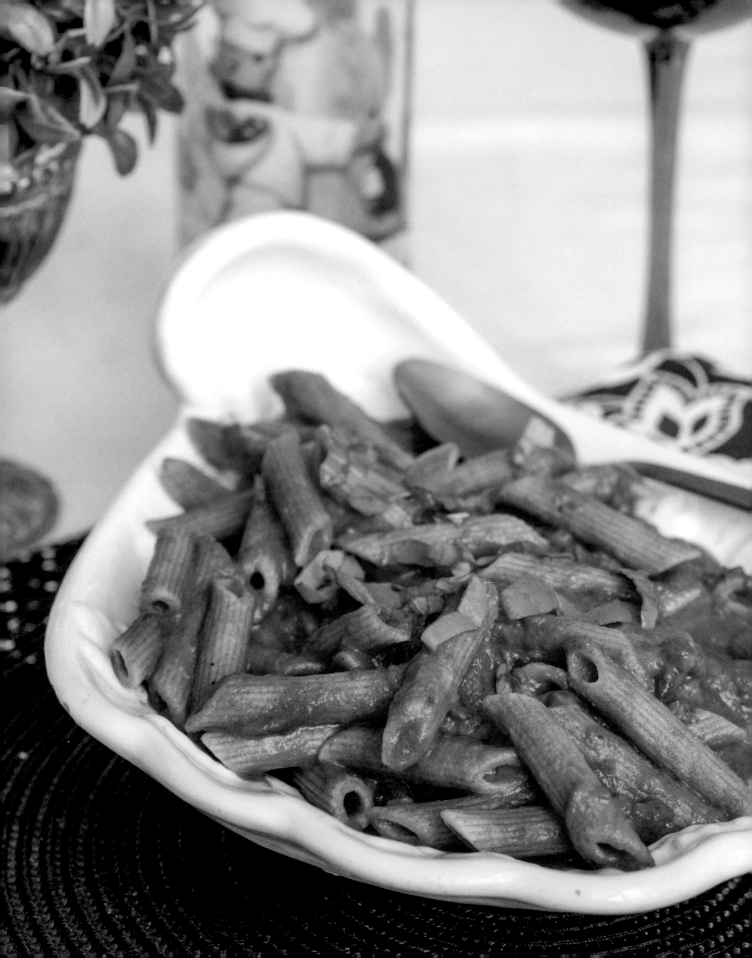

CHAPTER 13

meatless mondays

polenta pizza
with white sauce & mushrooms

MAKES one 9-inch deep-dish pizza (6 servings)
PREP TIME: 35 minutes, plus time to chill the crust   COOK TIME: 50 minutes

When I started eating clean two decades ago, pizza was one of the first foods I knew I had to give up. I would never, in a million years, have thought that pizza without cheese or wheat could one day be one of my favorite foods. But here it is! I have been making polenta pizza crust for ages now, and although this particular recipe calls for a white sauce, the crust is delicious with a more traditional red sauce too. Whether you are gluten-free, dairy-free, vegetarian, or none of the above, this pizza is sure to satisfy.

For the polenta crust:

4 cups vegetable broth

2 tablespoons extra-virgin olive oil, plus more for brushing

½ teaspoon dried oregano leaves

2 cups corn grits or polenta

For the white sauce:
(Makes about ½ cup)

2 cloves garlic, peeled

½ cup raw cashews, preferably soaked in water for 1 to 2 hours, then rinsed and drained (see Note)

½ cup water

⅛ teaspoon Himalayan pink salt

For the mushroom topping:

¼ cup extra-virgin olive oil

5 cloves garlic, minced

1 large shallot, finely chopped

1½ cups cremini mushrooms, coarsely chopped

1½ cups maitake mushrooms, coarsely chopped

1½ cups shiitake mushrooms, stemmed and coarsely chopped

Himalayan pink salt

½ teaspoon dried oregano leaves

⅓ cup finely chopped fresh parsley, for garnish

TO MAKE THE POLENTA CRUST:

1. Preheat the oven to 350°F. Line the bottom of a 9½-inch springform pan with parchment paper.

2. In a medium saucepan, bring the vegetable broth to a boil over high heat. Turn the heat down to medium and add the oil and oregano. Whisking continuously, pour in the grits and continue whisking for 5 to 7 minutes, until smooth and thick. Pour the batter into the prepared springform pan, put it in the freezer, and chill for 10 to 15 minutes.

3. Release the springform pan but keep the polenta crust on the base. Transfer the polenta crust to a baking sheet (this will make it easier to remove from the hot oven), brush the top with oil, and bake for 35 to 40 minutes, until lightly browned on top. Meanwhile, make the sauce and topping.

TO MAKE THE WHITE SAUCE: Put all of the ingredients in a blender or food processor and process until smooth and creamy. Set aside.

TO MAKE THE MUSHROOM TOPPING: Heat the oil in a large saucepan over medium heat. Add the garlic and shallot and sauté, stirring constantly, for about 30 seconds. Add the mushrooms and sauté until very soft, 10 to 12 minutes. Season lightly with salt and the oregano. Taste and add more oregano if desired.

TO ASSEMBLE THE PIZZA: Spoon the white sauce onto the top of the baked polenta crust. (Note: You will have some sauce left over. It is delicious on pasta or zoodles!) Top with the mushrooms and sprinkle the parsley on top. Serve warm.

NOTE _____

If you're using a high-powered blender, soaking the cashews is optional, but it does create a creamier texture. If you're using a conventional blender instead of a high-powered one, soaking the cashews is necessary to get the right texture.

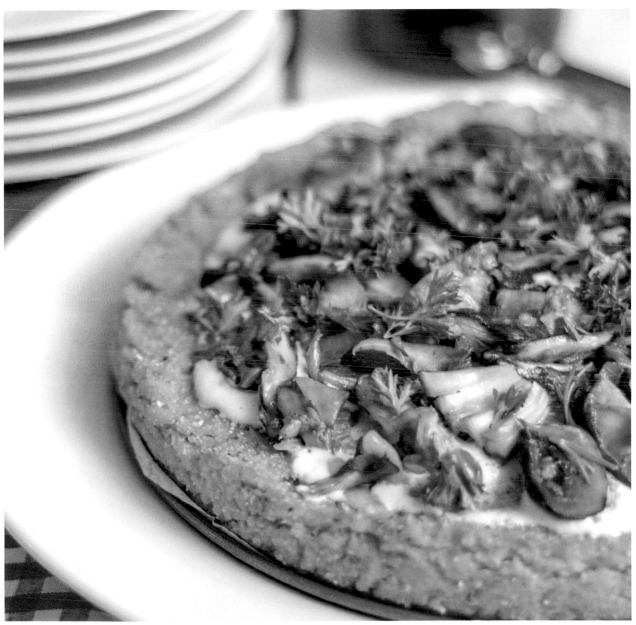

roasted vegetable lasagna

SERVES 10 to 12   PREP TIME: 45 minutes   COOK TIME: 1 hour 10 minutes

If your family is new to Meatless Monday, they might not be all that enthused at first. But I promise nobody will complain about no meat on Monday if you serve this rib-sticking roasted vegetable lasagna! I know the idea of making lasagna can be a bit intimidating if you have never done it, but this really is a super-simple dish to make. And the roasted vegetables give it an incredible depth of flavor. It's an extra step to roast them, but so, so worth it!

2 medium zucchini, cut lengthwise into ¼-inch-thick planks

1 medium eggplant, cut lengthwise into ¼-inch-thick planks

1 medium onion, sliced

1 tablespoon extra-virgin olive oil

½ teaspoon Himalayan pink salt, divided

½ cup pine nuts

1½ cups raw cashews, preferably soaked in water for 1 to 2 hours, then rinsed and drained (see Note)

1 cup water

2 cloves garlic, peeled

1 large egg

3 cups Tomato Sauce with Garlic & Italian Herbs (page 380) or store-bought marinara sauce

9 brown rice lasagna noodles, cooked according to package directions, rinsed with cold water, and drained

1 (14-ounce) package extra-firm tofu, drained, patted dry with paper towels, and sliced lengthwise into ¼-inch strips

SPECIAL TOOLS _____

Mini food processor

1. Preheat the oven to 400°F. Line 2 rimmed baking sheets with parchment paper. Arrange the zucchini, eggplant, and onion on the parchment paper and brush both sides lightly with the olive oil. Season with ¼ teaspoon of the salt. Roast the vegetables for 20 minutes, until tender but not mushy. Remove the vegetables from the oven and set aside to cool. Keep the oven on, but lower the temperature to 375°F.

2. Put the pine nuts in a mini food processor and pulse into crumb-sized pieces. Set aside.

3. In a blender, process the cashews, water, garlic, and egg until smooth and creamy. Set the cashew cream aside.

4. Assemble the lasagna in an ovenproof 9 by 13-inch casserole dish as follows:

    • Spread 1 cup of the tomato sauce on the bottom of the dish.

    • Arrange 3 noodles on top of the sauce.

    • Spread ½ cup of the tomato sauce over the noodles.

    • Arrange half of the roasted vegetables on top of the sauce.

    • Spread half of the cashew cream on top of the vegetables.

    • Arrange all of the tofu on top of the cashew cream.

    • Spread ½ cup of the tomato sauce on top of the tofu.

    • Arrange 3 noodles on top of the sauce.

    • Arrange the remaining roasted vegetables on top of the noodles.

    • Spread the remaining cashew cream on top of the vegetables.

    • Arrange the remaining 3 noodles on top of the cashew cream.

    • Pour the remaining 1 cup of tomato sauce on top of the noodles.

    • Scatter the pine nut crumbs over the top.

STORAGE INFORMATION ——————
Leftovers can be stored in a covered container in the refrigerator for up to 4 days. This lasagna also freezes beautifully for up to 3 weeks.

5. Bake the lasagna, uncovered, for 50 minutes, until the vegetable noodles can easily be pierced with a knife and the sauce is bubbling. Remove from the oven and let rest for at least 15 minutes so that the juices can settle back down. Serve warm.

NOTE ——————————————————————

If you're using a conventional blender instead of a high-powered one, be sure to soak the cashews first to ensure a smooth texture.

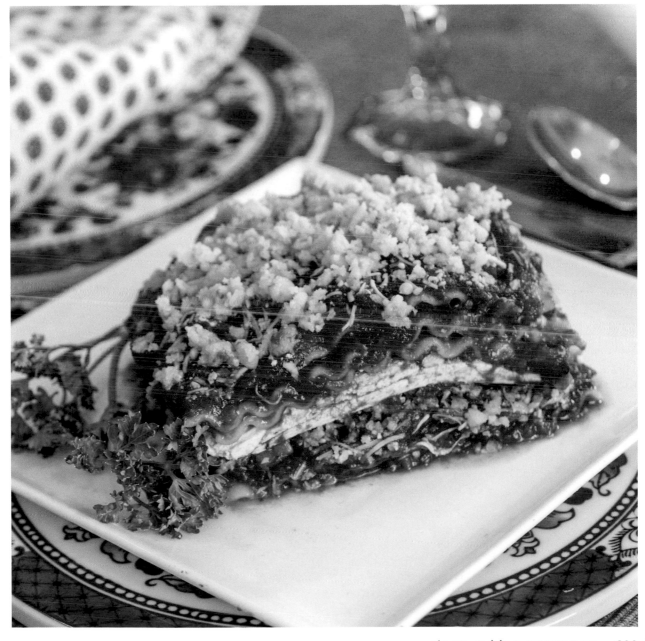

spinach & artichoke quiche

SERVES 6 to 8   PREP TIME: 20 minutes   COOK TIME: 1 hour 15 minutes

I first made this quiche for a sit-down bridal luncheon I hosted for twenty-one lovely ladies in honor of my dear friend Erin Lodeesen. Making quiche after quiche from scratch for twenty-one people is a bit of work, but if you are just serving a family of six, one quiche will do. And making one quiche is not at all difficult, especially if you have the crust made in advance. Add a simple side salad or Classic-Style Caesar Salad (page 158), and it's perfect for Meatless Monday!

---

1 (9-ounce) package frozen artichoke hearts

1 tablespoon plus 1 teaspoon extra-virgin olive oil, divided

¾ teaspoon Himalayan pink salt, divided

½ cup chopped shallots

3 cups baby spinach

2 tablespoons finely chopped parsley

1 prebaked Savory Crust (page 360)

5 large eggs

½ cup raw cashews, preferably soaked in water for 1 to 2 hours, then rinsed and drained (see Note)

½ cup water

1 tablespoon fresh lemon juice

STORAGE INFORMATION ————

Leftover quiche will keep in an airtight container in the refrigerator for 2 days. To reheat, allow the quiche to come to room temperature and then heat in a preheated 250°F oven for about 10 minutes.

1. Preheat the oven to 400°F.

2. Line a rimmed baking sheet with parchment paper. Place the frozen artichoke hearts on the parchment paper, then drizzle with 1 teaspoon of the olive oil and season with ¼ teaspoon of the salt. Roast for 35 to 40 minutes, until soft.

3. While the artichoke hearts are roasting, heat the remaining tablespoon of oil in a large skillet over medium heat. Add the shallots to the pan and sauté for 3 to 4 minutes, until soft. Season with ¼ teaspoon of the salt. Stir in the spinach and sauté until it just begins to wilt, about 30 seconds. Remove the pan from the heat and set aside.

4. Remove the artichoke hearts from the oven, but keep the oven turned on and the temperature at 400°F. Once the artichoke hearts are cool enough to handle, use kitchen shears to cut them into bite-sized pieces. Add the cut artichoke hearts and parsley to the skillet with the shallot-spinach mixture and gently toss the ingredients together. Transfer the vegetable mixture to the prebaked crust and spread it out evenly.

5. Put the eggs, cashews, water, lemon juice, and remaining ¼ teaspoon of salt in a blender. Process on high for at least 1 full minute, until the mixture is smooth and creamy. Pour the cashew-egg mixture over the vegetables.

6. Bake the quiche for 30 to 35 minutes, until the top is ever-so-slightly golden and the eggs are set. Let rest for at least 10 minutes, then slice and serve warm.

NOTE ————

If you're using a conventional blender instead of a high-powered one, be sure to soak the cashews before pureeing them to ensure a smooth texture.

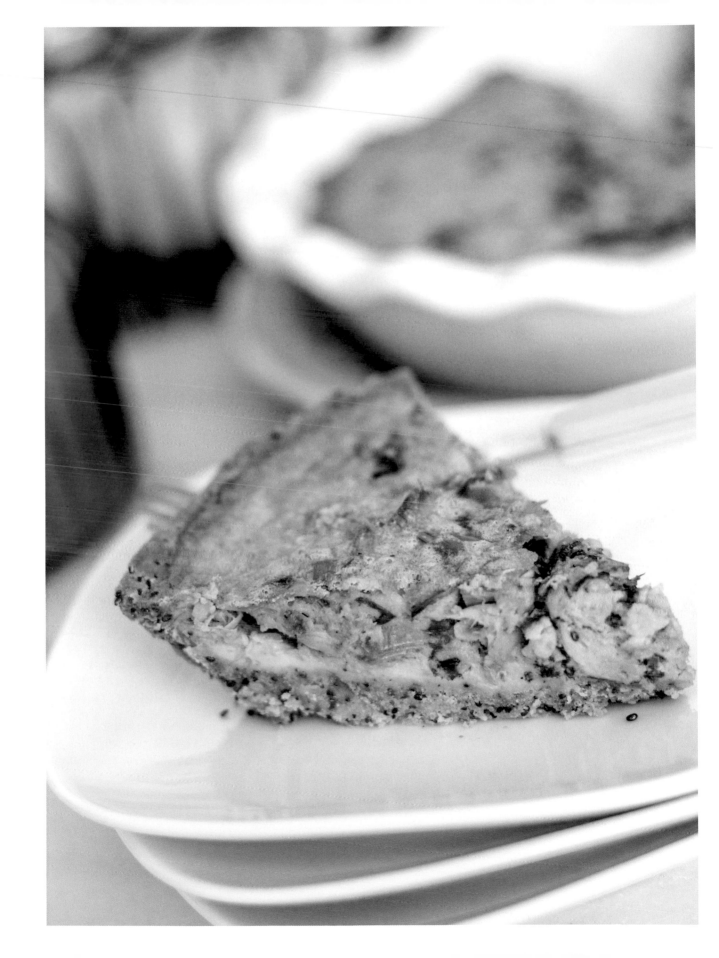

risotto with asparagus
& shiitake mushrooms

SERVES 6   PREP TIME: 20 minutes   COOK TIME: 40 minutes

In the late nineties, an article in the *New York Times* revealed that a serving of restaurant risotto has over 1,200 calories and 100 grams of fat. After reading the article, I decided if I was ever going to eat risotto again, I would have to learn to make it myself. For years, I made my risotto with quinoa (which is delicious!) instead of refined Arborio rice. But now that sprouted short-grain brown rice has become a staple in most natural food stores, I have started using it instead. Not only does sprouting make the nutrients in brown rice easier to absorb, but it dramatically reduces the risotto's cooking time. Best of all, the end result truly rivals the taste and texture of conventional risotto. This dish makes a great Meatless Monday entrée, but I also like to serve it as a side dish at holiday dinners.

1 pound asparagus, trimmed

4½ cups vegetable broth, divided

¼ cup pine nuts (see Notes)

2 tablespoons extra-virgin olive oil

¾ cup chopped onions

1 dozen shiitake mushrooms, stemmed and thinly sliced

3 cloves garlic, chopped

Himalayan pink salt and ground white pepper

1½ cups short-grain brown rice (preferably sprouted; see Notes)

½ cup white wine

NOTES _____

If you are using a conventional blender instead of a high-powered one, soak the pine nuts in water for 30 minutes, then rinse and drain them, before using.

If you cannot find sprouted short-grain brown rice, quick-cooking brown rice is an acceptable alternative.

1. Cut the tips off the asparagus and set aside (do not discard; you'll use them in step 6), then cut the stems into thirds. Place the asparagus stems in a saucepan with ½ cup of the vegetable broth. Bring to a boil over high heat. Turn the heat down to medium, cover, and cook until the asparagus is bright green and soft, about 5 minutes. Transfer the asparagus and cooking liquid to a blender, add the pine nuts, and process until smooth and creamy. Set the asparagus puree aside. Add the remaining 4 cups of vegetable broth to the same saucepan and bring to a boil, then turn the heat down to low and keep at a simmer (you'll use it in step 5).

2. Heat the oil in a large skillet over medium heat. When the oil is hot, add the onions, mushrooms, and garlic. Sauté until the onions are golden, about 10 minutes. Season with a few pinches each of salt and pepper.

3. Add the rice to the skillet and sauté, stirring constantly, for 1 minute.

4. Add the wine, turn the heat down to low, and simmer, stirring constantly and slowly, until the wine has been completely absorbed.

5. Add ½ cup of the hot vegetable broth and simmer, stirring continuously, until all of the liquid is absorbed. Repeat with the remaining hot vegetable broth, adding ½ cup at a time. The entire process should take 15 or 20 minutes.

6. Once all of the broth is added and absorbed into the rice, the rice should be tender but have a firm bite; if the rice is not yet tender, add hot water or hot broth ¼ cup at a time until the rice is soft. Add the reserved asparagus puree and uncooked tips. Stir well, turn the heat up to medium, and cook for about 1 minute. Season with additional salt and pepper to taste. Serve warm.

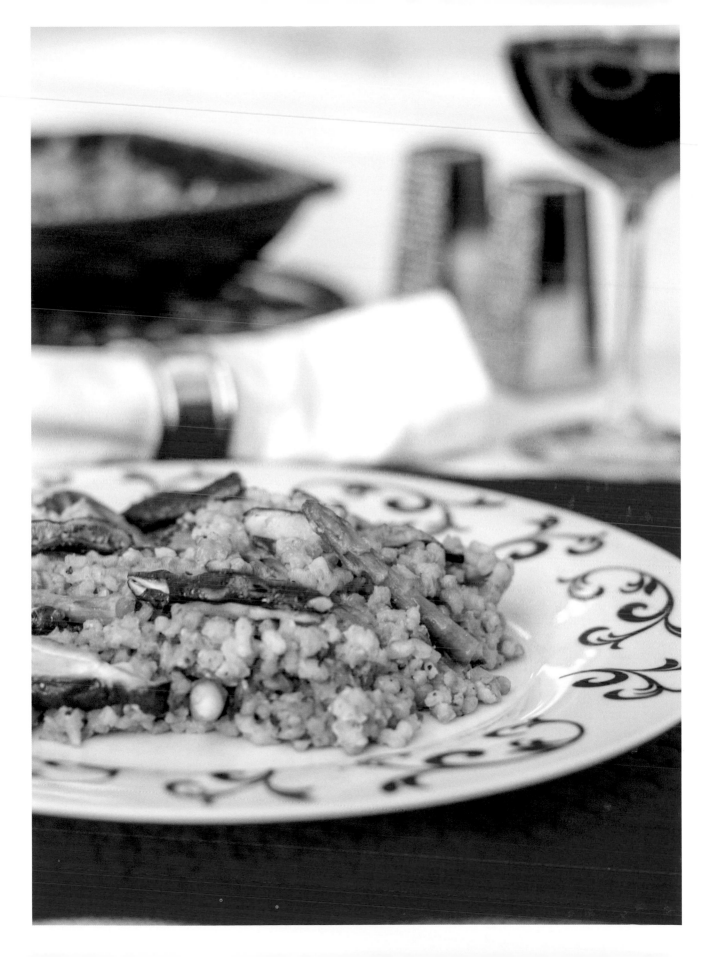

refried black bean tostadas

SERVES 4   PREP TIME: 10 minutes   COOK TIME: 8 minutes

This is one of our family's favorite dinners for Meatless Monday. If you have the refried black beans, tortillas, and sour cream made in advance, you can get this entrée on the table in less than twenty minutes. Serve it with a simple green salad and dinner is done!

8 Tortillas (page 366)

1 recipe Karen's Easy Refried Beans (page 272)

½ cup Clean Cuisine Sour Cream (page 372)

2 Hass avocados, peeled, pitted, and sliced

For garnish (optional):

Crushed red pepper

Halved cherry tomatoes

Chopped fresh cilantro

1. Preheat the oven to 400°F.

2. Lay the tortillas on 2 large rimmed baking sheets. Spread the refried beans on the tortillas in a thin layer. Transfer to the oven and warm for about 8 minutes.

3. Divide the tostadas evenly among 4 plates and top with the sour cream and avocado slices. Garnish with crushed red pepper, halved cherry tomatoes, and chopped cilantro, if desired.

MAKE IT VEGAN

Omit the honey in the sour cream.

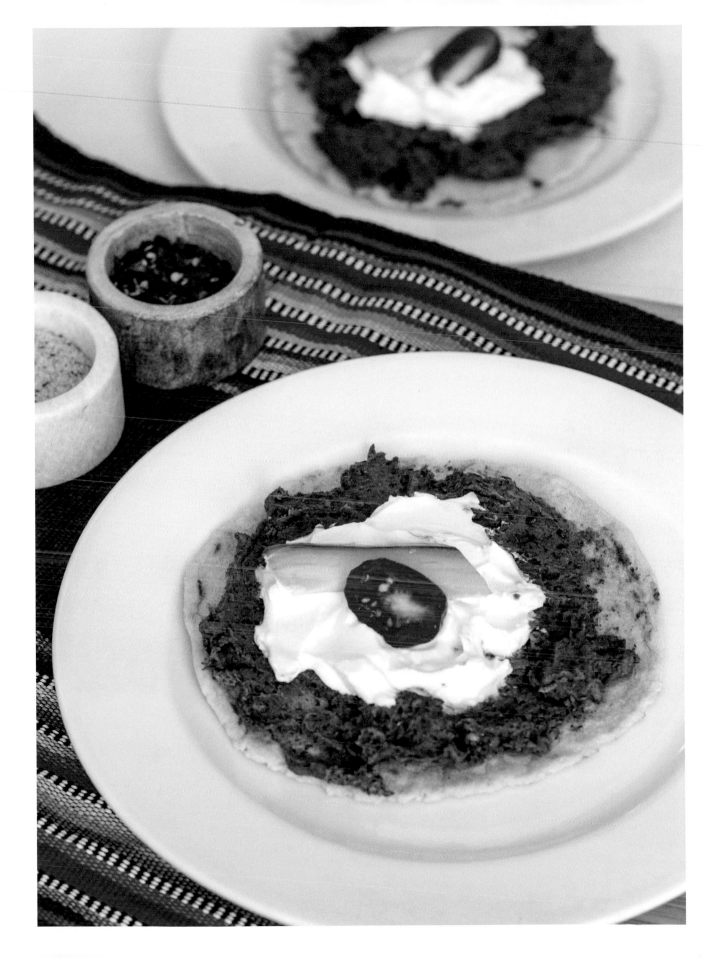

live to 100 vegetable chili

SERVES 6   PREP TIME: 30 minutes   COOK TIME: 1 hour 15 minutes

As far as I am concerned, all chili is good chili. But I know some chili fanatics are not going to like the idea of a vegetable chili, much less one loaded with beans! I grew up eating my mom's chili, which she loaded with beans (and topped with cottage cheese!), so to me, a chili without beans just isn't a real chili. But I also add beans to my chili for their incredible health benefits—residents of the world's Blue Zones, which have the highest concentrations of centenarians in the world, all eat beans as a dietary staple. (See page 36 for more on the amazing health benefits of beans.) So if you want to live to be one hundred, you might want to consider making this chili a weekly staple.

3 tablespoons extra-virgin olive oil

8 cloves garlic, chopped

2 yellow or red bell peppers, chopped

1 large onion, chopped

1 small eggplant, peeled and cut into ½-inch cubes

2 tablespoons chili powder

1 tablespoon dried oregano leaves

1 tablespoon ground cumin

½ teaspoon crushed red pepper

1 teaspoon Himalayan pink salt, divided

1 (26.46-ounce) box chopped tomatoes, with juices, or 1 (28-ounce) can diced tomatoes, with juices (see Note)

1 (15-ounce) can black beans, rinsed and drained

1 (15-ounce) can great northern beans, rinsed and drained

1 (15-ounce) can kidney beans, rinsed and drained

1 (15-ounce) can lentils, rinsed and drained

3 tablespoons fresh lime juice

Toppings (optional):

Chopped fresh cilantro

Sliced or mashed avocado

Clean Cuisine Sour Cream (page 372)

1. Heat the oil in a large saucepan over medium heat. When the oil is hot, add the garlic, peppers, onion, eggplant, spices, and ½ teaspoon of the salt. Cook, stirring occasionally, until the vegetables are golden, about 10 minutes.

2. Add the tomatoes, beans, and lentils. Turn the heat down to low, cover, and simmer, stirring occasionally, for 45 minutes to 1 hour, until the liquid is reduced and the chili is somewhat thickened.

3. Stir in the lime juice and remaining ½ teaspoon of salt and simmer, covered, for an additional 5 minutes. Taste to check for seasoning and add more salt if needed. Serve warm with any desired toppings.

NOTE

Pomi brand BPA-free boxed chopped tomatoes from Italy are particularly delicious in this dish.

MAKE IT VEGAN

Omit the honey in the sour cream.

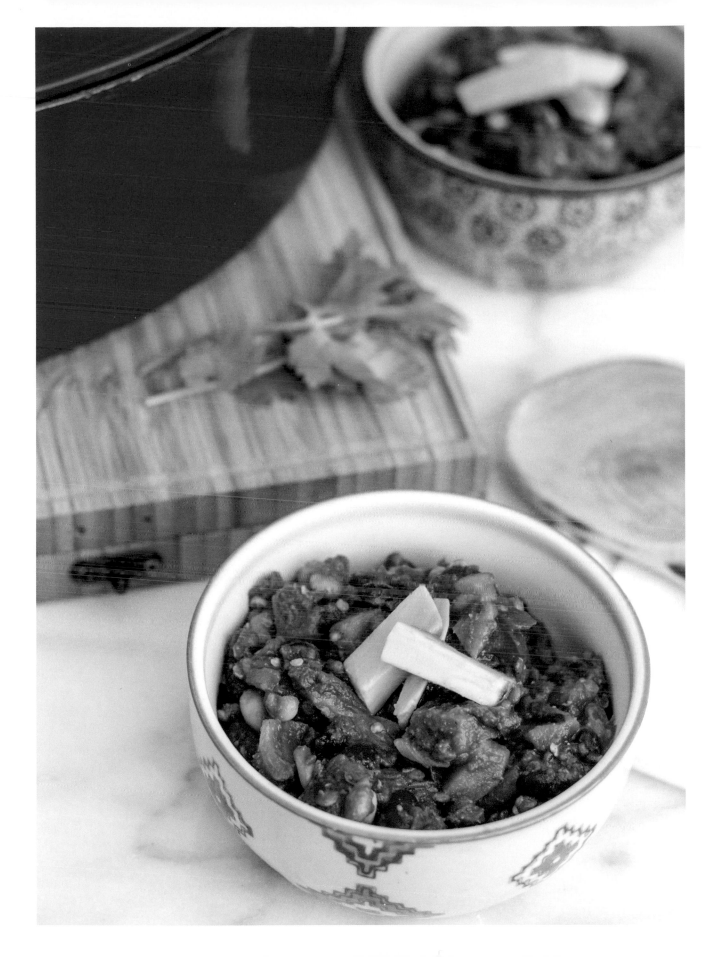

black bean burgers

MAKES 6 burgers   PREP TIME: 20 minutes   COOK TIME: 25 minutes

Over the years I have fiddled around with so many different bean burger recipes, and I'm not going to stretch the truth: not very many would win a cook-off. But this one is different. It's one seriously good burger! I've mixed in sautéed minced veggies, lime-soaked chia seeds, walnut crumbs, and toasted sprouted whole-grain bread for what I believe is the absolute best black bean burger ever—the texture and taste are amazing. Don't forget the ketchup (page 390), mayo (page 392), and mustard! And avocado slices are a great alternative to cheese.

2 tablespoons chia seeds

2 tablespoons fresh lime juice

½ cup raw walnuts

1 slice gluten-free whole-grain bread, toasted

4 cloves garlic, peeled

½ cup coarsely chopped shallots

½ cup peeled and coarsely chopped carrots (about 1 large carrot)

2 tablespoons extra-virgin olive oil, plus more for frying the burgers

2 (15-ounce) cans black beans, rinsed and drained

½ teaspoon Himalayan pink salt

¼ teaspoon ground cumin

For serving (optional):

Gluten-free whole-grain buns

Ketchup, homemade (page 390) or store-bought

Mayonnaise, homemade (page 392) or store-bought

Prepared yellow mustard

Sliced avocados

Sliced red onions

Sliced tomatoes

1. Put the chia seeds and lime juice in a small bowl and soak the chia seeds for at least 5 minutes to allow the seeds to swell.

2. Place the walnuts in a food processor and process into fine crumbs. Remove the walnut crumbs from the food processor and set aside. Place the toasted bread in the food processor and process into fine crumbs. Remove the breadcrumbs from the food processor and set aside.

3. Place the garlic and shallots in the food processor and pulse to finely chop them (be careful not to overprocess—they should be about the size of a pencil eraser). Remove the garlic and shallots from the food processor. Place the carrots in the food processor and pulse to finely chop (again, be careful not to overprocess; they should also be the size of a pencil eraser). Set the carrots aside.

4. Heat the oil in a large skillet over medium heat, then add the garlic and shallots and sauté for 3 to 4 minutes, until soft. Add the carrots and sauté for 3 to 4 minutes, until soft. Transfer the shallots and carrots to a large mixing bowl. Do not wash the pan.

5. Add the beans to the bowl with the sautéed vegetables. Use a potato masher to mash the beans with the vegetables (you can also use your clean hands). Add the lime-soaked chia seeds, walnut crumbs, breadcrumbs, salt, and cumin. Use your hands to mix the ingredients together. Spoon out ½ cup of the mixture and form it into a patty with your hands. Repeat with the remaining mixture; you should have 6 patties.

6. Lightly rub the same skillet with oil and heat over medium heat. Working in batches, fry the patties for 3 to 4 minutes per side, until a very thin crust appears and the burgers are warm. As you finish a batch, transfer the burgers to a paper towel or place in a preheated 200°F oven to keep warm. Serve warm with desired toppings.

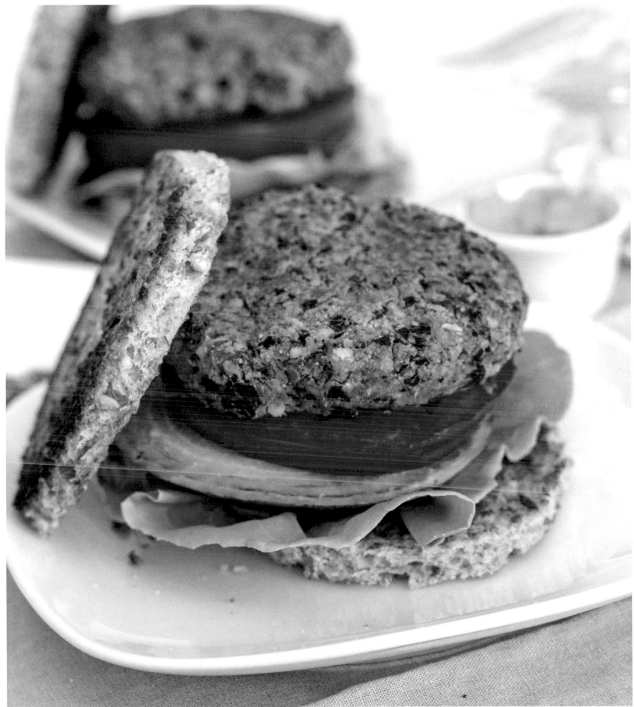

the legienza veggie burger

MAKES 6 burgers   PREP TIME: 20 minutes   COOK TIME: 50 minutes

Andy's cousin Tom Legienza and his wife, Kim, gave me the idea for this recipe when we were all out celebrating my mother-in-law's birthday one night. I made the comment that I never eat veggie burgers when I'm eating out because I have no idea what's in them. Kim then chimed in that she had the best-ever veggie burger recipe that I just had to make! And here it is, with just a few modifications to make it gluten-free.

2 medium sweet potatoes, halved lengthwise

3 tablespoons extra-virgin olive oil, divided, plus more for frying the burgers

½ cup raw walnut halves

½ cup finely chopped onions

3 cloves garlic, crushed to a paste

1 (15-ounce) can chickpeas, rinsed and drained

1 large egg, whisked

1½ teaspoons Himalayan pink salt

1 teaspoon garlic powder

1 teaspoon ground cumin

½ teaspoon chili powder

⅓ cup masa harina corn flour, plus up to 3 tablespoons more if needed

For serving (optional):

Gluten-free whole-grain buns

Mayonnaise, homemade (page 392) or store-bought

Pea sprouts or other sprouts

Sliced avocados

Sliced red onions

1. Preheat the oven to 400°F. Line a rimmed baking sheet with foil. Rub the cut sides of the sweet potatoes with 1 tablespoon of the olive oil and place cut side down on the baking sheet. Bake until soft and tender to the touch, about 30 minutes (the exact time depends on the size of the sweet potatoes). Once they're cooled, scoop out the sweet potato flesh, place it in a large mixing bowl, and mash with a potato masher. Set aside.

2. Place the walnuts in a food processor and process into fine crumbs. Set aside.

3. Heat the remaining 2 tablespoons of oil in a large skillet over medium heat. Add the onions and garlic and sauté until the onions are very soft, about 4 minutes. Transfer the cooked onions and garlic to the bowl with the mashed sweet potatoes.

4. To the bowl with the onions and sweet potatoes, add the chickpeas, walnut crumbs, and egg. Use a potato masher to mash the chickpeas and thoroughly mix all of the ingredients together. Mix in the salt, garlic powder, ground cumin, and chili powder. Mix in the masa harina. If the mixture doesn't easily stick together, add up to 3 tablespoons more masa harina, a tablespoon at a time, until the ingredients stick together.

5. Divide the mixture into 6 equal-sized portions. Using your hands, gently form each portion into a patty.

6. Lightly oil the bottom of the same skillet and heat over medium heat. Working in batches, cook the burgers for about 4 minutes per side, until lightly browned. Serve warm with buns and desired toppings.

These burgers freeze beautifully. To freeze, cook the burgers as directed, allow them to cool, and then place ½ inch apart on a tray or rimmed baking sheet and place in the freezer. Once they've had a chance to partially freeze, you can pile them in baggies or an airtight container to save for a future clean fast-food dinner! To reheat, microwave each thawed burger on high for about 1½ minutes.

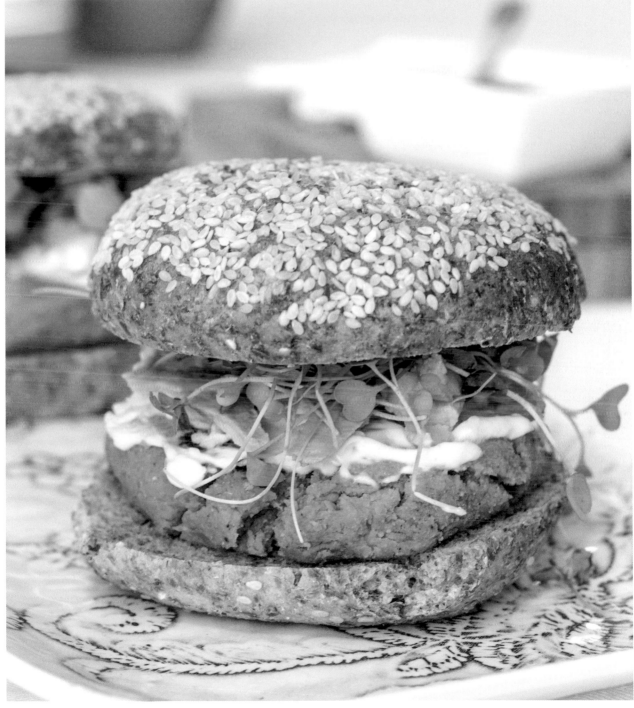

sweet potato & chickpea curry

SERVES 6 PREP TIME: 25 minutes COOK TIME: 30 minutes

This full-bodied, rib-sticking vegetarian curry is so rich and satisfying that nobody ever complains about the lack of meat. The ingredients list might look a little long, but don't let that intimidate you. This is one incredibly quick and easy dish! I frequently make it in the winter and serve it either straight up or over sautéed spinach or steamed sprouted short-grain brown rice (or both).

3 tablespoons extra-virgin coconut oil

5 cloves garlic, chopped

3 stalks celery, chopped

1 jalapeño pepper, seeded and finely chopped

1 large onion, chopped

1 red bell pepper, chopped

2 tablespoons grated fresh ginger

2 tablespoons curry powder

Himalayan pink salt and ground black pepper

2 large sweet potatoes, peeled and cut into ½-inch cubes

1 (15-ounce) can chickpeas, rinsed and drained

1 (13.5-ounce) can full-fat coconut milk

1 cup vegetable broth

1 (14.5-ounce) can diced tomatoes, drained

1 cup frozen petite green peas, thawed

Juice of 1 lime

1. In a large saucepan, heat the oil over medium-low heat. Add the garlic, celery, jalapeño, onion, bell pepper, and ginger. Cook, stirring occasionally, until the onion is translucent and the vegetables are soft, 5 to 6 minutes. Stir in the curry powder and cook, stirring constantly, until fragrant, about 30 seconds. Add a few pinches each of salt and pepper.

2. To the pan, add the sweet potatoes, chickpeas, coconut milk, and vegetable broth. Raise the heat to medium-high and bring just to a boil, then turn the heat down to low and simmer, uncovered, until the sweet potatoes are tender, 10 to 15 minutes.

3. Add the tomatoes and peas and cook for 3 to 4 minutes to soften the peas. Stir in the lime juice.

4. Remove the saucepan from the heat and let the curry sit for 15 to 20 minutes to allow the flavors to deepen. Season with additional salt and pepper to taste. Serve warm.

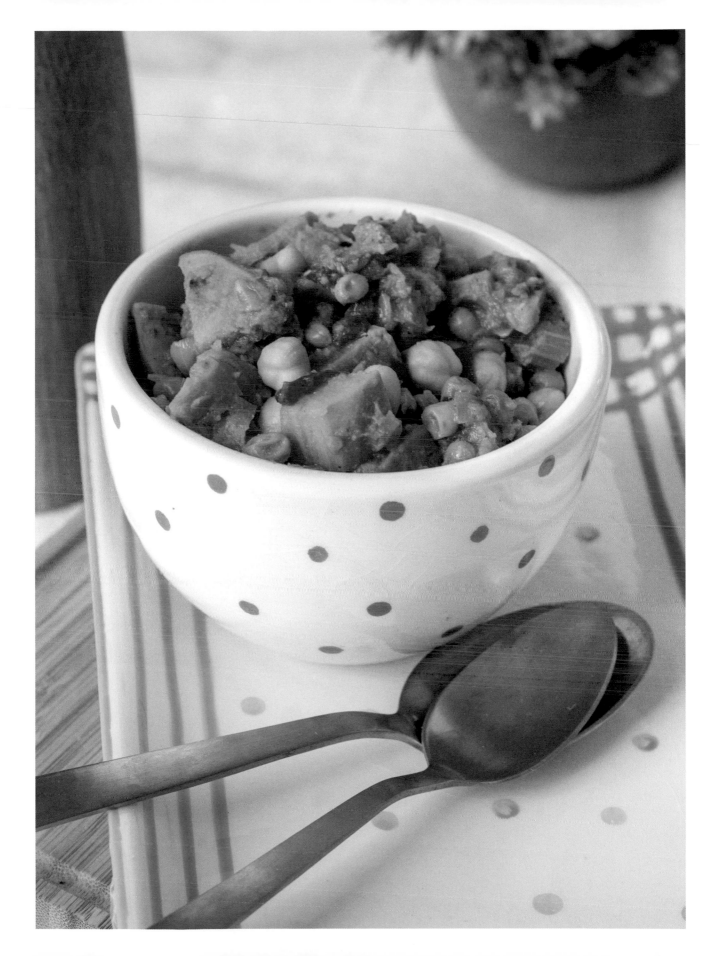

easy pad thai

SERVES 4   PREP TIME: 20 minutes   COOK TIME: 5 minutes

Faster than any takeout (yes, really!), this easy recipe is sure to become one of your absolute favorite weeknight dinners. It's made with a mildly sweet, savory, teensy bit salty, umami-flavored cashew cream and loads of veggie noodles. It's rich enough that you won't miss the meat!

For the sauce:

¾ cup raw cashews, preferably soaked in water for 1 to 2 hours, then rinsed and drained (see Note)

2 cloves garlic, chopped

½ cup water

2 tablespoons fresh lime juice

2 tablespoons raw honey

1½ tablespoons fish sauce

1 tablespoon gluten-free tamari (or unpasteurized soy sauce, if not gluten-free)

1 tablespoon Sriracha sauce

1 tablespoon unrefined toasted sesame oil

2 teaspoons grated fresh ginger

For the noodles and vegetables:

1 (8-ounce) package gluten-free brown rice noodles

3 cups zucchini noodles (about 1 large zucchini)

2 cups peeled and shredded carrots (about 4 large carrots)

1 cup bean sprouts

½ cup chopped fresh cilantro

2 scallions, sliced, for garnish (optional)

Crushed red pepper, for garnish (optional)

TO MAKE THE SAUCE: Put all the sauce ingredients in a blender or food processor. Process on high for about 1 full minute, until the ingredients are well blended and the sauce is smooth and creamy. It should be about the consistency of a thin yogurt. If you'd like it to be thinner, add more water, 2 tablespoons at a time. Set aside.

TO MAKE THE VEGETABLES AND NOODLES:

1. Bring a large pot of salted water to a boil. Add the rice noodles and simmer for 1 minute. Add the zucchini noodles, carrots, and bean sprouts and cook for 2 to 3 minutes, until the vegetables are soft but not mushy. Drain the noodles and vegetables and immediately transfer to a large skillet.

2. Add the sauce to the skillet and cook over medium heat for 1 to 2 minutes, until heated through, tossing until the noodles and vegetables are coated in the sauce. Turn off the heat and stir in the cilantro. Transfer to a serving plate and sprinkle on the scallions and crushed red pepper, if desired. Serve at once.

NOTE _____

If you're using a conventional blender rather than a high-powered one or a food processor, be sure to soak the cashews before pureeing them to ensure a smooth texture.

MAKE IT VEGETARIAN _____

Omit the fish sauce.

MAKE IT VEGAN _____

Omit the fish sauce and honey.

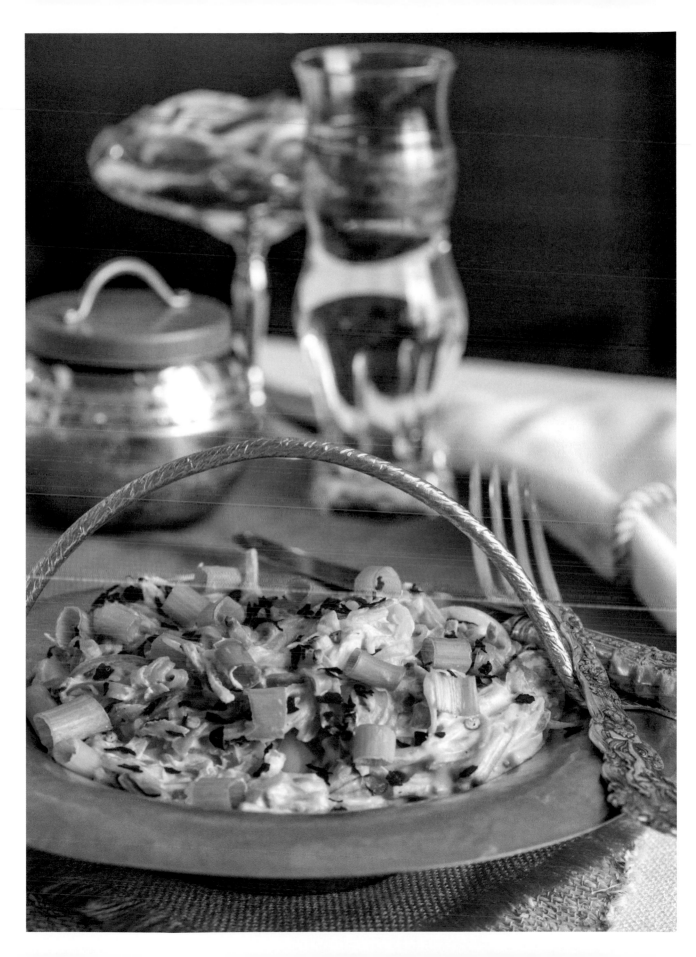

pasta alla vodka

SERVES 4 to 6   PREP TIME: 25 minutes   COOK TIME: 25 minutes

Until I cleaned up my diet, pasta alla vodka was one of my favorite dishes to order when dining out. Of course, I know now that conventional recipes are full of heavy cream and butter. Let's just say that pasta alla vodka is no longer on my list of most frequently ordered restaurant items! Luckily this clean version is super easy to make at home, and honestly, it's every bit as rich, decadent, and delicious as the conventional one. We mostly eat it for Meatless Monday, but it also makes a great dish for guests, especially when topped with pan-seared jumbo shrimp.

---

1 (35-ounce) can peeled San Marzano tomatoes (see Notes)

¼ cup extra-virgin olive oil

3 cloves garlic, sliced very, very thin

½ cup finely chopped onions

2 tablespoons tomato paste

½ teaspoon Himalayan pink salt

10 ounces gluten-free whole-grain penne pasta

¾ cup raw cashews, preferably soaked in water for 1 to 2 hours, then rinsed and drained (see Notes)

½ cup water

2 tablespoons gluten-free vodka

1 teaspoon coconut sugar

½ teaspoon crushed red pepper

Chopped fresh basil, for garnish

1. Put the tomatoes in a blender and process until smooth and creamy. Remove from the blender and set aside. Rinse out the blender jar.

2. Bring a large pot of salted water to a boil.

3. Meanwhile, heat the oil in a large saucepan over medium heat. Add the garlic and onions and sauté for 6 to 7 minutes, until the onions are soft. Stir in the tomato paste and season with the salt. Turn the heat down to low, add the pureed tomatoes, and simmer, stirring frequently, for 5 minutes.

4. Add the penne to the boiling water and cook according to package directions. Drain (but do not rinse!) and set aside.

5. In the blender, process the cashews, water, vodka, and coconut sugar on high speed until the mixture is smooth and creamy. Pour the vodka-cashew cream into the pan with the tomato sauce. Stir to combine and simmer, stirring occasionally, for 10 minutes. Add the crushed red pepper and season with additional salt to taste.

6. Add the cooked pasta to the sauce and toss to coat. Cook over low heat for 2 to 3 minutes. Transfer to a serving platter, garnish with fresh basil, and serve warm.

MAKE IT GRAIN-FREE _____

Use a chickpea (aka garbanzo bean) pasta.

NOTES _____

Using San Marzano tomatoes is very important for this recipe. San Marzanos are the most famous plum tomato to come out of Italy and are considered by many cooks to be the best tomatoes to use in a sauce. They have a mild, sweet flavor and low acidity. I personally prefer Cento brand organic San Marzano tomatoes. It is not easy to find the organic Cento variety at the supermarket, but if you use them as much as I do, then it's worth ordering them online.

If you're using a conventional blender instead of a high-powered one, be sure to soak the cashews before pureeing them to ensure a smooth texture.

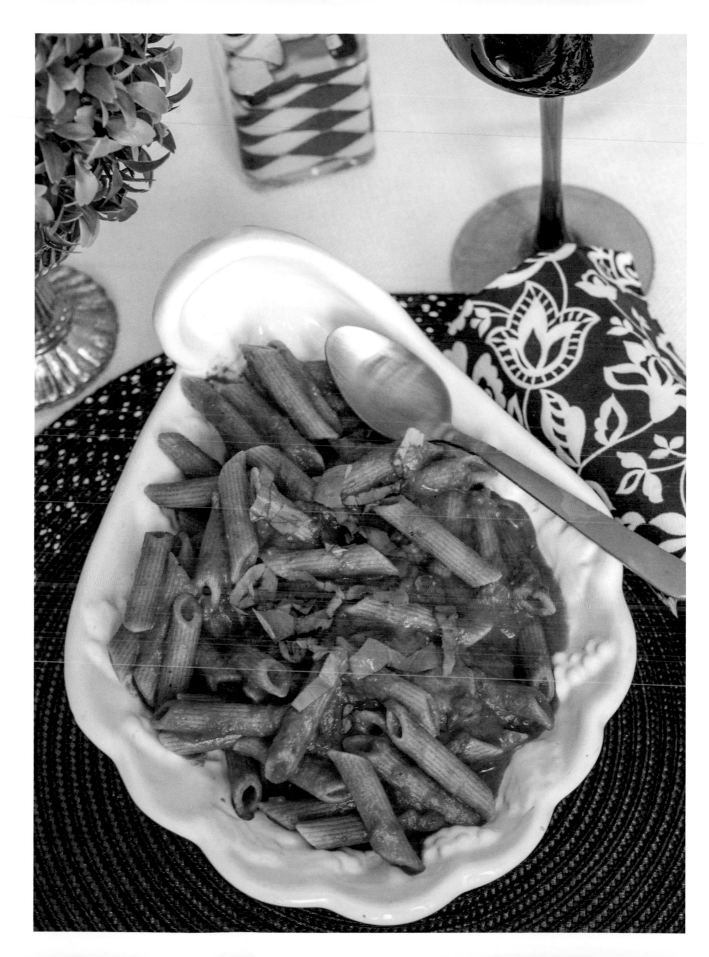

personal-size white pizzas with garlic & mushrooms

SERVES 4   PREP TIME: 20 minutes
COOK TIME: 20 to 28 minutes, depending on style of crust

This variation of Polenta Pizza with White Sauce & Mushrooms (page 230) uses a more traditional crust and richer, cheesy-tasting Alfredo sauce instead of a mild white sauce. I first got the idea for making a pizza with Alfredo sauce, garlic, and mushrooms from one of our family's favorite local plant-based restaurants, Christopher's Kitchen. Whenever we eat there, nine times out of ten one of us will order the white pizza. I realize the idea of a no-cheese pizza might not sound all that fun, but with the creamy Alfredo sauce, nobody will miss the cheese. And because this recipe uses Super-Easy Mini Pizza Crusts (page 364), you can make them with thick or thin crusts, and everyone gets their own decadent pizza pie!

---

4 formed (but unbaked) Super-Easy Mini Pizza Crusts (page 364)

3 tablespoons extra-virgin olive oil, plus more for the baking sheet

⅓ cup finely chopped shallots

2¼ cups stemmed and sliced shiitake mushrooms

2 teaspoons finely chopped garlic

½ teaspoon Himalayan pink salt

¼ teaspoon ground white pepper

1 cup Alfredo Sauce (page 382)

1 tablespoon fresh thyme leaves

1. Place an oven rack in the top position and preheat the oven to 475°F. Generously oil 2 baking sheets (or 4 personal-size pizza stones) and place the uncooked pizza crusts on them. Set aside.

2. Heat the oil in a large skillet over medium heat. Add the shallots and cook for 3 to 4 minutes, until soft. Add the mushrooms and cook for 3 to 4 minutes, until the mushrooms soften. Stir in the garlic, season with the salt and white pepper, and cook for 30 to 45 seconds, until the garlic softens just a bit.

3. Spoon ¼ cup of the Alfredo sauce on each pizza crust and spread it evenly over the top. Divide the mushroom topping evenly among the pizzas.

4. Place both baking sheets on the top rack of the oven. For thick-crust pizzas: Cook for 18 to 20 minutes, until the crust is crispy on the outside and soft on the inside. For thin-crust pizzas: Cook for 14 to 16 minutes, until the crust is crispy.

5. Remove the pizzas from the oven and scatter the fresh thyme over the tops. Let the pizzas rest for 5 minutes before serving. Serve warm.

NOTE

The photo of this pizza shows the thick-crust version of the mini pizza crusts.

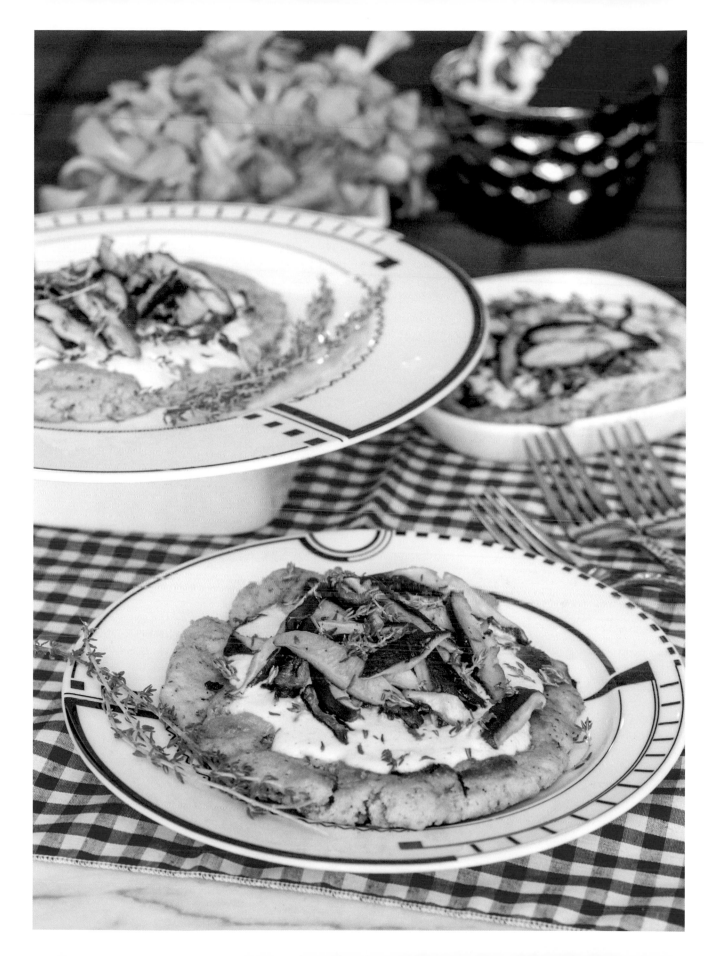

roman pizza

SERVES 4   PREP TIME: 20 minutes
COOK TIME: 25 to 30 minutes, depending on style of crust

On a family trip to Rome, we had a thin-crust pizza that was piled high with onions, peppers, and garlic and sprinkled with just a little bit of Parmesan cheese. It was much lighter than the veggie-scarce, cheese-rich pizzas we are accustomed to here in the States. It also had considerably more flavor. This dairy-free, grain-free version is very similar—believe it or not, you don't need Parmesan to make an authentic-tasting Italian-style pizza! The nut "cheese" used here lets you go dairy-free without feeling deprived. You can make this pizza with thin or thick crusts, but if you want to make a truly Roman-style pizza, go thin (as shown in the photo).

---

4 formed (but unbaked) Super-Easy Mini Pizza Crusts (page 364)

3 tablespoons extra-virgin olive oil

2 red bell peppers, thinly sliced

1½ medium onions, thinly sliced

5 cloves garlic, thinly sliced

¼ teaspoon Himalayan pink salt

1 cup Tomato Sauce with Garlic & Italian Herbs (page 380) or store-bought marinara sauce

1 cup Parmesan Nut "Cheese" (page 370)

1 teaspoon dried oregano leaves

½ teaspoon crushed red pepper

½ cup chopped fresh basil, for garnish

1. Place an oven rack in the top position and preheat the oven to 475°F. Generously oil the bottom of 2 baking sheets (or 4 personal-size pizza stones) and place the uncooked pizza crusts on them. Set aside.

2. Heat the oil in a large skillet over medium heat. Add the peppers and onions and sauté for 8 to 10 minutes, until the vegetables are soft. Add the garlic and salt and sauté for 1 minute, until the garlic softens just a bit.

3. Spoon ¼ cup of tomato sauce on each pizza crust and spread it evenly over the tops. Divide the peppers-and-onions mixture among the pizzas. Scatter the nut cheese, oregano, and crushed red pepper over the tops of the pizzas. Add more crushed red pepper to taste.

4. Place both baking sheets on the top rack of the oven. For thick-crust pizzas: Cook for 18 to 20 minutes, until the crusts are crispy on the outside and soft on the inside. For thin-crust pizzas: Cook for 14 to 16 minutes, until the crusts are crispy.

5. Remove the pizzas from the oven and scatter the fresh basil on them. Let the pizzas rest for 5 minutes before serving. Serve warm.

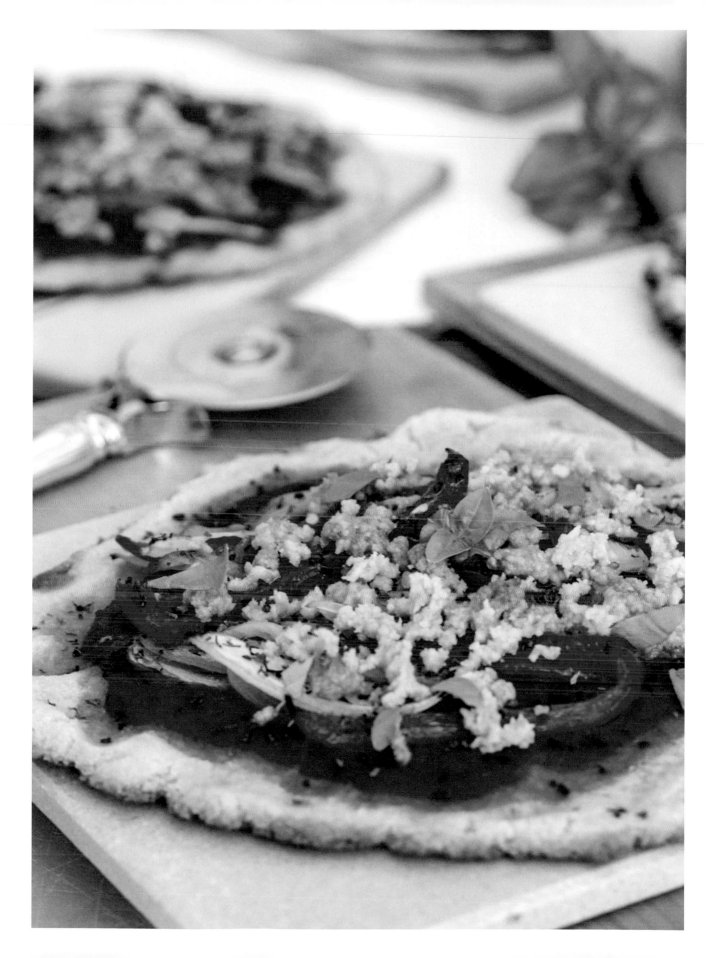

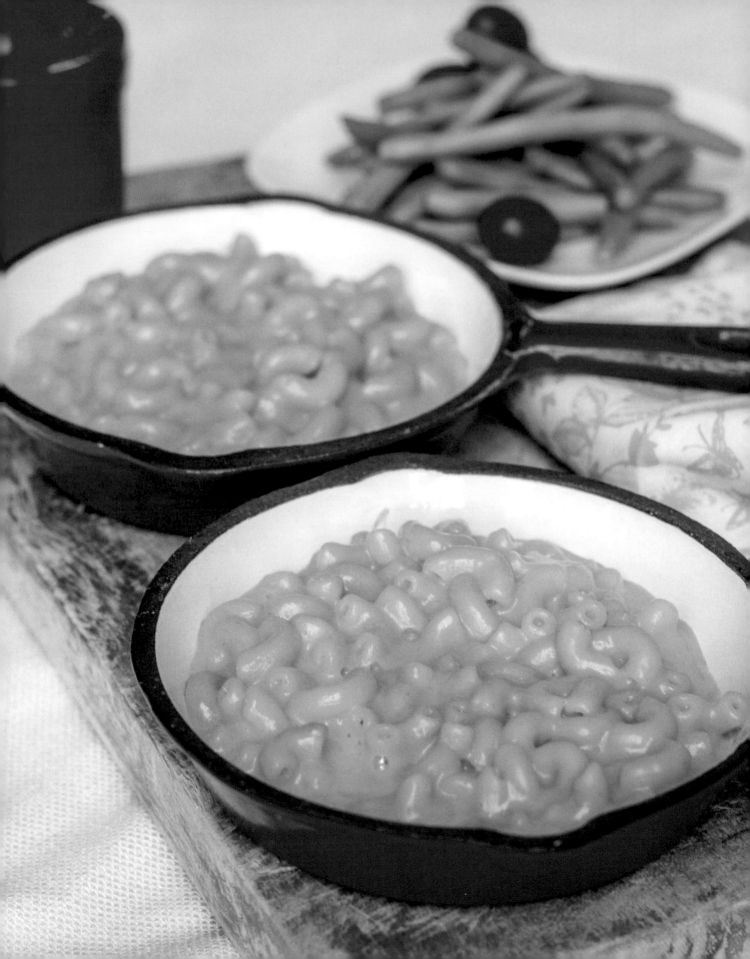

CHAPTER 14

simple sides

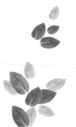

baked beans

SERVES 6 to 8   PREP TIME: 20 minutes   COOK TIME: 1 hour 35 minutes

If you are headed to a cookout of any type, you can't go wrong with baked beans! This dish also makes a delicious side for weeknight dinners. One of my favorite summertime suppers is grilled corn on the cob, turkey burgers, a simple green salad, and a big side serving of these baked beans. By the way, swirling ketchup into these baked beans at the very end tastes amazing (or at least I think so!).

2 tablespoons extra-virgin olive oil

2 cups chopped onions

5 cloves garlic, minced

¾ teaspoon Himalayan pink salt, divided

3 (15-ounce) cans navy beans, rinsed and drained

13 Deglet Noor dates, pitted (see Note)

1½ cups water

1¼ cups canned unflavored tomato sauce

¼ cup raw apple cider vinegar

2 tablespoons pure maple syrup

2 teaspoons dry mustard

2 teaspoons gluten-free Worcestershire sauce

1 teaspoon hot sauce, such as Tabasco

Sliced scallions, for garnish (optional)

1. Preheat the oven to 325°F.

2. Heat the oil in a large saucepan over medium heat. Add the onions and cook for 5 minutes, or until they start to soften. Add the garlic and ½ teaspoon of the salt and cook for 1 minute more.

3. Transfer the onion mixture to an ovenproof 8-inch square casserole dish. Stir in the beans and set the casserole dish aside.

4. In a blender, blend the dates, water, tomato sauce, apple cider vinegar, maple syrup, dry mustard, Worcestershire sauce, hot sauce, and remaining ¼ teaspoon of salt on high speed until the mixture is smooth.

5. Pour the sauce into the bean mixture and gently stir to combine. Cover and bake for 1½ hours, until thickened. Serve warm and garnished with sliced scallions, if desired.

NOTE

If you're using a conventional blender rather than a high-powered one, soak the dates in water for 15 to 30 minutes to soften them before pureeing.

MAKE IT VEGAN AND VEGETARIAN

Use a vegan Worcestershire sauce.

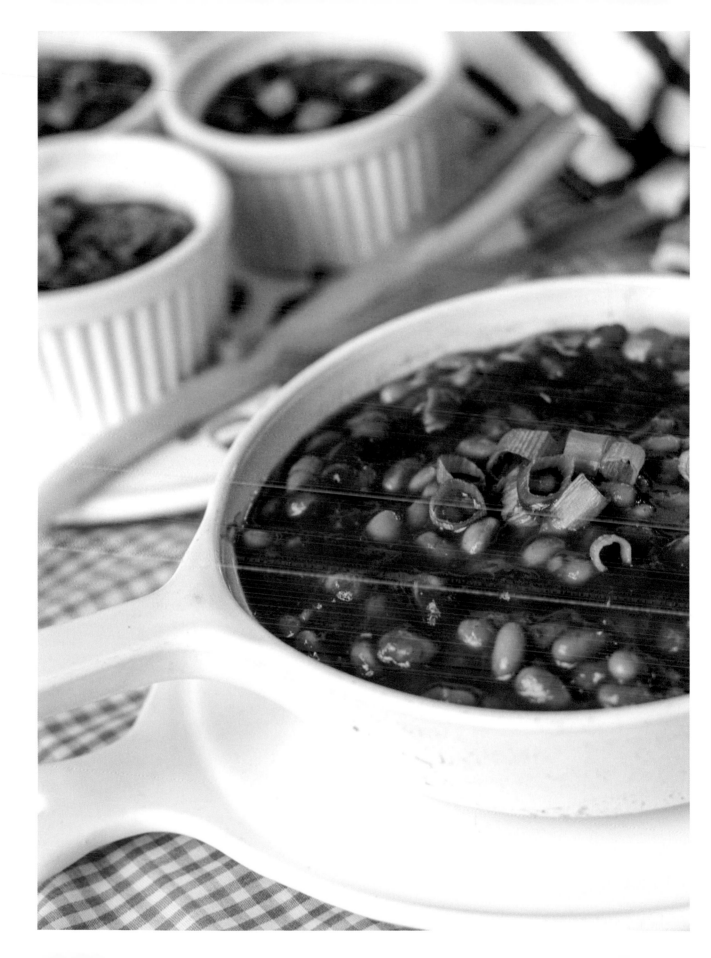

chinese-style cauliflower fried rice

SERVES 4 to 6   PREP TIME: 25 minutes   COOK TIME: 20 minutes

This dish was inspired by the many dinner parties my mom hosted when I was growing up. Fried rice was frequently on her menus. This fried rice has all of the main ingredients that Mom used in her dinner-party recipe—I've just substituted riced cauliflower for the white rice. When it's time for the taste test you won't believe it's cauliflower. You will seriously think you are eating stir-fried rice! By the way, it's not that I have anything at all against brown rice or whole grains; it's just that I am always looking for creative ways to eat more vegetables.

1 tablespoon plus 1 teaspoon extra-virgin olive oil or unrefined avocado oil, divided

2 large eggs, whisked

2 stalks celery, diced

1 medium carrot, peeled and diced

1 red bell pepper, diced

¼ cup finely chopped shallots

6 cloves garlic, minced

1 teaspoon grated fresh ginger

2 tablespoons gluten-free tamari (or unpasteurized soy sauce, if not gluten-free), plus more to taste

2 tablespoons Sriracha sauce, plus more to taste

1 medium head cauliflower (about 1½ pounds), riced (see right)

1 tablespoon unrefined toasted sesame oil

1 cup frozen petite green peas, thawed

½ cup chopped scallions

1. Heat 1 teaspoon of the oil in a large skillet or wok over medium-high heat. Add the eggs and cook until scrambled. Transfer the scrambled eggs to a plate and set aside.

2. Heat the remaining tablespoon of oil in the skillet over medium-high heat. Add the celery, carrot, bell pepper, shallots, garlic, and ginger and sauté for 5 to 6 minutes, until the vegetables are soft. Add the tamari and Sriracha sauce and cook until the liquid evaporates, about 2 minutes.

3. Add the riced cauliflower and sesame oil to the skillet. Cook, stirring constantly, for 4 to 5 minutes, until the cauliflower is soft. Season with more Sriracha or tamari if desired.

4. Stir in the scrambled eggs, peas, and scallions and cook until heated through. Serve warm.

HOW TO RICE CAULIFLOWER _____

Pull the leaves off a head of cauliflower and slice it in half lengthwise, through the stem. Break the cauliflower into large florets, rinse them well, and use a paper towel to pat them as dry as possible. Break the florets into smaller pieces, then put half of them in the bowl of a large food processor and pulse until finely chopped into pieces the size of grains of rice. Transfer the riced cauliflower to a bowl. Repeat the process with the remaining cauliflower. If you don't have a food processor, using the large shredding holes on a box grater works well too. One medium head of cauliflower should give you about 3½ cups of riced cauliflower.

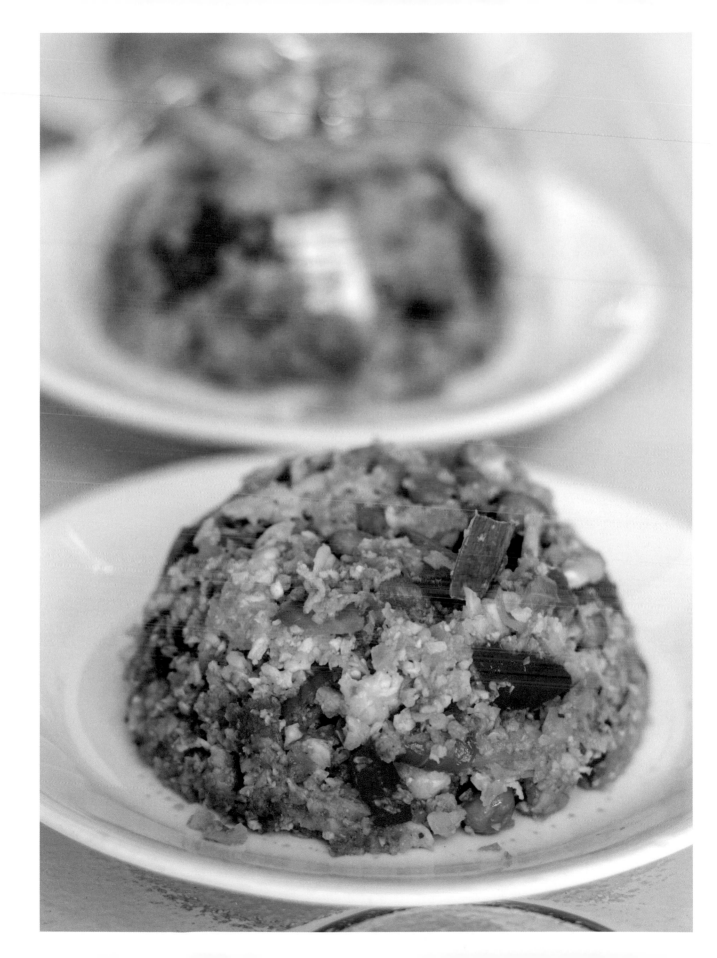

wild rice pilaf

SERVES 6 to 8   PREP TIME: 20 minutes   COOK TIME: 1 hour 20 minutes

This is one dish that frequently lands on our holiday table. Its distinctive nutty flavor, chewy texture, and purplish hue pair well with chicken, beef, and lamb dishes. Nutritionally, wild rice is as robust as the flavors it imparts: it contains almost twice the protein and fiber of brown rice and is also high in B vitamins, manganese, zinc, potassium, phosphorus, and magnesium. (By the way, wild rice is not a grain but the seed of a native North American marsh grass.) If you prefer a subtler flavor, include the (thawed) frozen corn. You can also try adding some cooked long-grain brown rice; simply stir it in after the wild rice has been cooked.

1 cup raw pecans, finely chopped

4 tablespoons extra-virgin olive oil, divided

½ teaspoon Himalayan pink salt, divided

½ cup diced celery

½ cup finely chopped shallots

½ cup peeled and diced carrots

4 cloves garlic, minced

1¼ cups wild rice

3½ cups vegetable broth

1 tablespoon fresh lemon juice

1 tablespoon fresh thyme leaves

1½ cups frozen corn, thawed (optional)

1. Preheat the oven to 375°F and line a rimmed baking sheet with parchment paper.

2. Transfer the chopped nuts to the parchment paper–lined baking sheet. Drizzle 1 tablespoon of the oil over them and sprinkle on ¼ teaspoon of the salt. Toss to coat and roast for 10 minutes, until fragrant. Remove the nuts from the oven and set aside.

3. Heat the remaining 3 tablespoons of oil in a large ovenproof casserole dish over medium heat. Add the celery, shallots, and carrots and sauté for 5 to 6 minutes, until the vegetables are soft. Add the garlic and sauté for 1 more minute, until softened slightly. Add the rice, toss to coat it in the oil and combine it with the vegetable mixture, and cook for 2 to 3 minutes, until heated through.

4. Stir in the broth and remaining ¼ teaspoon of salt and bring the broth to a boil. Stir in the lemon juice, cover, and transfer the casserole dish to the oven.

5. Bake for 50 to 55 minutes, until the liquid evaporates. Stir in the thyme, toasted nuts, and corn (if using). Serve warm.

MAKE IT GRAIN-FREE AND PALEO-FRIENDLY _____
Omit the corn.

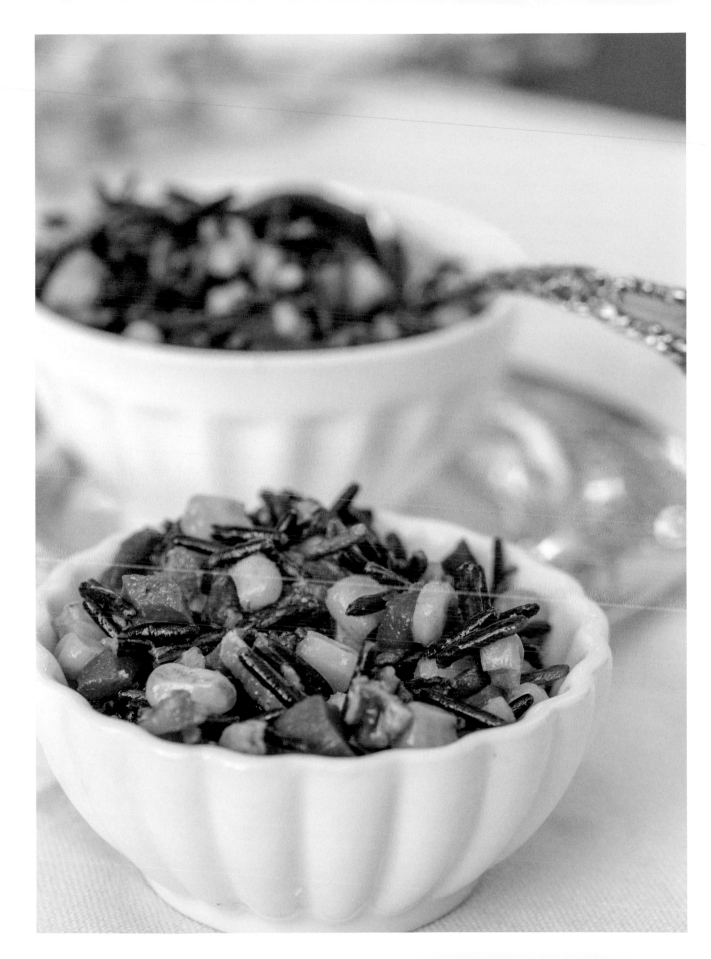

thanksgiving day green bean casserole

SERVES 6 to 8   PREP TIME: 25 minutes   COOK TIME: 30 minutes

I originally came up with this clean green bean casserole recipe for the Thanksgiving feature article of *Natural Health* magazine a few years back. I was asked to develop recipes for a whole-foods Thanksgiving feast using ten of Dr. Oz's favorite superfoods. The superfoods in this dish are pumpkin seeds and shiitake mushrooms. Although green bean casserole is often made just once a year, around the holiday season, there is no reason not to enjoy it all year long (in fact, green beans are in season half the year, summer through mid-fall).

1 tablespoon plus ¾ teaspoon Himalayan pink salt, divided

⅓ cup raw cashews, preferably soaked in water for 1 to 2 hours, then rinsed and drained (see Notes)

1 cup water

1½ pounds green beans, trimmed and broken into bite-sized pieces

2 tablespoons plus 1 teaspoon extra-virgin olive oil, divided

½ cup chopped shallots

1 tablespoon minced garlic

7 ounces shiitake mushrooms, stemmed and broken into bite-sized pieces (see Notes)

½ teaspoon ground white pepper, divided

3 tablespoons white wine

2 tablespoons cassava flour (or sprouted spelt flour if not gluten- or grain-free)

For the crumb topping:

½ cup raw pumpkin seeds

2 teaspoons extra-virgin olive oil

SPECIAL TOOLS _____

Mini food processor

1. Preheat the oven to 425°F. Lightly oil an ovenproof 9 by 13-inch baking dish. Set aside.

2. Prepare an ice bath by filling a large bowl with cold water and ice. Set aside.

3. Fill a large pot with water and add 1 tablespoon of the salt. Bring the water to a boil.

4. While the water is coming to a boil, make the cashew cream: Place the cashews and 1 cup of water in a blender and process until smooth and creamy. Set aside.

5. Add the green beans to the boiling water and cook for 5 to 6 minutes, until fork-tender. Drain the beans in a colander and immediately plunge them into the ice bath. Drain the beans again in a colander. Dry the beans with a kitchen towel or paper towels (don't skip this step!). Set aside.

6. Heat 1 tablespoon plus 1 teaspoon of the oil in a large skillet over medium heat. Add the shallots and sauté for 2 to 3 minutes. Add the garlic and sauté for another minute or so, until the shallots and garlic are soft. Add the mushrooms and sauté until soft, about 5 minutes. Season with ½ teaspoon of the salt and ¼ teaspoon of the white pepper. Add the wine and continue cooking until the liquid evaporates, about 2 minutes.

7. Remove the skillet from the heat. Add the cooked green beans to the skillet with the mushrooms and gently toss. Transfer the green bean–mushroom mixture to the prepared baking dish.

8. To the same skillet used to cook the mushrooms, add the remaining tablespoon of oil and the flour. Heat over low heat, whisking constantly, for 1 minute. Pour in the cashew cream very, very slowly while whisking and continue whisking until the mixture is creamy and smooth, about 2 minutes. Add the remaining ¼ teaspoon of salt and ¼ teaspoon of white pepper. Add this roux to the green bean–mushroom mixture and gently toss to coat. Set aside.

If you are using a conventional blender instead of a high-powered one, be sure to soak the nuts first to ensure a smooth consistency.

For this particular recipe, resist the urge to chop the mushrooms into military uniformity—breaking them up by hand not only gives the casserole an appealing rustic appearance but somehow it makes the whole thing taste better too. Trust me on this one!

9. To make the crumb topping, put the pumpkin seeds and oil in a mini food processor; process by pulsing about 10 times. Scatter the pumpkin seed crumbs on top of the green bean–mushroom mixture.

10. Bake, uncovered, for 10 minutes. Serve warm.

STORAGE INFORMATION _____
Green bean casserole will keep in a covered container in the refrigerator for up to 2 days.

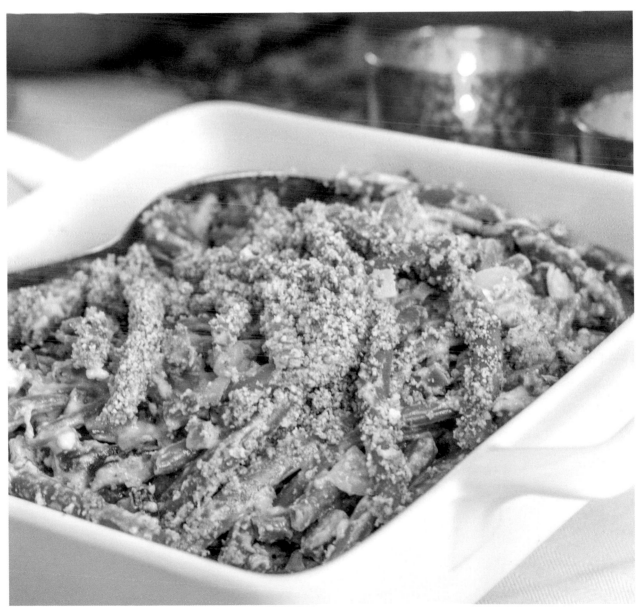

mac and cheese

SERVES 6   PREP TIME: 20 minutes   COOK TIME: 20 minutes

I worked really hard on this one, mostly for my son. He very much wanted me to come up with a clean mac and cheese that was actually worth eating. After multiple tweaks and numerous remakes, this is the best flavor-and-texture combination I think you can possibly get with a no-cheese mac and cheese. The sauce is amazing on baked potatoes, too!

8 ounces gluten-free whole-grain pasta shells, rigatoni, or elbow macaroni

1 tablespoon unrefined red palm oil or extra-virgin olive oil

⅓ cup chopped onions

½ cup peeled and chopped carrots

¾ cup frozen cubed butternut squash

½ teaspoon paprika

½ teaspoon turmeric powder

¼ teaspoon Himalayan pink salt

3 cloves garlic, chopped

½ cup raw cashews, preferably soaked in water for 1 to 2 hours, then rinsed and drained (see Note)

¼ cup coconut cream (see page 74)

1 tablespoon fresh lime juice

1 tablespoon unfortified nutritional yeast

1 teaspoon raw honey

1 teaspoon unseasoned rice vinegar

1. Bring a large pot of salted water to a boil. Add the pasta and cook according to the package directions. Drain, reserving 1 cup of the cooking water. Put the cooked pasta back in the cooking pot and set aside.

2. Heat the oil in a large saucepan over medium heat. Add the onions and carrots and sauté until the vegetables are soft, about 5 minutes. Add the frozen butternut squash and sauté until it completely thaws, about 5 minutes. Season the vegetables with the paprika, turmeric, and salt.

3. Transfer the vegetable mixture to a blender or food processor and add the reserved 1 cup of pasta cooking water. Process for 1 full minute, or until smooth and creamy. Add the garlic, cashews, coconut cream, lime juice, nutritional yeast, honey, and vinegar. Process on high speed until well blended. Taste and add more salt if necessary.

4. Pour the sauce into the pot with the pasta and warm over medium heat, stirring constantly, for about 3 minutes, until warmed through. Serve warm.

VARIATION: SUNDAY MAC AND CHEESE
To make a fancier version with a nutty herb crumble topping, put ½ cup raw pecans or raw walnuts and ½ cup fresh parsley leaves (loosely packed) in a mini food processor and pulse until the ingredients are well blended and in crumb-sized pieces. Sprinkle the topping on each portion of mac and cheese just before serving.

NOTE
If you are using a conventional rather than a high-powered blender or a food processor, be sure to soak the nuts first to ensure a smooth consistency.

MAKE IT VEGAN
Omit the honey.

MAKE IT GRAIN-FREE
Use a chickpea (garbanzo bean) pasta.

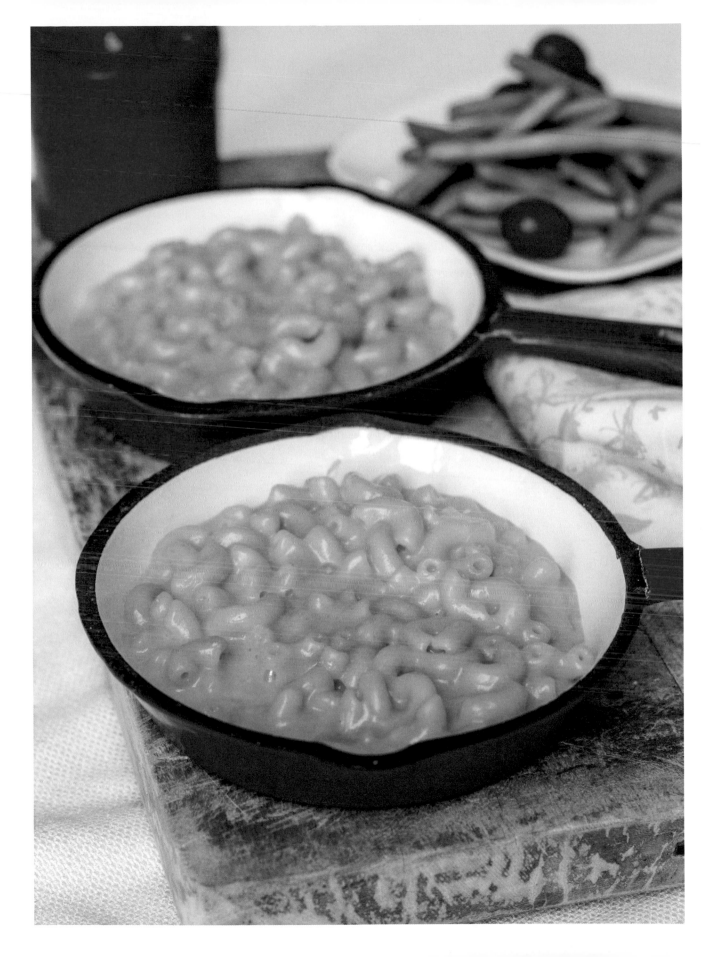

joe's perfect broccoli rabe

SERVES 4   PREP TIME: 10 minutes   COOK TIME: 25 minutes

Even though it is so simple, this broccoli rabe is one of the most popular recipes on our blog. I first started eating broccoli rabe at restaurants over a decade ago, but every time I tried to make it at home it turned into a major (and very bitter!) fail. Luckily for me, our dear family friend Joe Riti was kind enough to teach me the perfect way to make it. Joe is a master of Italian cooking who grew up eating broccoli rabe by the pound—his mom even packed him broccoli rabe and mozzarella sandwiches for his school lunch! One quick note: The recipe calls for a whole bulb of garlic. That is not a mistake.

---

1 large bunch broccoli rabe (about 1 pound) (see Notes)

3 tablespoons extra-virgin olive oil, divided

Cloves from 1 bulb garlic, coarsely chopped (see Notes)

7 tablespoons water, divided

Himalayan pink salt

½ teaspoon crushed red pepper

1. Trim the thick, tough stems from the broccoli rabe, then rinse and pat very dry.

2. Heat 2 tablespoons of the oil in a large skillet over medium heat. Add the chopped garlic and sauté briefly, for 30 to 45 seconds, until warm.

3. Add the broccoli rabe, toss to coat it in the oil and garlic, and turn the heat down to medium-low. Cook, stirring occasionally, until the broccoli wilts, about 5 minutes. Add the remaining tablespoon of oil and 1 tablespoon of the water and season lightly with salt and crushed red pepper. Add more crushed red pepper to taste.

4. Continue to cook the broccoli rabe for 20 minutes, or until it is very, very wilted. Every 3 minutes or so, add an additional tablespoon of water to the pan, stirring after each addition. Adjust the seasoning to taste and serve.

NOTES _____

When buying broccoli rabe, look for bunches with large dark green leaves without any yellowing or wilting. Any stalks with small buds that look like loose broccoli heads should be equally green and fresh looking.

I use a mini food processor to make chopping several cloves of garlic easier.

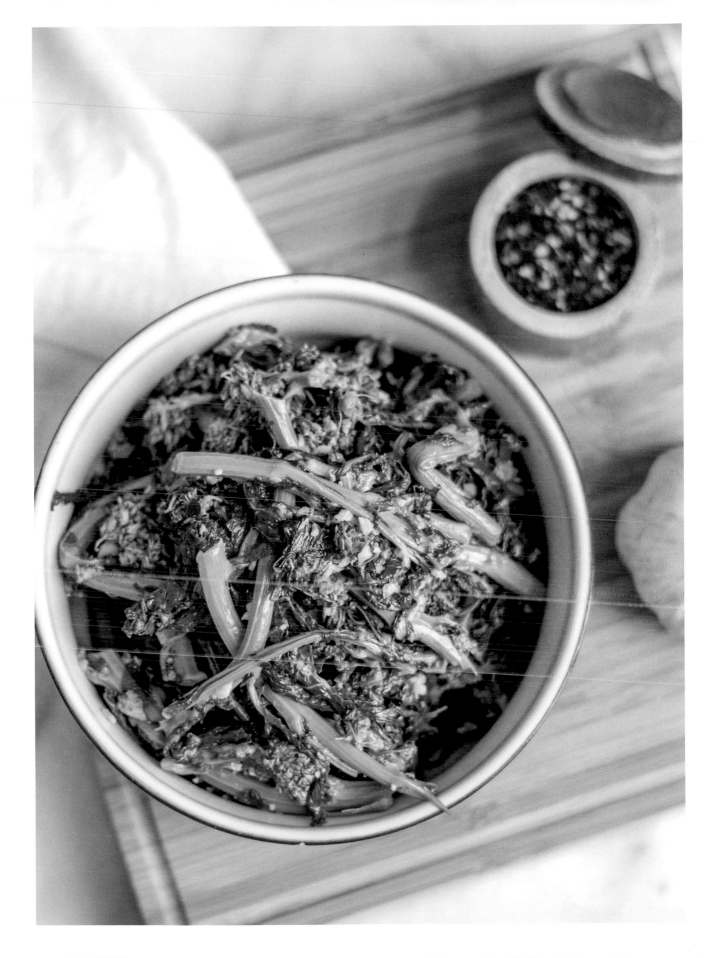

an easier ratatouille

SERVES 8   PREP TIME: 25 minutes   COOK TIME: 2 hours

Pixar's Oscar-winning 2007 film *Ratatouille* made the traditional French vegetable dish incredibly enticing. I vividly remember watching the movie with my son, Blake, when he was just six years old. As we walked out of the theater, Blake talked enthusiastically about how much fun it would be to make ratatouille. So we headed straight to the store to buy all of the ingredients for a recipe I found online. I had never made the dish before, and what an ordeal! The recipe called for cooking each vegetable in a separate pot and then layering everything in a bigger pot and cooking it all with fresh tomatoes. Yes, it tasted amazing, but I just don't have the patience to stand in the kitchen hovering over—and then cleaning—pots all day! This is a simplified version that calls for baking the vegetables instead. It's delicious on everything from beans to baked potatoes, chicken, fish, whole grains, on toast, or even on its own.

---

3 red bell peppers, seeded and cut into ¼-inch strips

2 medium onions, halved lengthwise and sliced into ¼-inch-thick half-moons

8 tablespoons extra-virgin olive oil, divided

3 medium zucchini, cut into ¼-inch slices

2 medium eggplant, cut into 1-inch cubes

6 sprigs fresh thyme

3 sprigs fresh rosemary, plus more for garnish if desired

Himalayan pink salt

1 bulb garlic

2 (14.5-ounce) cans diced tomatoes, drained

STORAGE INFORMATION _____

Ratatouille will keep in a covered container in the refrigerator for up to a week.

1. Preheat the oven to 350°F. Line 2 rimmed baking sheets with parchment paper.

2. Spread the peppers and onions onto one of the prepared baking sheets and drizzle with 2 tablespoons of the oil. Spread the zucchini and eggplant onto the second prepared baking sheet, top with the thyme and rosemary, and drizzle with 3 tablespoons of the oil. Season all of the vegetables with salt and gently toss them in the oil to coat.

3. Use a sharp knife to slice the top off the bulb of the garlic. Place the bulb in a small ovenproof dish. Drizzle 2 tablespoons of the oil on top of the garlic and season with salt.

4. Transfer the pepper-onion baking sheet, the zucchini-eggplant baking sheet, and the garlic to the oven. Bake the onions and peppers for 35 minutes. Bake the zucchini and eggplant for 40 minutes. Bake the garlic for 1 hour.

5. Remove the vegetables from the oven and squeeze the garlic into a Dutch oven (or other large, heavy ovenproof pot). Transfer the rest of the vegetables to the Dutch oven.

6. Stir in the tomatoes and the remaining tablespoon of oil. Season lightly with salt. Place in the oven and bake for 1 hour, stirring every 20 minutes. Spoon into individual bowls and garnish with rosemary sprigs, if desired. Serve warm or at room temperature.

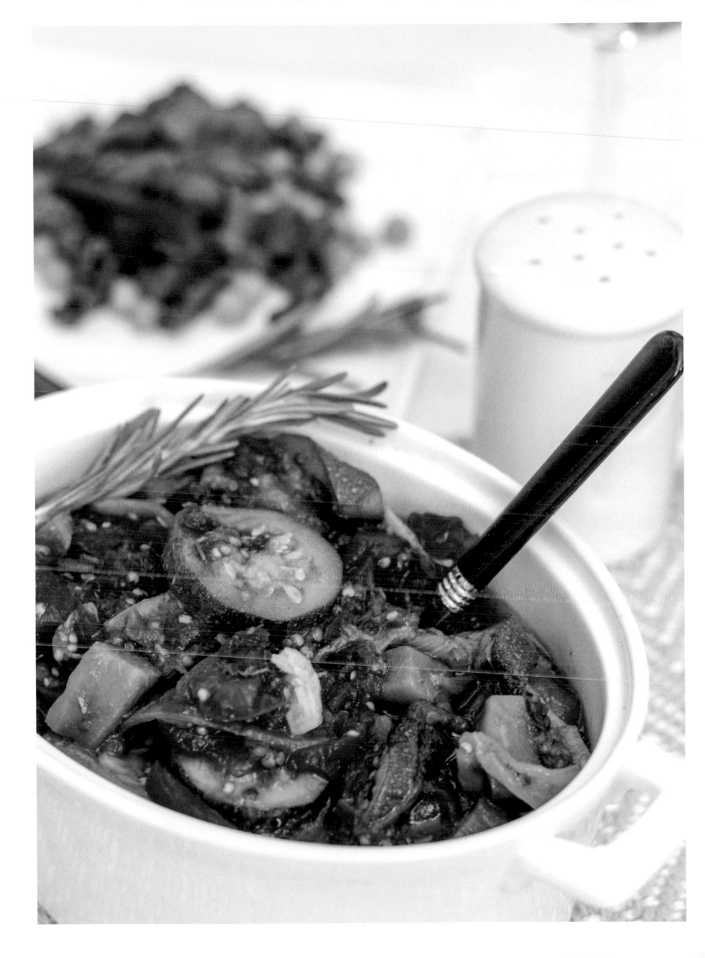

karen's easy refried beans

MAKES about 2 cups   PREP TIME: 10 minutes   COOK TIME: 20 minutes

Karen Herrera, a dear friend of mine from Honduras, shared this recipe for refried beans with me years ago, and I cannot think of a single way to improve it. These beans are incredibly satisfying and very helpful at filling up our always-hungry teenage son! I serve them with eggs for breakfast, spread them on toast for lunch, use them for tostadas (see the recipe on page 238), serve them alongside roasted chicken and carrots for an easy dinner, use them as a dip for vegetables, and often just eat them straight up. It's such a simple recipe, but it is one of our family favorites! Note: You can easily swap pinto beans for black beans in this recipe.

---

3 (15-ounce) cans black beans (do not drain; see Note)

1 large clove garlic, peeled

½ cup chopped onions

½ teaspoon Himalayan pink salt

3 tablespoons extra-virgin olive oil or unrefined avocado oil

For garnish (optional):

Crushed red pepper

Fresh cilantro leaves

1. Open the cans of beans and pour the liquid from all the cans into a 1-cup measuring cup. Reserve half of the liquid (½ cup) and discard the rest.

2. Put the beans, reserved bean liquid, garlic, onions, and salt in a food processor. Process until the mixture is smooth and creamy.

3. Heat the oil in a large skillet over medium heat. Add the bean mixture to the skillet and stir to combine the beans with the oil. Cook the beans, stirring frequently, until thickened, 15 to 20 minutes. Season with additional salt to taste. Garnish with a little cilantro and/or crushed red pepper, if desired. Serve warm.

STORAGE INFORMATION _____

Refried black beans will keep for up to 4 days if stored in a covered container in the refrigerator.

NOTE _____

This is the only recipe in the book in which the beans do not require draining and rinsing (as discussed on page 68).

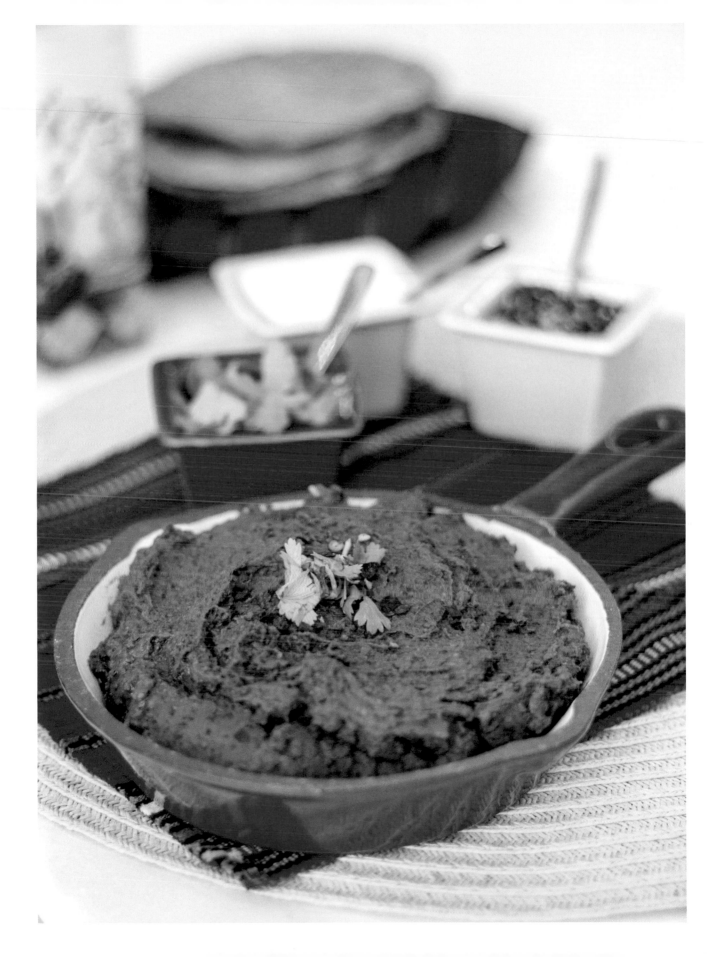

sweet potato chili fries

SERVES 4   PREP TIME: 15 minutes, plus time to soak the fries   COOK TIME: 25 minutes

When my son, Blake, was younger, my husband's surgical call schedule was much more demanding than it is these days, and many a night he had to eat dinner at the hospital. On those nights I would take a break from cooking a big dinner, but I still wanted Blake and me to eat well. Dinner for us on "call night" often consisted of these fries with scrambled eggs and sautéed spinach. It was such an easy meal to put together and always so satisfying. Oh, and don't forget the ketchup (page 390)! If you're feeling fancy, garnish the fries with chopped fresh herbs—whatever you have on hand.

2 medium sweet potatoes

4 teaspoons brown rice flour, divided

2 tablespoons extra-virgin olive oil or unrefined macadamia nut oil, divided, plus more for the baking sheets

1 teaspoon chili powder, divided

1 teaspoon Himalayan pink salt, divided

1 teaspoon onion powder, divided

1. Peel the sweet potatoes and cut them into thin fry-shaped pieces. Try to cut them into equal-sized pieces so they will bake evenly. Soak the pieces in cold water for 30 minutes. Remove them from the water and pat dry with paper towels.

2. Preheat the oven to 425°F and lightly coat 2 large baking sheets with oil.

3. Add half of the sweet potato fries to a very large resealable plastic bag. Sprinkle 2 teaspoons of the flour over the potatoes, seal the bag, and shake to coat the fries in the flour. Transfer the sweet potatoes to a mixing bowl and add 1 tablespoon of the oil, ½ teaspoon of the chili powder, ½ teaspoon of the salt, and ½ teaspoon of the onion powder. Toss to coat the fries in the seasoning. Spread the fries on one of the prepared baking sheets in a single layer, not touching. Repeat with the remaining sweet potatoes, flour, oil, chili powder, salt, and onion powder; spread them on the second baking sheet.

4. Put the fries in the oven and bake for 15 minutes, then flip the fries and bake for another 10 minutes, or until lightly browned. Remove the fries from the oven and sprinkle on a bit more salt, if desired. Let the fries sit for about 5 minutes before serving.

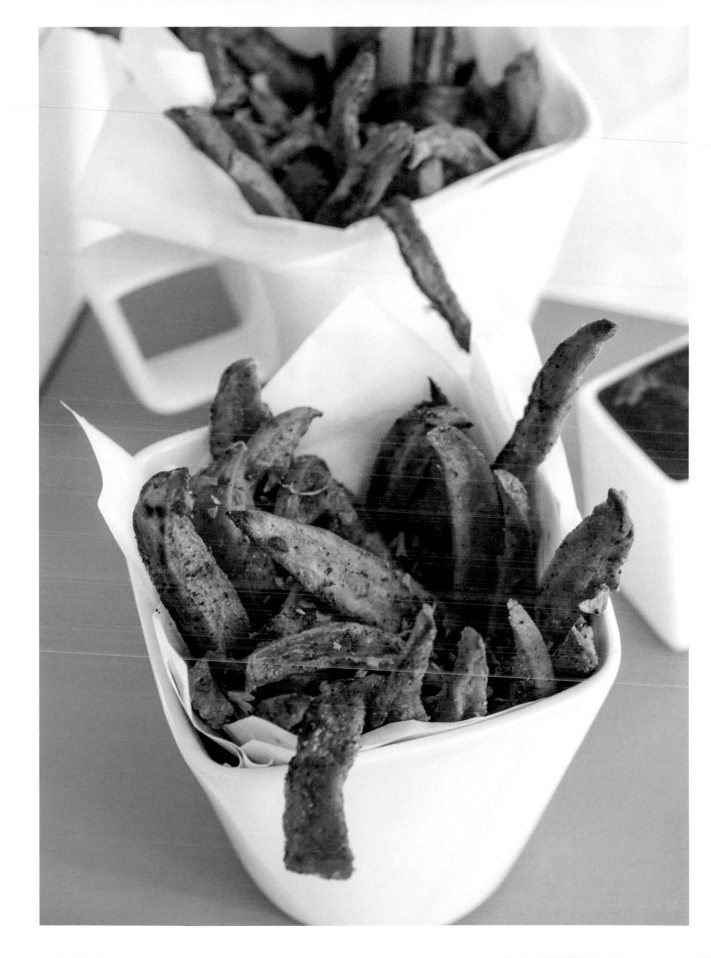

zucchini boats

MAKES 6 boats   PREP TIME: 20 minutes   COOK TIME: 50 minutes

A vegetable dish and whole-grain dish all in one, zucchini boats are something I frequently fall back on when I'm trying to make a special dinner for company. But there's no need to wait for company to make these jumbo stuffed jewels! Fun and festive, zucchini boats make eating your vegetables a little more exciting.

3 medium zucchini, halved lengthwise

1 teaspoon Himalayan pink salt, divided

3 tablespoons extra-virgin olive oil, divided

¾ cup finely chopped onions

½ cup coarsely chopped tomatoes

2 cloves garlic, crushed to a paste

¼ teaspoon ground black pepper

1 cup steamed short-grain brown rice (preferably sprouted)

½ cup pine nuts

1 slice gluten-free whole-grain bread, toasted and broken into bite-sized pieces

1. With a sharp teaspoon, remove the seeds and some of the pulp (do not discard) from each zucchini half to create shells about ¼ inch thick; be careful not to break through the zucchini shells. Coarsely chop the seeds and pulp. Arrange the shells next to each other in a large ovenproof baking dish and sprinkle with ½ teaspoon of the salt. Set aside.

2. Heat 2 tablespoons of the oil in a large saucepan over medium heat. Add the zucchini pulp, onions, tomatoes, garlic, the remaining ½ teaspoon of salt, and the black pepper. Cook, stirring every now and then, for 10 minutes, or until most of the liquid has evaporated. Stir in the cooked rice, remove from the heat, and set aside to cool.

3. Preheat the oven to 400°F.

4. Place the pine nuts, toasted bread pieces, and remaining tablespoon of oil in a food processor and pulse to process into crumbs.

5. Empty each zucchini shell of any accumulated liquid. Fill them with the zucchini-onion-tomato stuffing so that it slightly overlaps the rims of the shells. Sprinkle the pine nut–breadcrumb topping on top of each zucchini boat.

6. Bake for 40 minutes, or until the topping is golden brown. Allow to rest for at least 10 minutes before serving.

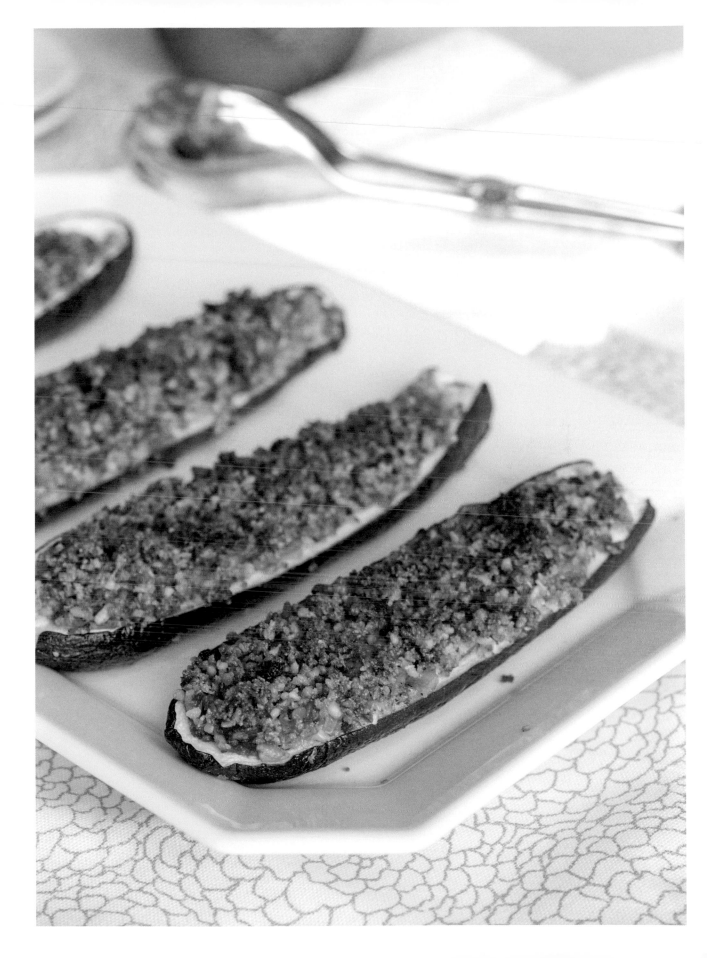

stuffed tomatoes

SERVES 6   PREP TIME: 5 minutes, plus 15 minutes to drain   COOK TIME: 13 minutes

This is one of my favorite uses for leftover rice. I use my Wild Rice Pilaf (page 262), but you could really use any leftover rice or grain. As long as the grain or rice is already fully cooked, you can stuff it in a tomato and end up with a beautiful side dish in minutes. (Note: If you follow a grain-free diet, wild rice is a great option; despite its name, wild rice is actually considered a seed.) The most important component of this recipe is super-fresh, firm, and ideally vine-ripened tomatoes. If you start with ultra-fresh tomatoes and don't overcook them, your stuffed tomatoes are pretty much guaranteed to turn out perfectly. You don't need to fret or fuss about much more than that.

6 ripe tomatoes (2½ to 3 inches in diameter)

Himalayan pink salt and ground black pepper

3 cups Wild Rice Pilaf (page 262)

For the topping:

¼ cup plus 2 tablespoons Parmesan Nut "Cheese" (page 370) or ground pecans

1. Preheat the oven to 400°F. Line a rimmed baking sheet with parchment paper. Set a wire rack on a second rimmed baking sheet.

2. Slice the tomatoes in half horizontally and scoop out the pulp and seeds. Lightly pat the insides of the tomatoes with a paper towel to remove the excess moisture and lightly salt the insides. Rest the tomato halves upside down on the wire rack for 10 to 15 minutes to drain any remaining juices.

3. Arrange the tomatoes on the parchment paper–lined baking sheet, cut side up, and season the insides lightly with salt and pepper.

4. Divide the rice pilaf among the tomatoes. Sprinkle the nut cheese on top of each tomato and transfer to the oven.

5. Bake the tomatoes for 10 to 13 minutes, until they are just softened (be careful not to overcook!). Remove the tomatoes from the oven and allow to cool for at least 10 minutes before serving. Serve warm or at room temperature.

MAKE IT GRAIN-FREE AND PALEO-FRIENDLY ⸻
Omit the corn from the wild rice pilaf.

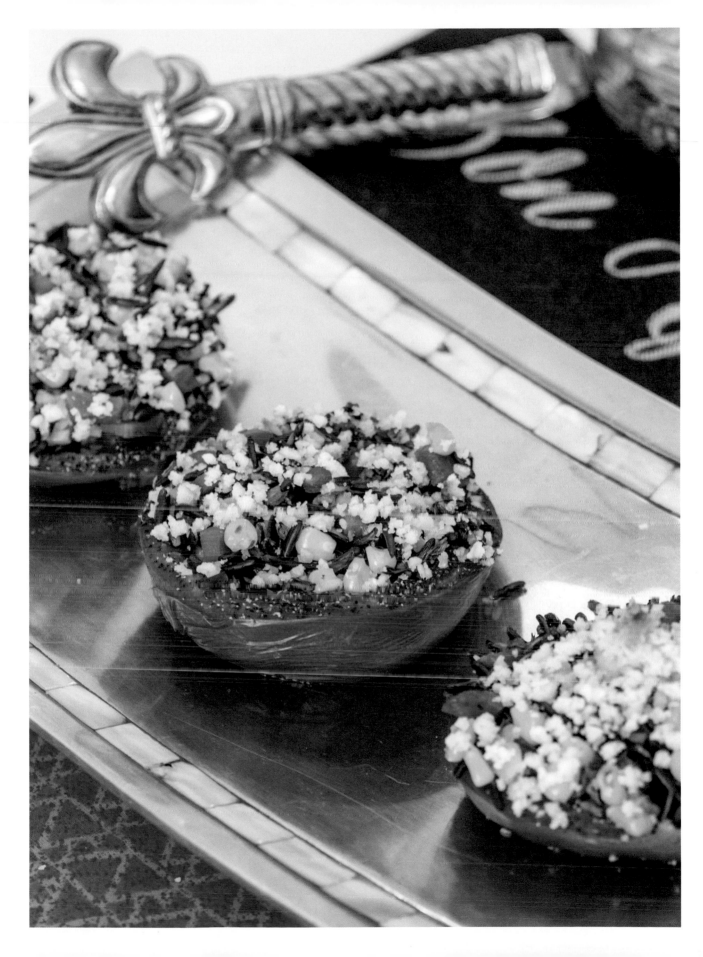

three-bean salad

SERVES 6 to 8   PREP TIME: 20 minutes

I can't tell you how many times I had this salad for lunch while writing this book. It's such a basic recipe that I almost didn't include it, but I figured sometimes super-basic recipes are the ones we all need the most! It's also incredibly satisfying; if you serve it over a bed of greens with sliced avocado on top, then you've practically got a meal. And believe it or not, it is to die for when smashed and then pan-fried between two sprouted-corn tortillas.

For the dressing:

2 teaspoons chopped garlic

⅓ cup extra-virgin olive oil or unrefined avocado oil, divided

3 tablespoons fresh lemon juice

1 tablespoon Italian seasoning

1 teaspoon Dijon mustard

1 teaspoon manuka honey or other raw honey

¾ teaspoon Himalayan pink salt

½ to 1 teaspoon anchovy paste (optional)

1 (15-ounce) can cannellini beans, rinsed and drained

1 (15-ounce) can chickpeas, rinsed and drained

1 (15-ounce) can kidney beans, rinsed and drained

⅔ cup chopped celery

⅔ cup chopped green bell peppers

⅔ cup chopped red bell peppers

⅔ cup chopped red onions

1. To make the dressing, put the garlic and 1 tablespoon of the oil in a medium-sized microwave-safe dish. Microwave for 1 minute, until the garlic softens. To the dish, add the remaining oil, lemon juice, Italian seasoning, Dijon mustard, honey, salt, and anchovy paste (if using). Whisk until the ingredients are well blended.

2. In a large serving bowl, combine the cannellini beans, chickpeas, kidney beans, celery, green bell peppers, red bell peppers, and red onions. Drizzle in the dressing and toss to thoroughly mix. Season with additional salt and Italian seasoning, if desired. Let the salad sit at room temperature for at least 30 minutes before serving to allow the flavors to develop.

MAKE IT VEGETARIAN
Omit the anchovy paste.

MAKE IT VEGAN
Omit the anchovy paste and honey.

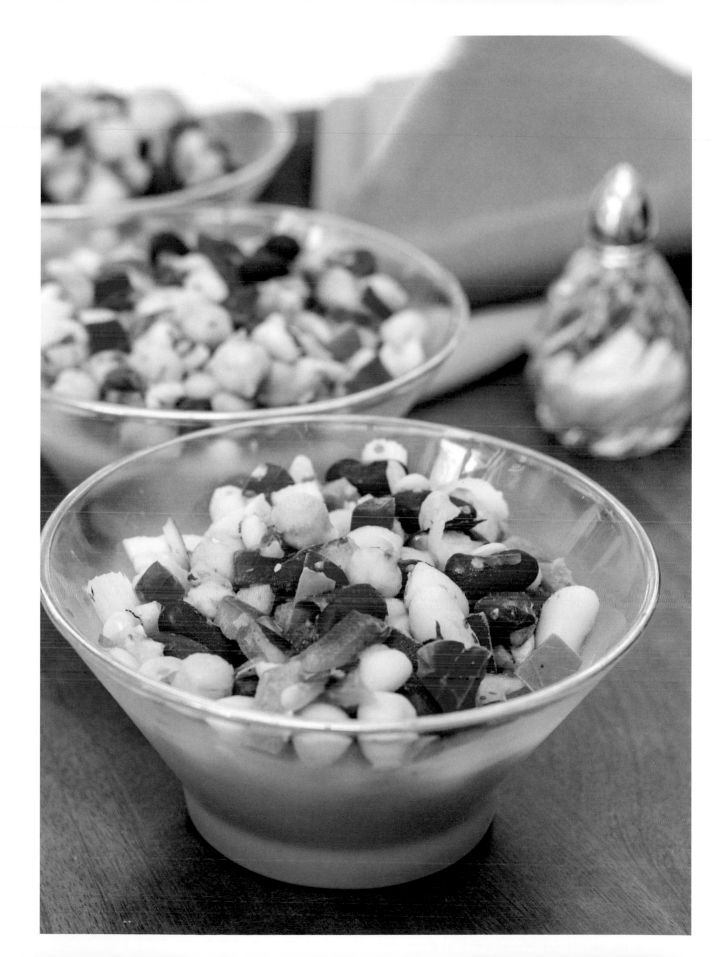

picnic-style potato salad

SERVES 8   PREP TIME: 20 minutes, plus time for the potatoes to cool
COOK TIME: 20 minutes

We live on an inlet, and when our son was younger, we frequently took our WaveRunner from the back of our house to a nearby island for summer evening picnic dinners. Nine times out of ten, this potato salad would be in our cooler. We have since sold the WaveRunner, so we no longer eat this on island dinner picnics, but we do serve it a lot for summer barbecues. It's a super-easy salad to make, but it is important to pick the right potatoes! Potatoes are divided into three general categories based on their texture: starchy, all-purpose, and waxy. For the best potato salad, choose waxy potatoes, such as Red Bliss potatoes, new potatoes, or fingerling potatoes. I use Red Bliss for this recipe, but the other two will also work.

---

3 pounds red potatoes (aka Red Bliss potatoes)

¾ cup raw cashews, preferably soaked for 1 to 2 hours, then rinsed and drained (see Note)

½ cup plus 3 tablespoons water

1 tablespoon fresh lemon juice

1 teaspoon manuka honey or other raw honey

¼ teaspoon Himalayan pink salt

6 cloves garlic, crushed to a paste

3 scallions, coarsely chopped

3 stalks celery, chopped

½ cup chopped fresh parsley

3 tablespoons fresh thyme

2 teaspoons Dijon mustard

Ground black pepper

1. Bring the potatoes to a boil in a large pot of salted water. Turn the heat down to medium-low and simmer until the potatoes are tender, about 17 minutes. Drain and let stand until cool enough to handle, about 20 minutes.

2. While the potatoes cool, in a blender or food processor, process the cashews, water, lemon juice, honey, and salt on high speed until smooth and creamy. Set the cashew cream aside.

3. Cut the potatoes into bite-sized pieces and place them in a large mixing bowl. Add the garlic, scallions, celery, parsley, thyme, and Dijon mustard. Mix in the cashew cream. Season with salt and pepper to taste. Serve at room temperature or chilled.

NOTE ───────────────
If you're using a conventional blender instead of a high-powered one or a food processor, be sure to soak the nuts first to ensure a smooth texture.

STORAGE INFORMATION ───────────────
Potato salad can be stored in a covered container in the refrigerator for up to 2 days.

MAKE IT VEGAN ───────────────
Omit the honey.

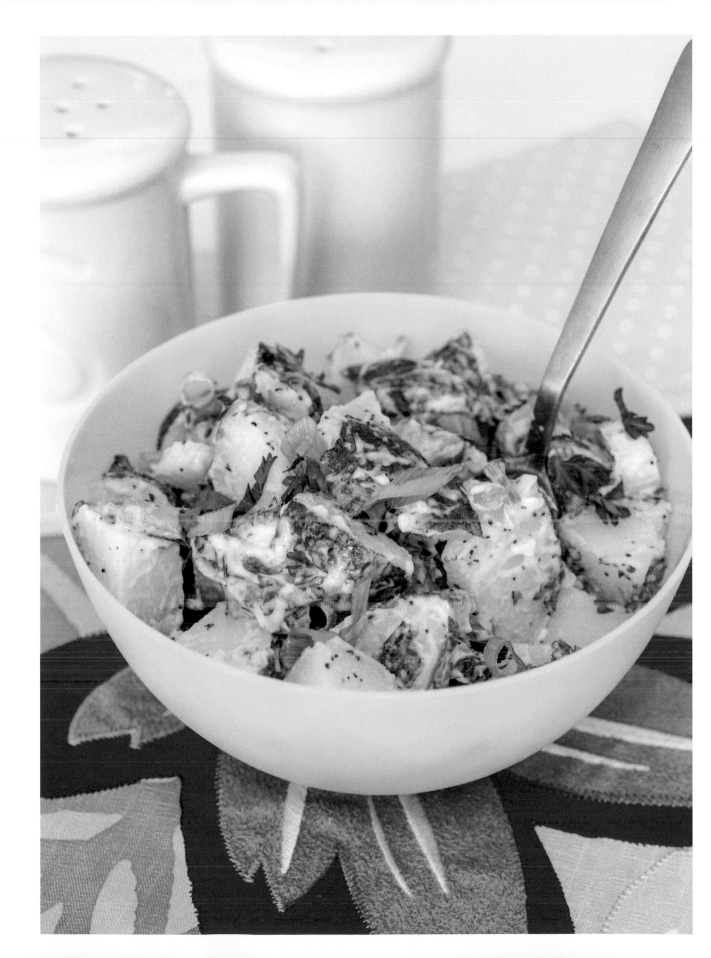

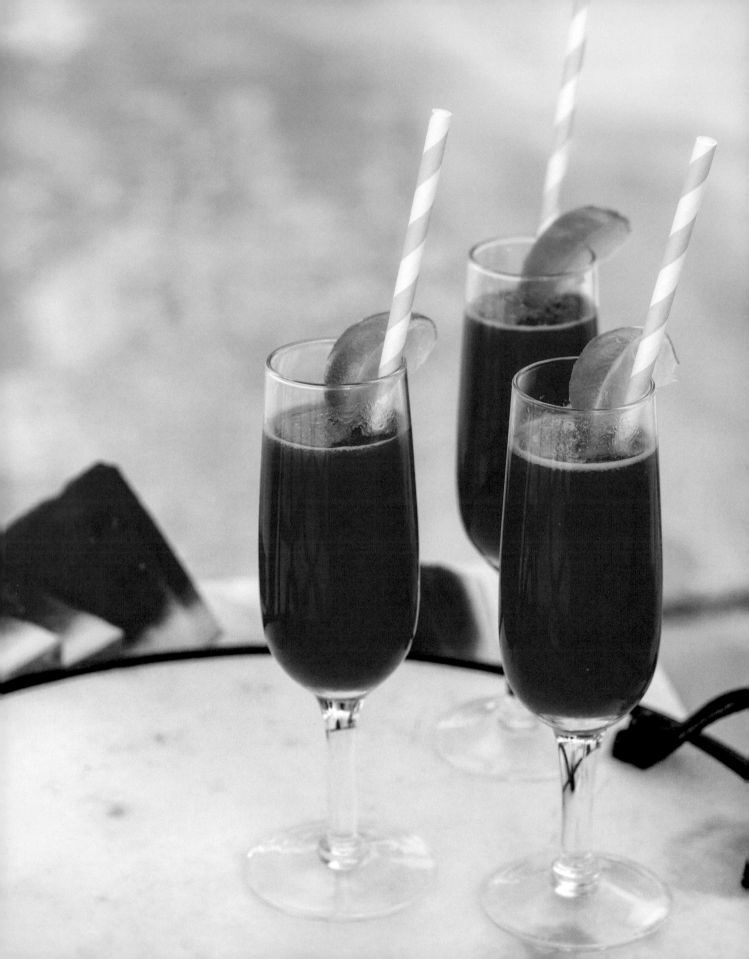

CHAPTER 15

juices, elixirs, and cocktails

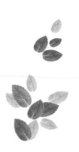

detoxifying green juice

SERVES 2   PREP TIME: 10 minutes

Sipping this tart, tangy, and light juice is an invigorating way to start the day. It also makes for a great midafternoon pick-me-up—it's as revitalizing as a cup of coffee, with none of the caffeine crash. Unlike conventional juice, my juice is made with whole fruits and vegetables, so you still get all of the fiber found in the whole food. This recipe does call for removing the fiber-rich skins from the apples and cucumbers, though, just because it makes for a smoother juice. But even without the skins, you are still getting fiber from the pulps of the cucumber and apple. I also added a second superfood vegetable (in addition to cucumbers): watercress. With more than fifteen essential vitamins and minerals—more iron than spinach, more calcium than milk, and more vitamin C than oranges—watercress is a powerhouse of nutrition and a great addition to any detox regimen.

---

1 cup cold water

Juice of 1 lemon

1 cup frozen pineapple chunks

1 (½-inch) piece fresh ginger, peeled and coarsely chopped (see Note)

1 cucumber, peeled and seeded (see Note)

Pinch of Himalayan pink salt

1 cup watercress

1 crisp apple, peeled and cored (see Note)

1 cup ice cubes

1 tablespoon manuka honey or other raw honey (optional)

Put all of the ingredients in a blender in the order given in the ingredients list. Process on high speed until the ingredients are well blended and the mixture is smooth. Divide between two 12-ounce glasses and serve at once.

NOTE _____

If you're using a conventional blender rather than a high-powered one, grate the ginger and coarsely chop the cucumber and apple before adding them to the blender.

STORAGE INFORMATION _____

Leftovers can be stored in the refrigerator for up to 1 day; stir well before serving.

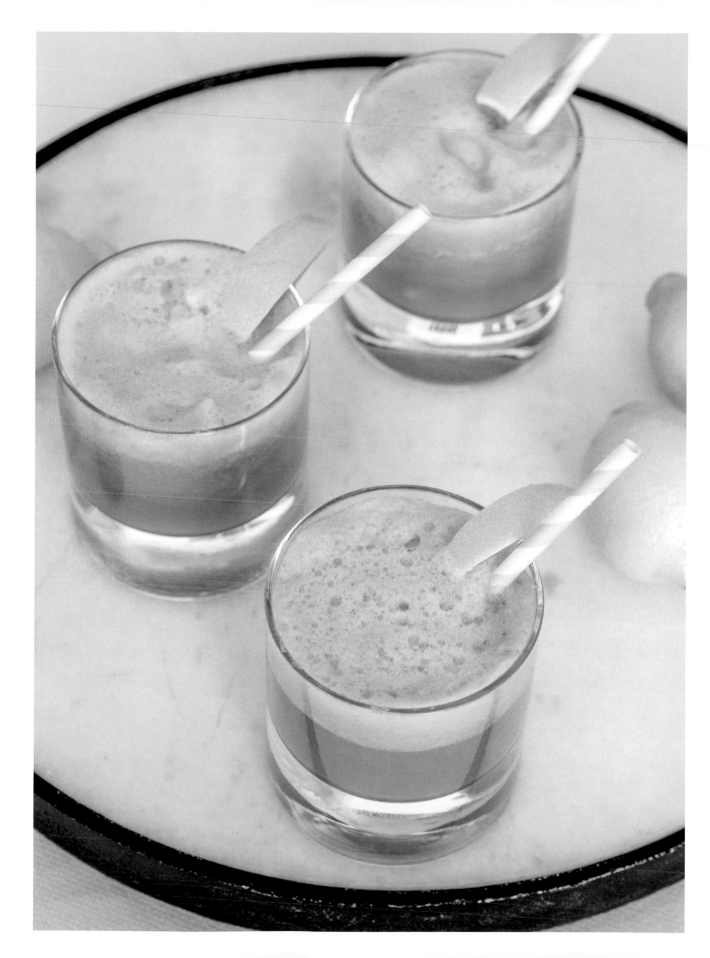

whole watermelon juice

SERVES 4   PREP TIME: 10 minutes, plus time to chill

Since it feels like summer where we live for about ten months of the year, this refreshing whole juice is a staple for us. Unlike conventional juice, whole juice is made with the whole fruit or vegetable and therefore contains the good stuff, including the fiber (which has potent anti-inflammatory benefits) and all of the antioxidants and phytonutrients. (See page 32 for more on juice.) This watermelon juice definitely got my son through many sweaty soccer nights, 5K runs, and cross-country practices. I always packed it in a thermos and brought it along to his various sport events because it was such a nutritious, replenishing sports drink.

---

1 medium watermelon, seeded and chopped (about 6 cups), very cold, divided

1 tablespoon fresh lime juice, divided

Pinch of Himalayan pink salt

Lime wedges, for garnish (optional)

Put 3 cups of the watermelon and 1½ teaspoons of the lime juice in a blender and process on high speed until smooth. Add the remaining 3 cups of watermelon, remaining 1½ teaspoons of lime juice, and the salt and process again until smooth. Refrigerate for at least 2 hours. When chilled, divide among four 8-ounce glasses and serve immediately. Garnish with lime wedges, if desired.

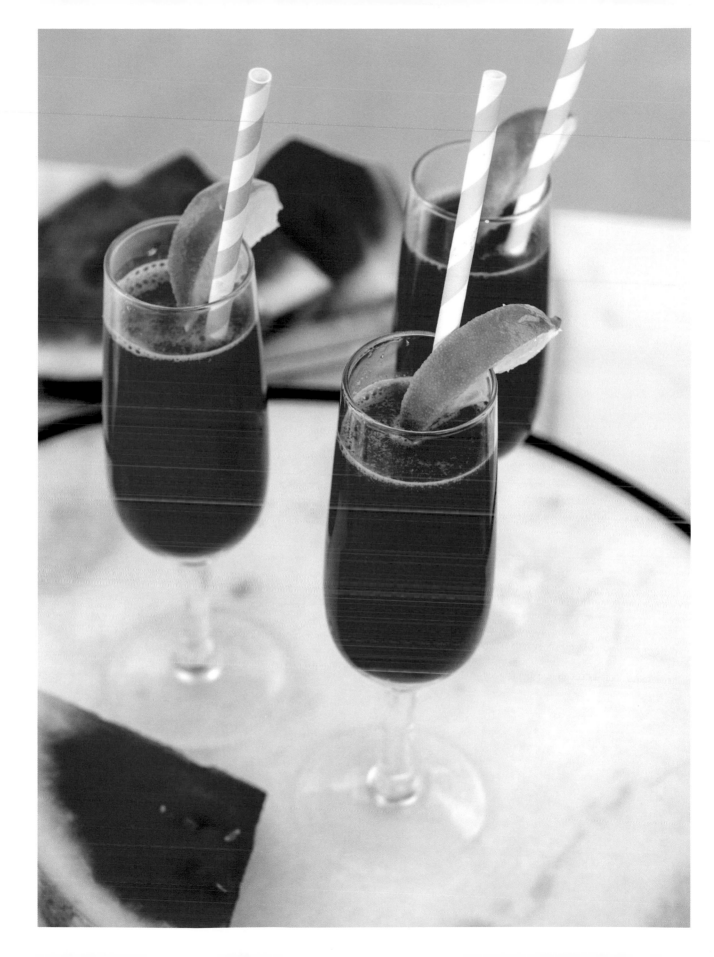

golden chai

SERVES 4   PREP TIME: 7 minutes   COOK TIME: 5 minutes

On a family ski trip, I enjoyed a cup of golden chai every day after hitting the slopes. If you have ever gone skiing (and you are also over the age of forty!), then you know how sore you feel at the end of the day. Having my cup of chai as soon as we got back to our hotel was the one thing I looked forward to as I left the slopes. It made me feel better almost immediately. Made with both ginger and turmeric, this warming chai has incredibly potent anti-inflammatory properties. By adding the black pepper and a bit of healthy fat (from the coconut milk and hemp seeds), the anti-inflammatory properties of turmeric are fully activated.

1½ cups water

½ cup full-fat coconut milk

10 Deglet Noor dates, pitted (see Note)

2 tablespoons hemp seeds

1 tablespoon grated fresh ginger

2 teaspoons fresh lemon juice

1½ teaspoons turmeric powder, plus more for garnish if desired

1 teaspoon ground cinnamon

¼ teaspoon cardamom

⅛ teaspoon ground black pepper

1. Put all of the ingredients in a blender in the order given in the ingredients list. Process until smooth and creamy.

2. Pour the mixture into a small saucepan and bring to a simmer. Divide among four 4-ounce cups. Serve warm. Garnish with extra turmeric, if desired.

NOTE

If you're using a conventional blender rather than a high-powered one, soak the dates in water for 15 to 30 minutes to soften them before pureeing.

STORAGE INFORMATION

Golden chai will keep in a covered container in the refrigerator for 3 to 4 days. Shake before reheating.

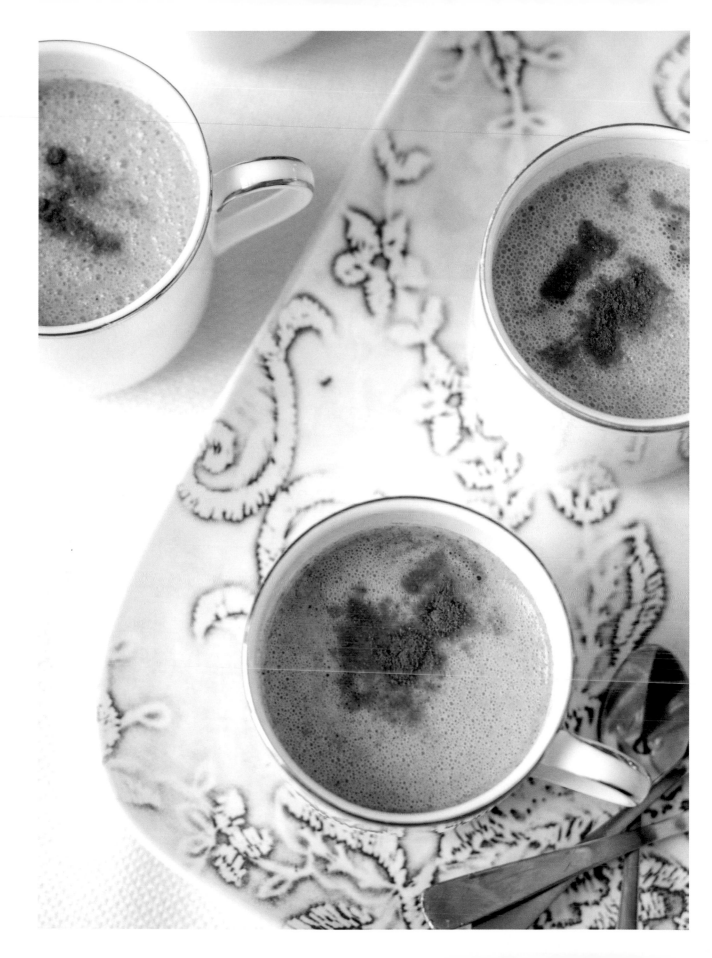

frozen avocado margaritas

SERVES 4   PREP TIME: 10 minutes

Hands down, this is my favorite Sunday brunch drink. I had my first avocado margarita at the Avocado Grill in downtown West Palm Beach while celebrating my forty-first birthday with one of my best girlfriends from childhood, Christine Legris. The next weekend I got to work re-creating a whole-foods version with no refined sugar. Once you try it, you won't want brunch without it!

6 ounces silver (aka blanco) tequila made with 100% agave (see right)

2 tablespoons medium- or coarse-grind Himalayan pink salt

1 lime wedge

⅓ Hass avocado, peeled and pitted

8 medjool dates, pitted (see Note)

¾ cup fresh lime juice

½ cup frozen pineapple chunks

⅓ cup chopped fresh cilantro

2 teaspoons seeded and chopped jalapeño pepper

1 or 2 pinches cayenne pepper

2 cups ice

1. Toss the salt on a small plate. Rub the rims of four 6-ounce margarita glasses with the lime wedge and dip each glass in the salt. Set the glasses aside.

2. In a blender, process the tequila, avocado, dates, lime juice, pineapple, cilantro, jalapeño pepper, and cayenne pepper until smooth and creamy. Add the ice and process again until smooth. Divide among the salt-rimmed glasses. Serve cold.

NOTE

If you're using a conventional blender rather than a high-powered one and your dates are on the dry side, soak them in water for 15 to 30 minutes to soften them before pureeing (very moist, succulent medjool dates do not require soaking).

TEQUILA IS BETTER FOR YOU THAN YOU THOUGHT!

I'm not going to tell you tequila is a superfood, but it does have some unique beneficial attributes. But not all tequila is created equal. The very best and healthiest tequila is made from 100 percent blue agave with no additives, and blanco is the purest type of 100 percent blue agave tequila. After a meal, 100 percent blue agave tequila can be a good digestif. The agave plant contains high amounts of inulin, which is a prebiotic known to aid the digestive system by promoting good bacteria. Tequila made with 100 percent agave also contains agavins, a kind of sugar that might help with weight loss. Unlike agave syrup, agavins won't raise blood sugar levels. Agavins also help produce a hormone (GPP-1) that is known to keep the stomach fuller longer. Again, I'm not saying tequila is a superfood, but it might not be quite as bad as you thought. Just remember to get the good stuff! Here are three kinds of tequila I recommend:

- *123 Certified Organic Tequila Blanco*
- *Patrón Silver*
- *Casamigos Tequila Blanco*

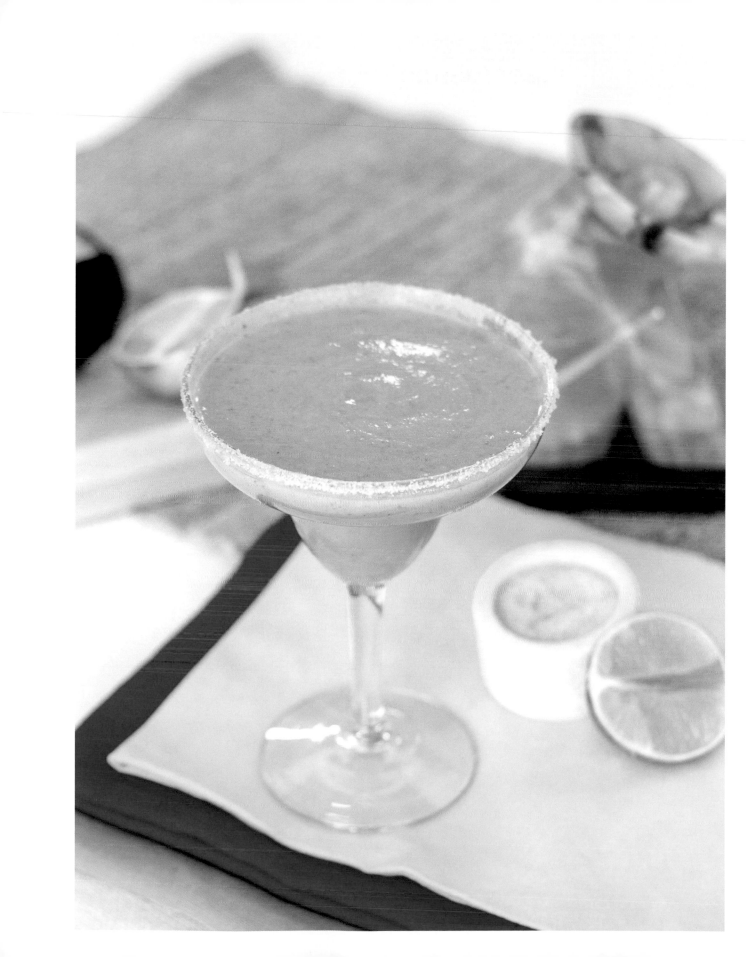

bloody marys for a crowd

MAKES 2½ quarts (10 servings)   PREP TIME: 30 minutes, plus time to chill
COOK TIME: 45 minutes

Not too many things excite people at brunch as much as seeing a build-your-own Bloody Mary bar. Once you've made the tomato juice base (which can be prepared and refrigerated two days in advance or frozen up to two weeks in advance), the rest is easy-peasy! I like my Bloody Marys loaded, so much so that they often look like I've got a salad in my glass. But if you are setting up a build-your-own Bloody Mary bar, you can offer as many or as few fixings as you like (see the facing page for ideas). Of course, you don't need to add alcohol if you just want to sip a super-healthy mocktail while you wait for the main course. Or have two—add some shrimp (my absolute favorite Bloody Mary add-in) to the second and call it lunch!

---

1 tablespoon extra-virgin olive oil

5 cups water

5 medium-large tomatoes, chopped

4 cloves garlic, peeled

1 medium beet, trimmed and chopped (leave skin on)

1 medium carrot, peeled and chopped

½ medium onion, chopped

1½ teaspoons gluten-free Worcestershire sauce

1 teaspoon Himalayan pink salt

½ teaspoon ground black pepper

4 medjool dates, pitted (see Note)

2 small cucumbers, peeled, cored, and chopped

¼ cup chopped fresh basil

¼ cup fresh lime juice

1 tablespoon prepared horseradish (optional)

For serving (optional):

Ice cubes

10 ounces gluten-free vodka

Garnishes (see facing page)

1. Heat the oil in a large saucepan over medium heat. Add the water, tomatoes, garlic, beet, carrot, onion, Worcestershire sauce, salt, and pepper. Cook for 35 to 45 minutes, until the vegetables are soft, stirring occasionally. Remove the vegetables from the heat and set aside to cool.

2. Once they're cooled to room temperature, transfer about 2 cups of the vegetables to a blender and puree on high speed until smooth. Continue adding the vegetables 2 cups at a time, pureeing after each addition, until all the vegetables have been pureed. To the vegetable puree in the blender, add the dates, cucumbers, basil, lime juice, and horseradish (if using). Process on high speed until the mixture is smooth.

3. Transfer the vegetable puree to a large pitcher and stir with a wooden spoon several times. Chill the Bloody Mary mix in the refrigerator for at least 4 hours before serving. (Note: The Bloody Mary mix can be prepared in advance and refrigerated for up to 2 days or frozen for up to 2 weeks.)

4. To serve, fill a tall 8-ounce glass with ice, if desired. Pour in 8 ounces of the Bloody Mary mix and 1 ounce of vodka, if desired, and stir well. Add the garnish(es) of your choice.

NOTE _____

If you're using a conventional blender rather than a high-powered one and your dates are on the dry side, soak them in water for 15 to 30 minutes to soften them before pureeing (very moist, succulent medjool dates do not require soaking).

MAKE IT VEGAN AND VEGETARIAN _____

Use a vegan Worcestershire sauce.

Choose as many (or as few) of the following garnishes as you like to create the ultimate clean Bloody Mary bar. Cocktail spears are also a nice addition.

PRODUCE AND PICKLED FOODS:

Baby corn

Celery stalks

Cornichons

Cucumber slices

Fresh parsley sprigs

Grape tomatoes

Lemon slices or wedges

Lime slices or wedges

Marinated artichoke hearts

Marinated pearl onions

Naturally fermented kosher pickle spears

Olives

Pickled beans and asparagus

Pickled beets, cauliflower, or carrots

Scallions

PROTEIN:

Cooked shrimp (tail on)

Hard-boiled eggs

Raw, freshly shucked oysters

FLAVOR BOOSTERS:

Garlic salt

Garlic powder

Lemon pepper

Old Bay Seasoning

Smoked paprika

SPICY KICKERS:

Kimchi

Prepared horseradish

Sriracha sauce

Tabasco sauce

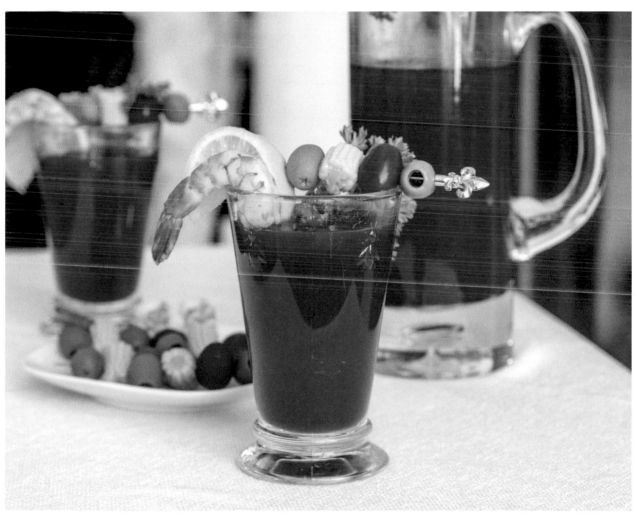

lemon-lime dateorade

I can't understand how sports drinks have become so popular that many people think they are actually an important component of a successful workout. The truth is, the vast majority of sports drinks are basically sugar water with some added electrolytes and artificial food dyes. Sure, you need water, and you should definitely replenish electrolytes, especially if you have been sweating. But nobody benefits from sugar and artificial food dyes! And it turns out you can get a great ratio of electrolytes from good old fruits and vegetables. But you also need liquid, so the idea of a "sports drink" does make sense if it contains water plus whole fruits and/or vegetables. This rejuvenating drink is made with dates, which are rich in electrolytes, especially potassium and magnesium, and contains sodium (another electrolyte) from an unrefined source (Himalayan pink salt), plus antioxidants from the lemon and lime juice. It's a nutritious and electrolyte-rich post-workout drink, and it's tasty, too. Even kids think so!

5 medjool dates, pitted (see Note)

3¾ cups water

¼ cup fresh lemon juice

¼ cup fresh lime juice

¼ teaspoon Himalayan pink salt

2 to 3 drops food-grade lemon essential oil, or 1 to 1½ teaspoons pure lemon extract (optional)

Ice, for serving (optional)

Fresh lemon slices, for garnish (optional)

Put all the ingredients except the ice and lemon slices in a blender and process until the dates are completely pureed. Divide among four 8-ounce glasses filled with ice, or pour into a pitcher and refrigerate for at least 4 hours to chill before serving. Garnish with lemon slices before serving, if desired.

STORAGE INFORMATION

Dateorade can be made up to 5 days in advance. It is best to process it again in the blender for about 30 seconds just before serving.

NOTE

If you're using a conventional blender rather than a high-powered one and your dates are on the dry side, soak them in water for 15 to 30 minutes to soften them before pureeing (very moist, succulent medjool dates do not require soaking).

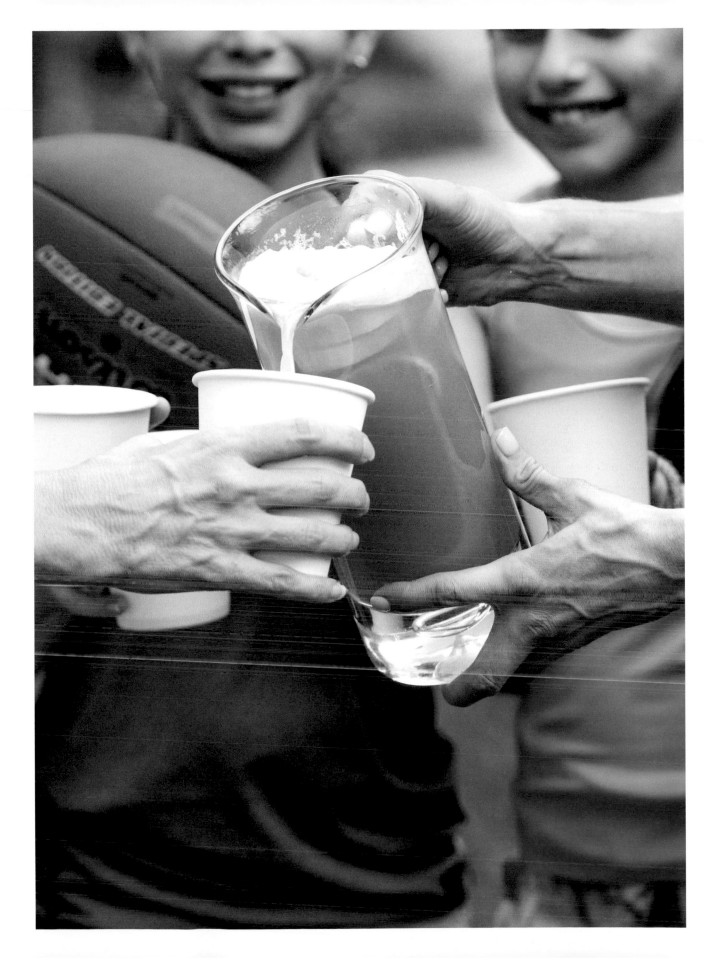

frozen raspberry-mango daiquiris

SERVES 2   PREP TIME: 10 minutes

Here in hot and sunny South Florida, chilled cocktails are always a big hit when my husband and I entertain friends. And this tart, tangy, and sweet combination of raspberry and mango always hits the spot! Since this recipe can easily be made kid-friendly by eliminating the rum, it makes for a versatile party staple, especially in the summer months.

3 ounces light rum

1 very ripe mango, peeled, pitted, and chopped (about 1¼ cups)

½ cup frozen raspberries

⅓ cup coconut water

¼ cup fresh lime juice

2 tablespoons pure maple syrup

1 cup ice cubes

For garnish (optional):

Fresh raspberries

Lime twists

Mango cubes

Place all the ingredients except the ice and garnishes in a blender and process until smooth and creamy. Add the ice and process again until no longer chunky. Divide between two 6-ounce glasses. Garnish with fresh raspberries, lime twists, and/or mango cubes, if desired, and serve immediately.

VARIATION: VIRGIN FROZEN RASPBERRY-MANGO DAIQUIRIS _____
Replace the rum with an equal amount of coconut water.

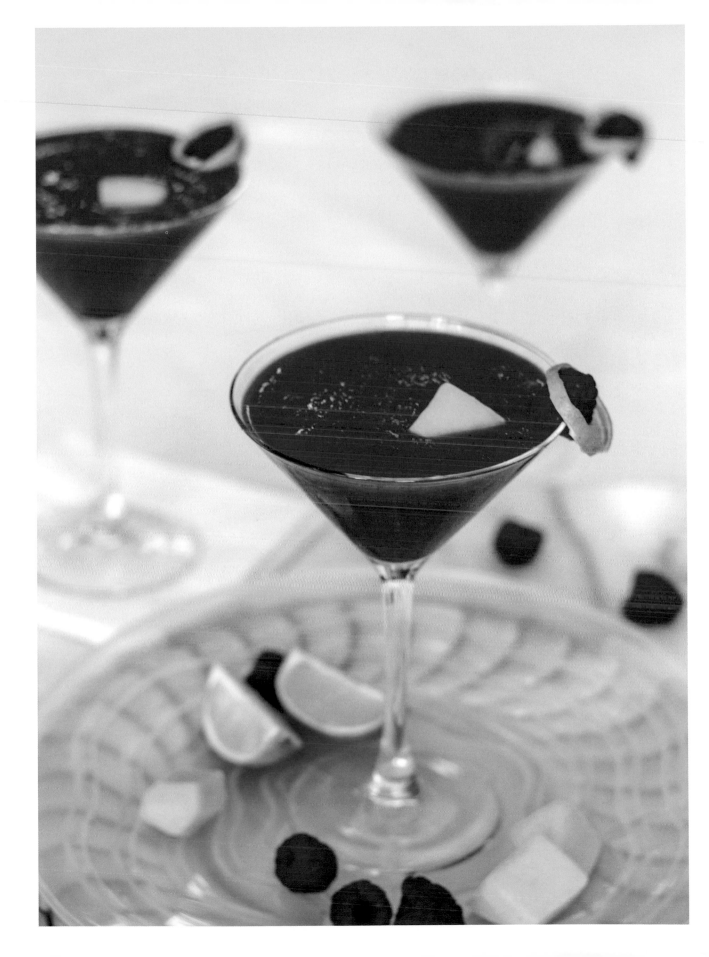

palm beach pineapple sangria

SERVES 4   PREP TIME: 10 minutes, plus time to chill

I couldn't do a cookbook without including a recipe inspired by my hometown, Palm Beach, and this pineapple sangria is it! It's a great cocktail for hot and sunny days, and it pairs perfectly with just about any seafood dish. Unlike conventional sangria recipes, this one is not particularly sweet, but you can definitely taste the pineapple and citrus. If you like a sweeter sangria, simply add a bit more honey.

3 cups chopped fresh pineapple (about 1 pineapple), divided

3 cups Sauvignon Blanc or other dry white wine (see Note)

3 to 4 tablespoons manuka honey or other raw honey

2 lemons, sliced

2 limes, sliced

1 orange, sliced

2 cups sparkling water, cold

For garnish (optional):

Fresh lemon slices

Fresh mint sprigs

Fresh orange slices

1. In a blender, puree 2 cups of the pineapple, the Sauvignon Blanc, and the honey until the mixture is smooth and lump-free. Pour the mixture into a serving pitcher. (Note: The pureed pineapple mixture is foamy at first but settles down once refrigerated.)

2. Add the remaining 1 cup of chopped pineapple and the lemon, lime, and orange slices. Cover and refrigerate for at least 12 hours or up to 48 hours.

3. Just before serving, pour in the cold sparkling water and stir everything together with a wooden spoon. Pour into four 6-ounce serving glasses and garnish with fresh mint, lemon slices, and/or orange slices, if desired. Serve cold.

NOTE

I like to use organic wines as much as possible (see page 44 for more on organic natural wine). For this recipe, I used organic Bonterra Sauvignon Blanc.

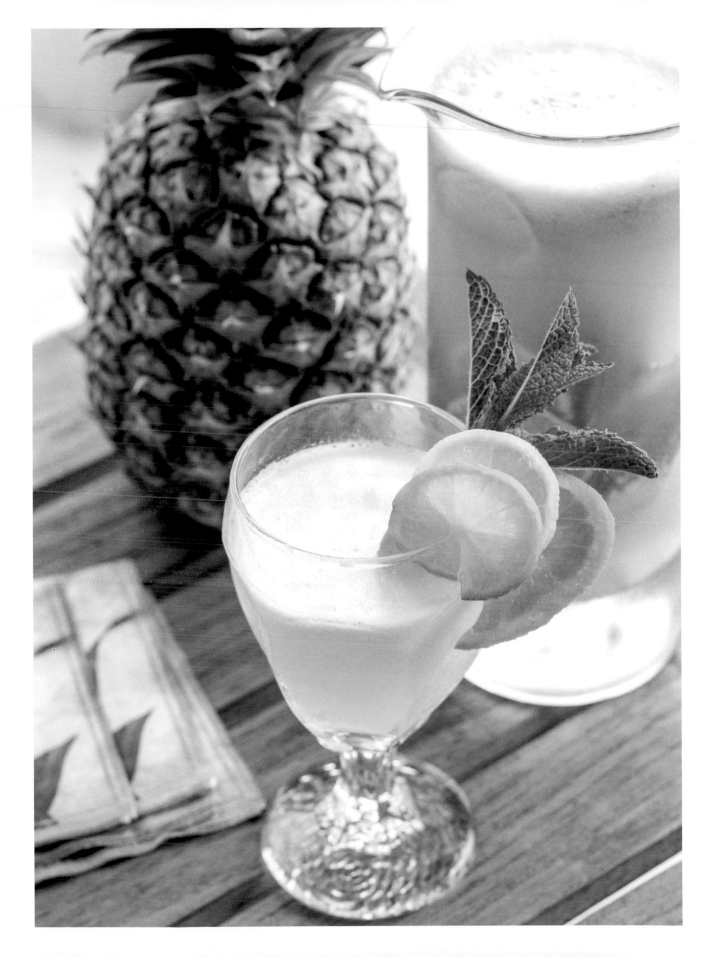

turmeric lemon toddy

When I was growing up, if either of my parents had insomnia or a bad cold, my dad would make his hot toddy remedy. It consisted of hot water, lemon juice, honey, and vodka, and it worked like a charm. I have used the basics of my dad's toddy recipe here but worked in a few additions: turmeric, for its anti-inflammatory benefits, and ground black pepper, to boost the absorption of the turmeric. Although it is an optional ingredient, I also like to add the superfood camu in the form of camu powder (see page 71). With a whopping ten times the amount of vitamin C found in an orange, just one teaspoon of camu powder will give you 760 percent of your daily recommended amount of vitamin C! And unlike refined vitamin C supplements, camu powder is a whole food, which means it contains everything your body needs to absorb and utilize the vitamin C.

⅓ cup fresh lemon juice

⅓ cup water

2 teaspoons raw honey

1 teaspoon turmeric powder

½ teaspoon camu powder (optional)

Pinch of ground black pepper

Pinch of Himalayan pink salt

2 ounces gluten-free unflavored vodka

1. Heat the lemon juice and water in a small saucepan or teapot over medium heat just until the liquid begins to boil. Remove the saucepan from the heat and stir in the honey until it dissolves. Add the turmeric, camu powder (if using), black pepper, and salt and stir to combine.

2. Pour the turmeric-lemon mixture into two 4-ounce cups and add an ounce of vodka to each. Serve warm.

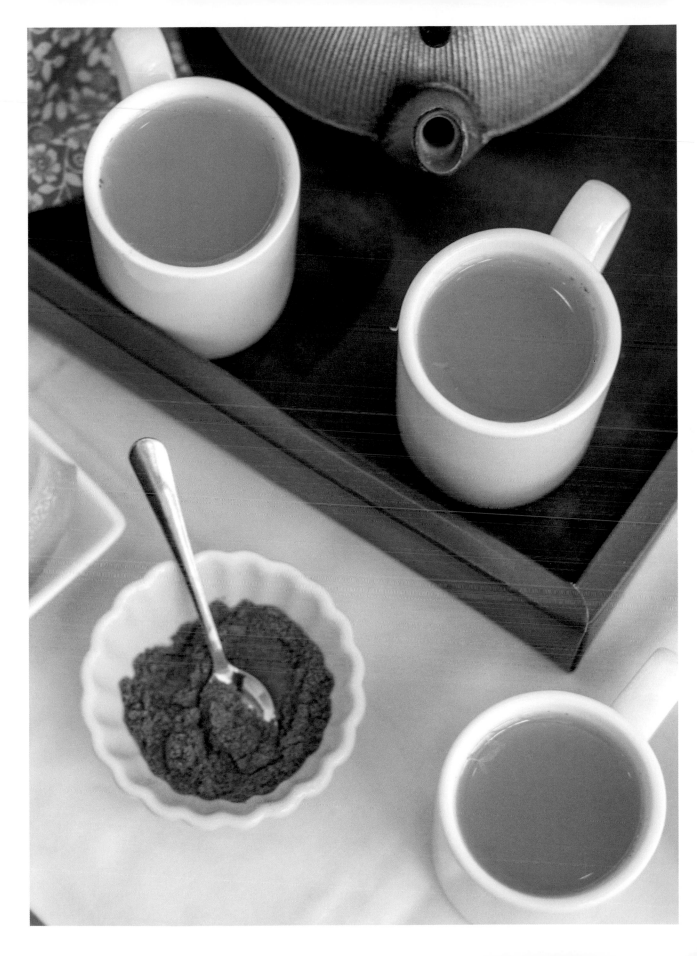

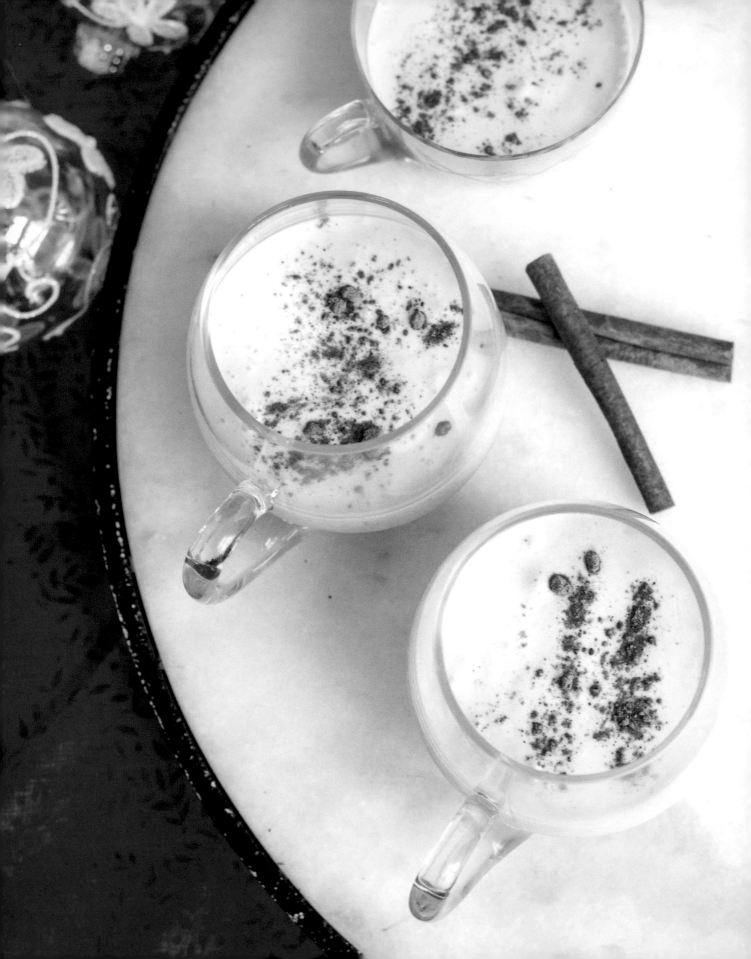

CHAPTER 16

no-milk shakes

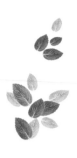

the best strawberry no-milk shake

SERVES 2   PREP TIME: 10 minutes

The first time I made this shake, I didn't measure anything. I just threw together a bunch of ingredients when making my husband a healthy shake after his workout. He doesn't usually rave about the post-workout shakes I make for him; he just dutifully drinks them down. But he couldn't stop saying how much he loved this one! I had to try to remember what was in it and test it a few times to get it just right. It's the best strawberry shake ever, if I do say so myself.

⅓ cup raw almonds, preferably soaked for 4 to 8 hours, then rinsed and drained (see Notes)

1 cup cold water

1½ cups frozen strawberries

3 medjool dates, pitted (see Notes)

1 tablespoon fresh lemon juice

½ teaspoon pure vanilla extract

½ cup ice cubes

2 fresh strawberries, for garnish (optional)

Place all of the ingredients except the ice and fresh strawberries in a blender in the order given in the ingredients list. Process on high until smooth and creamy. Add the ice and process again until smooth. Divide between two 8-ounce glasses, garnish each with a fresh strawberry, if desired, and serve immediately.

NOTES

If you're using a high-powered blender, soaking the almonds is optional, but it does create a creamier texture. If you're using a conventional blender instead of a high-powered one, soaking the almonds is necessary to get the right texture.

If you're using a conventional blender rather than a high-powered one and your dates are on the dry side, soak them in water for 15 to 30 minutes to soften them before pureeing (very moist, succulent medjool dates do not require soaking).

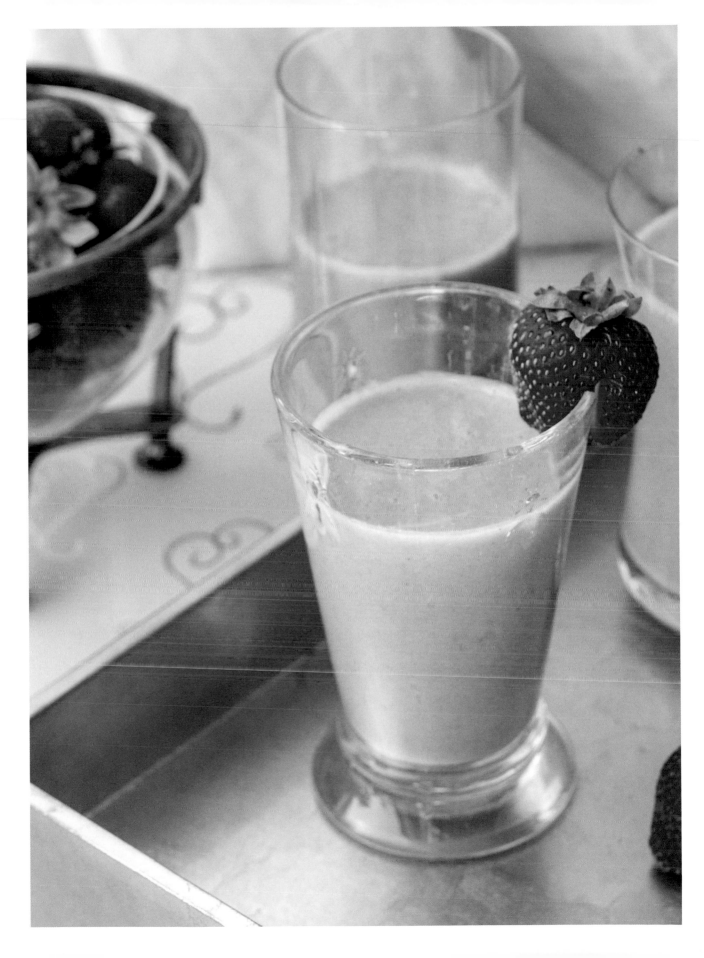

chocolate no-milk shake

SERVES 2   PREP TIME: 10 minutes

Shhh. Don't tell anyone this chocolate shake is made with cauliflower. Everyone finally seems to accept the idea that greens can be added to smoothies and shakes, but cauliflower isn't quite there yet (though I think once you taste this chocolate shake, you may start looking for more cauliflower shake recipes!). When it comes to using cauliflower in shakes or smoothies, frozen is the way to go. I have tested this shake recipe and several others using fresh cauliflower, and the results are not nearly as tasty. I think that is because frozen cauliflower is blanched just before it is frozen, and the combination of blanching and freezing mellows out the flavor a bit and makes for a better texture when pureed into a shake.

1½ cups water

⅓ cup gluten-free old-fashioned rolled oats

1 frozen banana, chopped

¾ cup frozen cauliflower florets

5 medjool dates, pitted (see Note)

¼ cup raw walnuts

2 tablespoons cacao powder

1 tablespoon pure maple syrup

1 teaspoon pure vanilla extract

Pinch of Himalayan pink salt

1½ cups ice cubes

Cacao nibs, for garnish (optional)

Put all of the ingredients except the ice and cacao nibs in a blender in the order given in the ingredients list. Process on high speed until smooth and creamy. Add the ice and process again until well blended. Divide between two 8-ounce glasses, garnish with cacao nibs, if desired, and serve immediately.

NOTE

If you're using a conventional blender rather than a high-powered one and your dates are on the dry side, soak them in water for 15 to 30 minutes to soften them before pureeing (very moist, succulent medjool dates do not require soaking).

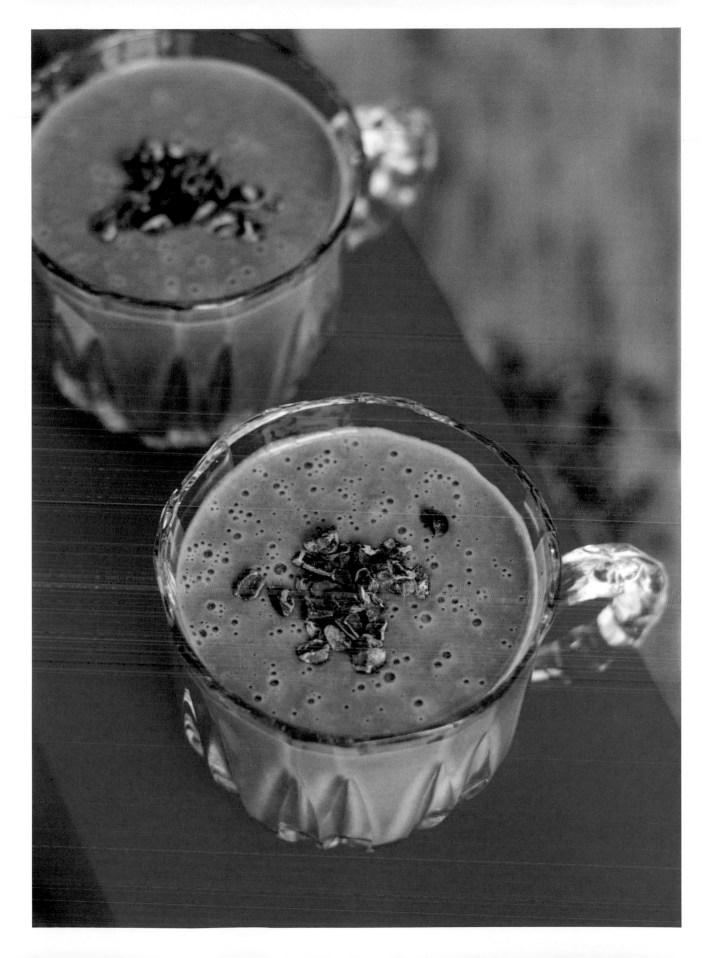

blackberry-lemon cobbler no-milk shake

SERVES 2   PREP TIME: 15 minutes

I always get new recipe ideas when we travel, and this one was inspired by a family trip to New York City. We went to the Big Apple with my nieces (who had never been to the city!), and when I asked them where they wanted to eat, Black Tap was at the top of their dining wish list. Black Tap is one of the city's hot spots, serving up giant milkshakes that are apparently a very big deal these days—especially with preteen girls on Instagram. When we got home, I came up with this recipe as a #NoRegrets clean alternative. It could very well end up being your favorite no-milk shake of all time! PS: You'll need a spoon to eat it.

2 cups frozen blackberries, partially thawed

½ cup plus 3 tablespoons water, divided

2 tablespoons plus 2 teaspoons fresh lemon juice, divided

2 tablespoons pure maple syrup

¼ cup gluten-free old-fashioned rolled oats

¼ cup raw walnuts

½ teaspoon pure lemon extract

3 medjool dates, pitted (see Notes)

Pinch of Himalayan pink salt

½ cup ice cubes

1. Put the blackberries, ¼ cup of the water, 2 teaspoons of the lemon juice, and the maple syrup in a blender. Process on high for about 1 minute, or until the ingredients are well blended. (Note: You may need to add 1 or 2 more tablespoons of water if the blackberries are not thawed enough.) Transfer the blackberry puree to a separate container and rinse the blender jar.

2. Put the remaining ¼ cup plus 3 tablespoons of water, remaining 2 tablespoons of lemon juice, oats, walnuts, lemon extract, dates, and salt into the clean blender jar and process on high speed until the mixture is smooth and creamy, about 1 minute. Add the ice and process again until smooth, about 20 seconds.

3. Using a spoon, divide half of the blackberry puree between two 10-ounce glass mugs or two mason jars. Pour equal amounts of the walnuts-and-oats mixture on top of the blackberry puree. Spoon half of the remaining blackberry puree on top of each glass. Drink at once!

NOTES

If you're using a conventional blender rather than a high-powered one and your dates are on the dry side, soak them in water for 15 to 30 minutes to soften them before pureeing (very moist, succulent medjool dates do not require soaking).

This recipe makes two large smoothies but could easily serve three in smaller 6-ounce glasses.

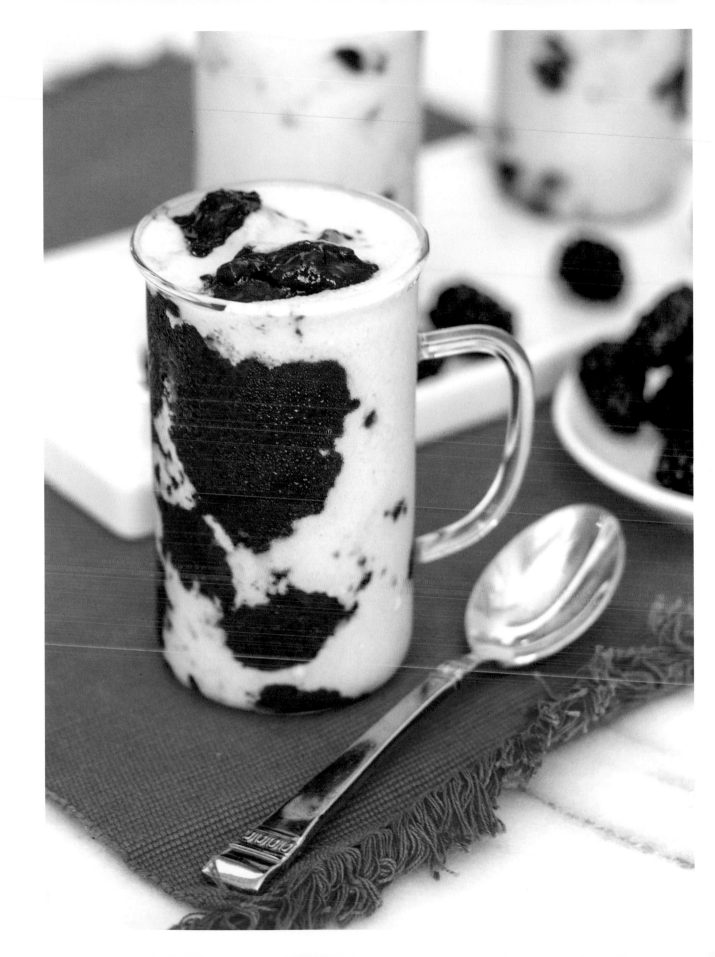

mint chocolate chip no-milk shake

SERVES 2 PREP TIME: 10 minutes

The legendary Girl Scout cookie called Thin Mints was the inspiration for this one! The shake is very rich and creamy, which makes it rather filling. If you want to thin it out a bit, it's best to add a bit more ice rather than more water. You can also freeze this shake in an ice pop mold to make mint chocolate chip ice pops.

¾ cup coconut cream (see page 74)

¾ cup spinach

¾ cup water

⅓ packed cup fresh mint leaves, plus more for garnish if desired

1 tablespoon pure maple syrup

⅛ teaspoon pure peppermint extract

4 medjool dates, pitted (see Note)

Pinch of Himalayan pink salt

1½ cups ice cubes

⅓ cup unsweetened cacao nibs, plus more for garnish if desired

1. Put all of the ingredients except the ice and cacao nibs in a blender and process on high speed until smooth and creamy. Add the ice and process again until smooth.

2. Stir in the cacao nibs; do not blend again. Divide the shake between two 8-ounce glasses and serve immediately, garnished with a fresh mint leaf or two and some cacao nibs, if desired.

NOTE

If you're using a conventional blender rather than a high-powered one and your dates are on the dry side, soak them in water for 15 to 30 minutes to soften them before pureeing (very moist, succulent medjool dates do not require soaking).

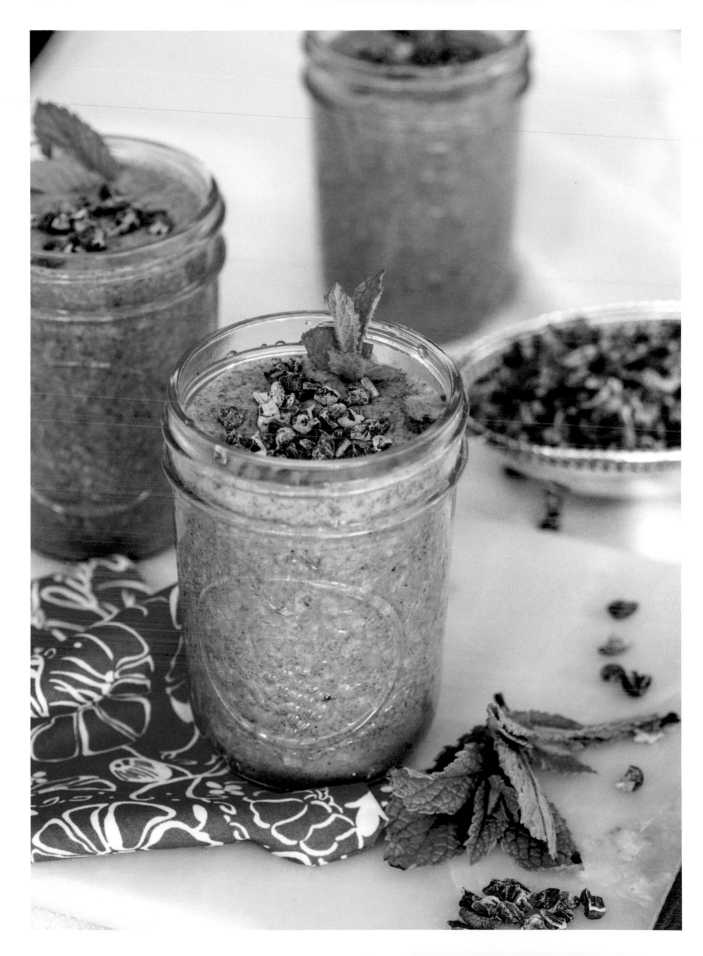

red velvet no-milk shake

SERVES 2   PREP TIME: 5 minutes

I came up with this recipe the day before Hurricane Irma was forecast to hit South Florida. It had been five days of preparing for what we all thought might be a Category 5 hurricane, and let's just say that, despite all of my mood-boosting tricks (fish oil, turmeric, etc.), nobody in the house was very happy. I had roasted some beets the night before and planned to use them to make a clean red velvet cake—yes, I still test recipes even when a hurricane is on its way!—but I was out of eggs and every single grocery store in town was already closed for the hurricane. I decided to turn my cake idea into a shake, and it was the only thing that went right that day!

1 small roasted beet, chopped (about ½ cup), chilled or at room temperature (see right)

1 cup frozen cherries, plus more (thawed) for garnish if desired

½ cup cacao powder

½ cup coconut cream (see page 74)

1 cup chilled water

1 cup ice cubes

8 medjool dates, pitted (see Note)

½ teaspoon pure vanilla extract

1 teaspoon gelatinized maca root powder (optional)

1 tablespoon pure maple syrup (optional)

Pinch of Himalayan pink salt

Puffed gluten-free whole-grain cereal, for garnish (optional)

Put all of the ingredients except the cereal in a blender in the order given in the ingredients list. Process on high until smooth and creamy. Divide between two 6-ounce glasses. Garnish with the puffed cereal and/or additional cherries, if desired. Serve at once.

NOTE

If you're using a conventional blender rather than a high-powered one and your dates are on the dry side, soak them in water for 15 to 30 minutes to soften them before pureeing (very moist, succulent medjool dates do not require soaking).

MAKE IT GRAIN-FREE
Omit the cereal topping.

HOW TO ROAST BEETS
Scrub the beets and wrap them separately in foil. Place them on a rimmed baking sheet and roast in a preheated 400°F oven for 40 to 45 minutes, until fork-tender. Remove the beets from the oven and allow them to cool until easy to handle (but still warm), then slip off the skins.

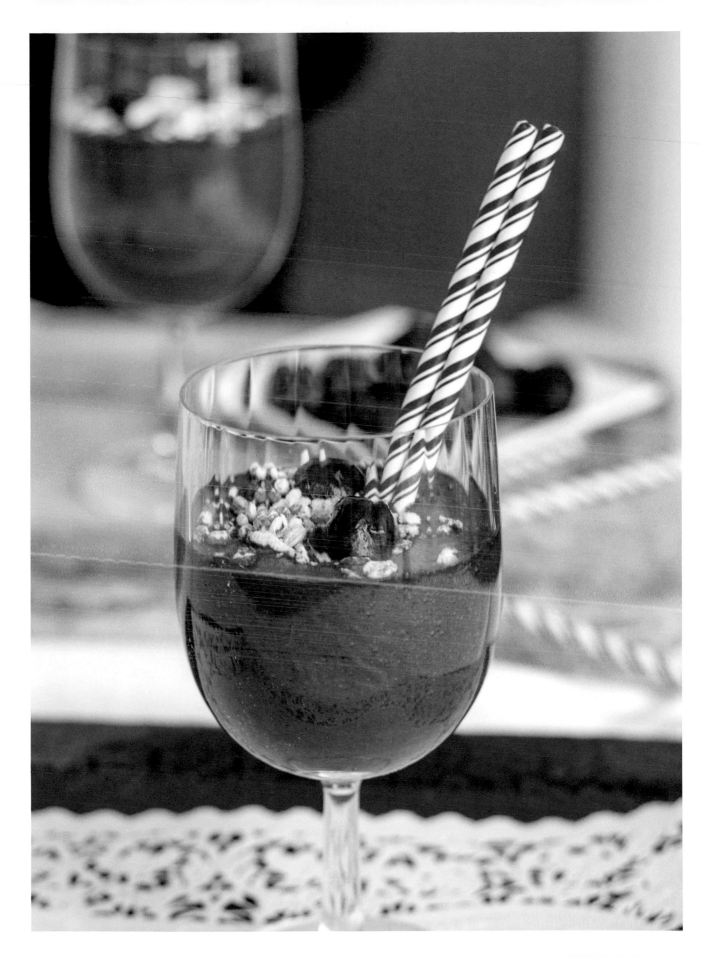

orange cream no-milk shake

SERVES 4   PREP TIME: 5 minutes

Creamsicles are classic American comfort food. At least they were for me! They were one of my favorite store-bought treats growing up. Once I started eating clean, I discovered that there was a very special something-something about a Creamsicle that I just couldn't replicate, no matter how many times I tried. So I gave up. But then one day, while I was making shakes, I accidentally discovered the secret: clementines! A cross between a sweet orange and a mandarin orange, clementines are a small, very sweet, and usually seedless fruit. Using clementines gives this clean shake that special flavor I remember from childhood.

4 very cold clementine oranges, peeled

4 medjool dates, pitted

⅓ cup coconut cream (see page 74)

1 tablespoon pure vanilla extract

2 teaspoons fresh lemon juice

1 to 2 teaspoons manuka honey or other raw honey

1 teaspoon grated clementine orange zest

2 cups ice cubes

Put all of the ingredients except the ice in a high-powered blender and process on high speed until smooth and creamy. Add the ice and process again until smooth. Divide among four 6-ounce glasses and serve at once.

NOTE

Because of the fiber in the clementines, I recommend using a high-powered blender for this shake.

SPECIAL TOOLS

High-powered blender

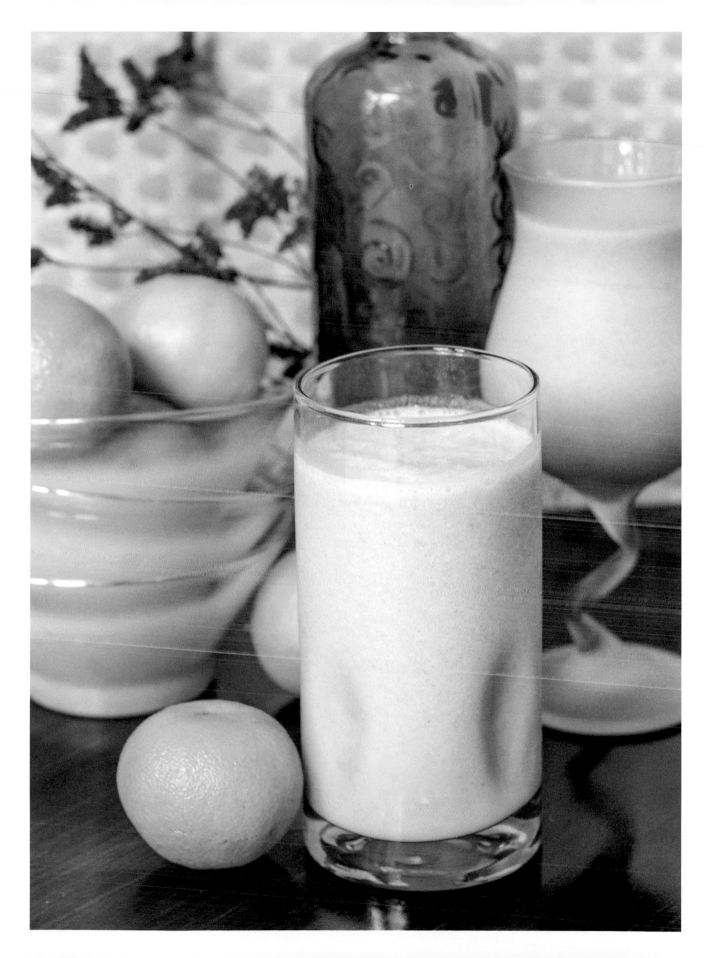

roasted peach cobbler no-milk shake

SERVES 2   PREP TIME: 10 minutes   COOK TIME: 22 minutes

My favorite summer shake! You will definitely want to make this one when peaches are ripe and juicy. I have tried to make it a few times with not-so-ripe peaches, and the results just are not the same. But if you have really ripe peaches in season, this shake takes the cake! Roasting the peaches brings out their natural sweetness. Nobody will even notice there's a whole cup of cauliflower slipped in! PS: No time to roast peaches? No worries! See the notes below for how to use frozen peaches instead.

2 peaches (see Notes)

½ cup water

1 cup frozen cauliflower florets

5 or 6 medjool dates, pitted (see Notes)

1 teaspoon ground cinnamon

2 tablespoons fresh lemon juice

½ cup raw pecans

1 tablespoon plus 1 teaspoon pure maple syrup (optional)

2 cups ice cubes

Chopped raw pecans, for garnish (optional)

1 stick cinnamon, for garnish (optional)

1. To roast the peaches, preheat the oven to 400°F. Slice the peaches in half and remove the pits (leave the skins on). Place the peaches cut side up on a rimmed baking sheet and roast for about 22 minutes, until fork-tender. Remove from the oven and let cool to room temperature.

2. Put the cooled roasted peaches and the rest of the ingredients in a blender, in the order given in the ingredients list. Process on high until smooth and creamy. Divide between two 8-ounce cups, garnish with chopped pecans and a cinnamon stick, if desired, and serve right away.

NOTES

If you don't have access to fresh, ripe peaches or don't have time to roast them, you can still make one super-delicious smoothie using frozen, but fully thawed, sliced peaches. To replace the two roasted peaches, you will need one 10-ounce bag of frozen sliced peaches.

If you're using a conventional blender rather than a high-powered one and your dates are on the dry side, soak them in water for 15 to 30 minutes to soften them before pureeing (very moist, succulent medjool dates do not require soaking).

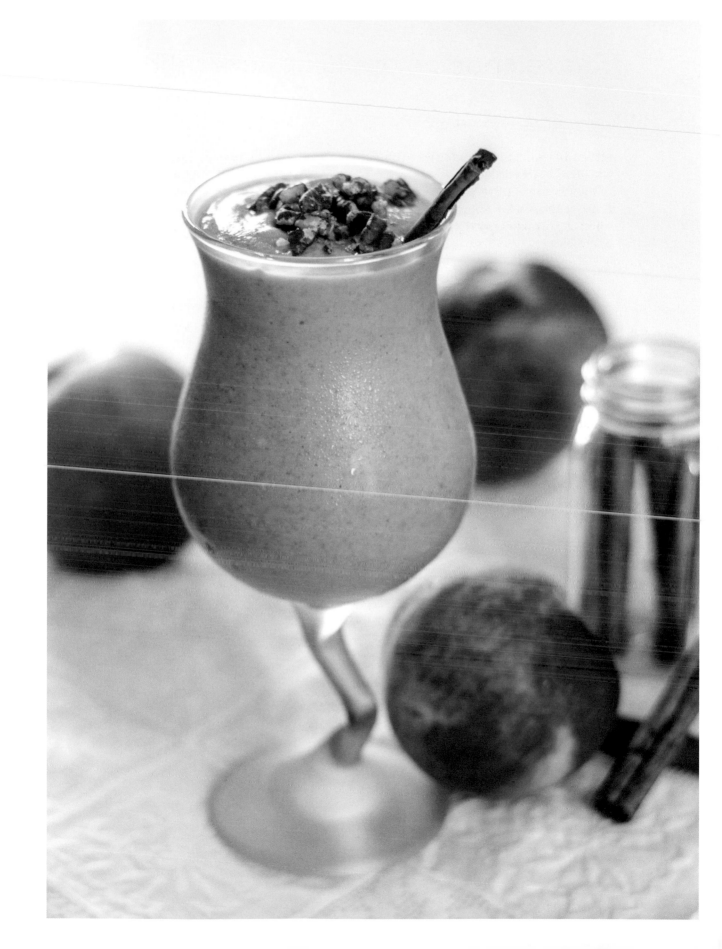

hot cinnamon apple no-milk shake

SERVES 2   PREP TIME: 10 minutes   COOK TIME: 5 minutes, plus time to cool

Where we live in South Florida, a sixty-degree day is sweater weather. It doesn't get cold very often, but when it does, I like to have a hot drink. I first made this one for my son when he was in elementary school, and it is still one of his favorites! The fragrant cinnamon not only boosts flavor but also has anti-inflammatory, antioxidant, and antiaging benefits. The phytonutrients found in cinnamon also stabilize blood sugar levels, prevent fat-storing in-sulin spikes, and, most amazingly, turn on genes within the body that produce highly pro-tective anti-inflammatory substances. And if all that isn't enough to make you want to start putting cinnamon on everything you eat, it can even boost the appearance of your skin and help protect against premature sun damage (which is especially helpful if you are exposed to sun year-round, as I am). But you can't just sprinkle on a teeny-tiny dash of cinnamon; you need to eat at least ¼ teaspoon a day or so in order to really get the benefits. This recipe has ½ teaspoon per serving, so it is definitely enough to make a difference!

---

2 apples, cored and cut into chunks (leave the skin on)

1¾ cups water, divided

¼ cup raisins

1 teaspoon ground cinnamon

½ cup raw walnuts

1 tablespoon fresh lemon juice

Pinch of Himalayan pink salt

For garnish (optional):

Chopped raw walnuts

Diced apples

Ground cinnamon and/or cinnamon sticks

1. Place the apple chunks, 1 cup of the water, the raisins, and the cinnamon in a small saucepan and heat over medium-high heat until the water boils and the apples soften, about 5 minutes. Remove the saucepan from the heat and let the apples and the water cool for about 5 minutes (see Note).

2. Transfer the cooled apple-raisin mixture (including the liquid) to a blender along with the remaining ¾ cup of water, the walnuts, lemon juice, and salt. Process on high speed for 1 full minute, until the mixture is smooth and creamy.

3. Transfer the mixture back to the saucepan and heat for about 1 minute, or until warm. Pour into two 6-ounce coffee mugs and garnish with the chopped walnuts and apples and a dusting of cinnamon and/or cinnamon sticks, if desired. Drink warm.

NOTE _____

WARNING: If you have a glass blender jar, you need to be extra careful to let the ingredients cool almost to room temperature before you put them in the blender; otherwise, the glass jar could explode and cause serious injury.

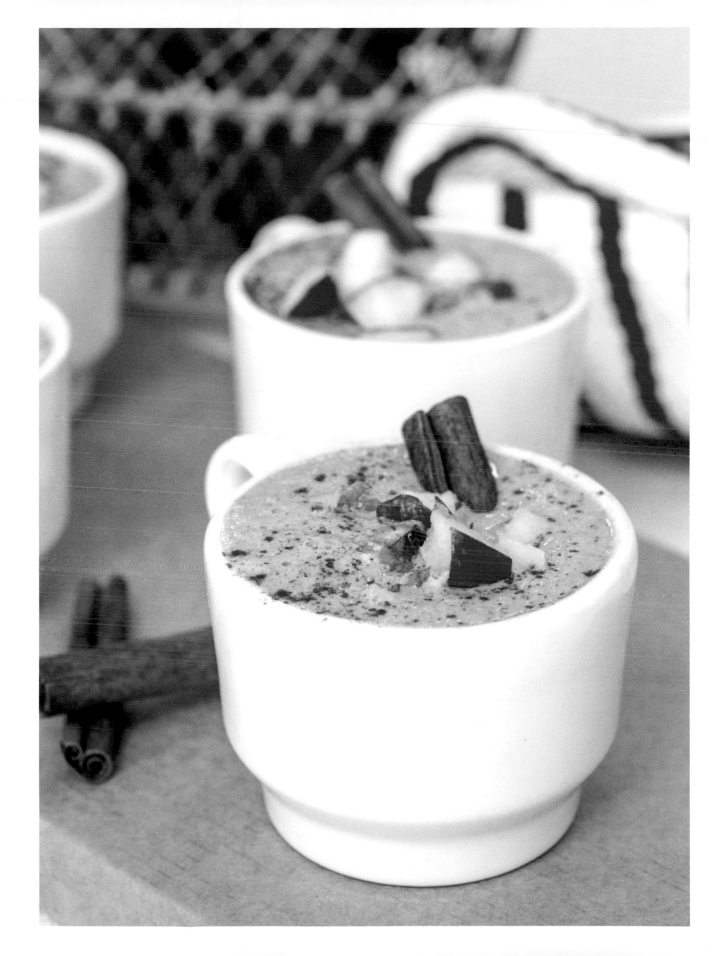

egg nog no-milk shake

SERVES 4   PREP TIME: 7 minutes

As soon as we wrap up Thanksgiving, I start making this shake for the holiday season! I realize it may seem very bah-humbug of me to suggest eliminating the key ingredients (dairy, eggs, and sugar) that make egg nog so deliciously decadent. But even *Bon Appétit* featured a recipe for dairy-free egg nog a few years back. Even when you push the envelope and eliminate the ingredients you think must surely be essential—not to mention add a few that are most definitely not traditional (like cauliflower!)—you still end up with a rich and decadent treat that should bring back fond memories for any fellow egg nog lover.

---

1 cup very cold water

½ cup plus 2 tablespoons cold full-fat coconut milk

3 to 5 medjool dates, pitted (see Notes)

2 tablespoons pure maple syrup

¼ cup raw almonds, preferably soaked for 4 to 8 hours, then rinsed and drained (see Notes)

1 frozen banana, cut into bite-sized pieces

½ cup frozen cauliflower florets

¾ cup ice cubes

½ teaspoon ground cinnamon

2 teaspoons pure vanilla extract

¼ teaspoon ground nutmeg

⅛ teaspoon ground cloves

Pinch of Himalayan pink salt

2 ounces Disaronno Originale or other amaretto liqueur (optional; see Notes)

For garnish (optional):

Cinnamon sticks or ground cinnamon

Ground nutmeg

Place all of the ingredients except the garnishes in a blender in the order given in the ingredients list. Process until smooth and creamy. Divide among four 8-ounce glasses, garnish with cinnamon sticks, ground cinnamon, and/or ground nutmeg, if desired, and serve at once.

STORAGE INFORMATION

This shake can be stored in a covered container in the refrigerator for up to 2 days. Shake well before serving.

NOTES

If you're using a conventional blender rather than a high-powered one and your dates are on the dry side, soak them in water for 15 to 30 minutes to soften them before pureeing (very moist, succulent medjool dates do not require soaking).

If you're using a high-powered blender, soaking the almonds is optional, but it does create a creamier texture. If you're using a conventional blender instead of a high-powered one, soaking the almonds is necessary to get the right texture.

A splash (or two!) of Disaronno adds a touch of magic to any egg nog recipe. Although classic spiked egg nog typically includes brandy, rum, or bourbon, I prefer the sweet almond flavor of amaretto. I am especially fond of the Italian-made Disaronno Originale. If you are buying it only for the egg nog recipe, you can just pick up a few miniature bottles. However, I always keep a large bottle stashed in our home bar; it's the perfect liqueur to pour over fresh fruit (peaches are my favorite in the summer, baked apples in the fall and winter) as a super-simple and elegant dessert for entertaining.

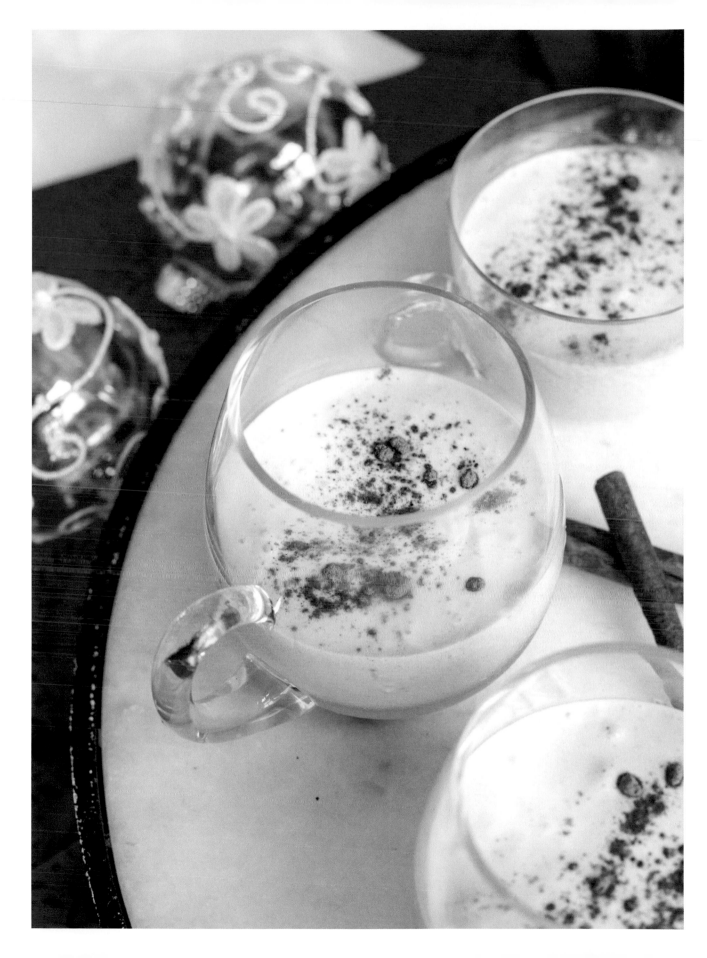

cherry almond no-milk shake

SERVES 1   PREP TIME: 5 minutes

This is my go-to shake when I am low on fresh produce in the house, especially after returning from a trip. I always have frozen cherries and frozen cauliflower on hand, though, along with all of the other ingredients, so this is always a quick, easy, and satisfying shake to make in a pinch. I can't tell you how many times I have sipped this one while unpacking! And don't worry, I promise you will not taste even a hint of cauliflower.

1 cup water

¼ cup raw almonds, preferably soaked for 4 to 8 hours, then rinsed and drained (see Notes)

¾ cup frozen cauliflower

¾ teaspoon pure almond extract

1 cup frozen cherries

3 medjool dates, pitted (see Notes)

¾ cup ice cubes

Pinch of Himalayan pink salt

Chopped raw almonds, for garnish (optional)

Place all the ingredients except the garnish in a blender in the order given in the ingredients list. Process on high speed until smooth and creamy. Pour into a 12-ounce or larger glass, garnish with chopped almonds, if desired, and serve at once.

NOTES

If you're using a high-powered blender, soaking the almonds is optional, but it does create a creamier texture. If you're using a conventional blender instead of a high-powered one, soaking the almonds is necessary to get the right texture.

If you're using a conventional blender rather than a high-powered one and your dates are on the dry side, soak them in water for 15 to 30 minutes to soften them before pureeing (very moist, succulent medjool dates do not require soaking).

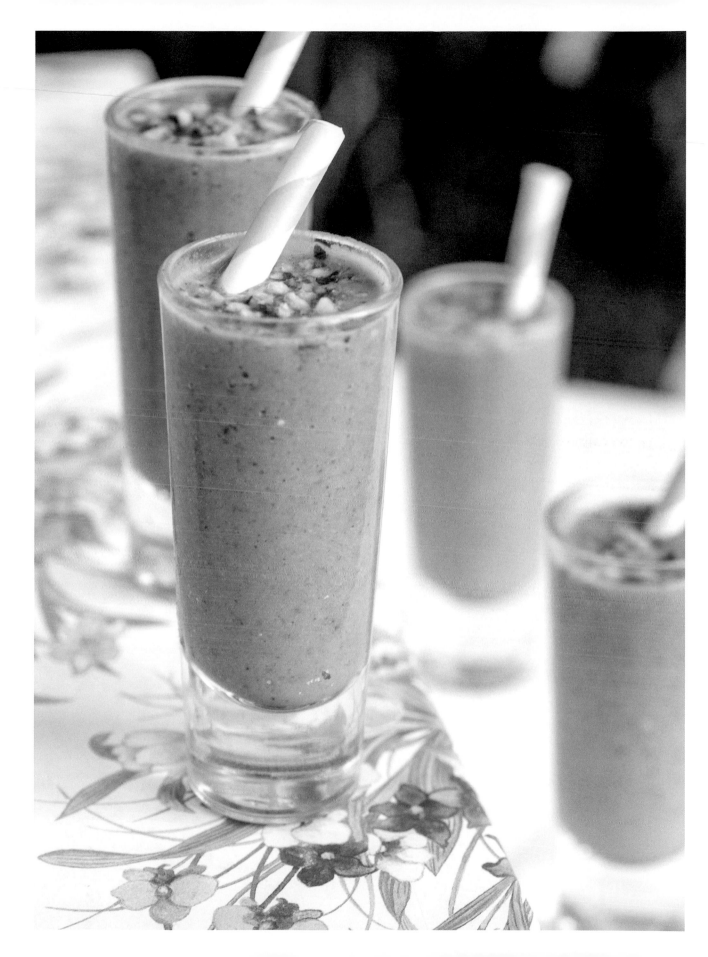

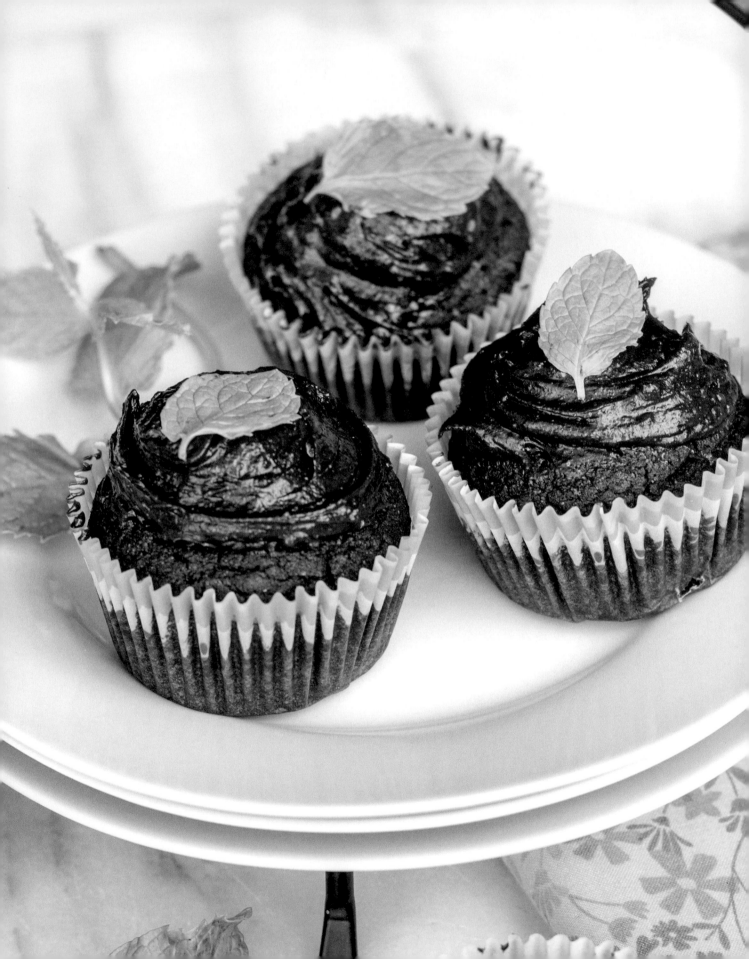

CHAPTER 17

no-regrets
sweet treats

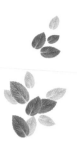

raspberry-lemon panna cotta

SERVES 4   PREP TIME: 10 minutes, plus time to chill   COOK TIME: 5 minutes

An easy Italian custard, panna cotta is one of those simple, classic desserts I wish I had learned to make years ago. After our family trip to Italy one summer, I came home on a big panna cotta kick. Over the course of a few months I made just about every flavor of panna cotta possible. This raspberry-lemon combination is my favorite. Not only does it make for an easy, elegant, and delicious dessert, it's incredibly healthy. In fact, you could easily serve this panna cotta as a make-ahead breakfast instead of yogurt.

For the custard:

2½ cups full-fat coconut milk, divided

2½ teaspoons unflavored gelatin (see Note, page 122)

2 drops food-grade lemon essential oil, or 2 teaspoons pure lemon extract

¼ cup plus 2 tablespoons pure maple syrup

1 tablespoon fresh lemon juice

2 pinches Himalayan pink salt

For the raspberry topping:

2 cups fresh raspberries

2 tablespoons coconut sugar

1 drop food-grade lemon essential oil, or 1 teaspoon pure lemon extract

2 tablespoons grated lemon zest, for garnish

1. To make the custard, put ½ cup of the coconut milk in a small bowl. Whisk in the gelatin and lemon essential oil. Allow the mixture to sit for 5 minutes.

2. Meanwhile, in a small saucepan, warm the remaining 2 cups of coconut milk, the maple syrup, lemon juice, and salt over low heat until tiny bubbles start to form, about 3 minutes, whisking occasionally with a fork. Remove the mixture from the heat and let sit for 5 minutes.

3. Whisk the coconut-gelatin mixture slowly into the warm coconut–maple syrup mixture until completely smooth and the gelatin is dissolved. Divide the mixture evenly among 4 small bowls or fancy glasses (5 or 6 ounces each) and refrigerate for at least 4 hours, or until firm.

4. When the panna cotta is ready to serve, make the raspberry topping: Place the raspberries, coconut sugar, and lemon essential oil in a medium-sized bowl and gently toss together (be careful not to smash the raspberries). Spoon the raspberry mixture on top of the panna cotta and sprinkle with the lemon zest. Serve chilled. (Note: Once the custards are topped with the berries, they should be eaten the same day.)

STORAGE INFORMATION _____
Panna cotta can be stored in a covered container in the refrigerator for up to 1 day.

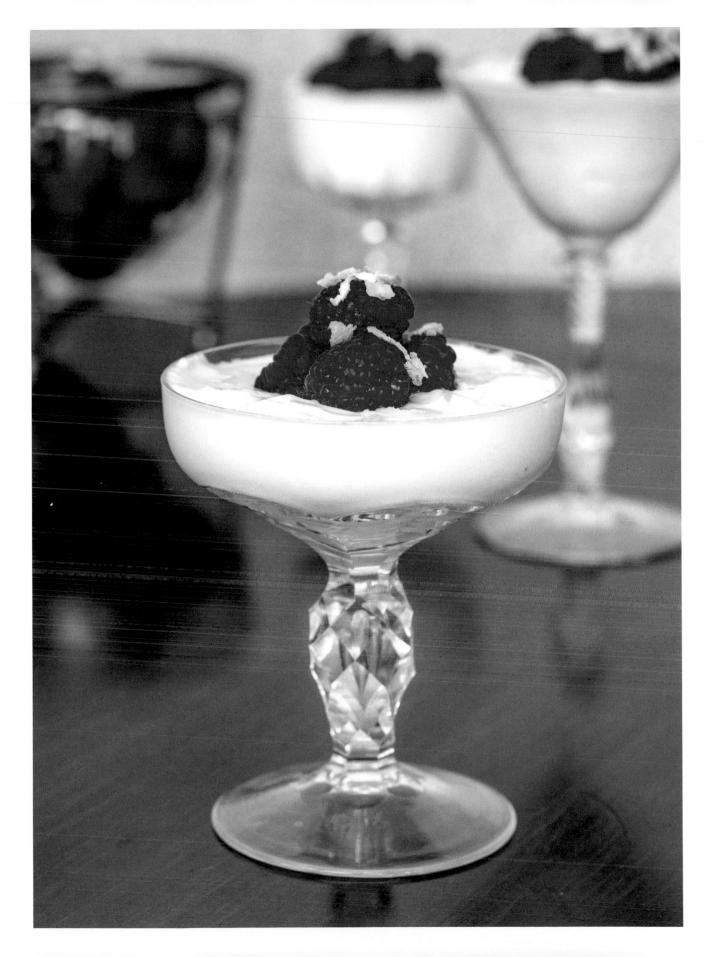

gingerbread spice cake

MAKES one 9-inch loaf cake (10 servings)   PREP TIME: 20 minutes
COOK TIME: 50 to 55 minutes

As soon as October rolls around, I start thinking of this gingerbread spice cake, which tastes just like gingerbread cookies. But unlike typical gingerbread cookies, this cake is super moist. Over the years, I have tweaked the recipe to make it healthier and tastier. This is the first gluten-free version I have ever made, but it's my favorite one so far! And I have to say, three-day-old gingerbread spice cake makes the best Christmas-morning French toast ever—just dip thick slices of cake into a mixture of almond milk, eggs, and vanilla, then cook them in a coconut-oiled skillet over medium-high heat. So good!

1 cup cassava flour (or sprouted spelt flour if not gluten- or grain-free)

¾ cup gluten-free oat flour

¼ cup brown rice flour

¼ cup ground flax seeds

1 teaspoon baking soda

1 teaspoon ground cinnamon

¼ teaspoon ground allspice

¼ teaspoon Himalayan pink salt

¼ cup plus 1 tablespoon extra-virgin coconut oil, melted, plus more for the pan

½ cup plus 2 tablespoons coconut sugar

1 large egg

1 cup thawed frozen butternut squash puree or roasted and pureed butternut squash

½ cup full-fat coconut milk

¼ cup blackstrap molasses

¼ cup unsweetened applesauce

1 tablespoon grated fresh ginger

1 tablespoon pure vanilla extract

1. Preheat the oven to 375°F. Coat a 9 by 5-inch loaf pan with coconut oil.

2. In a large bowl, whisk the flours, ground flax seeds, baking soda, cinnamon, allspice, and salt until blended.

3. In a blender, process the coconut oil, coconut sugar, and egg until smooth and creamy. Add the butternut squash puree, coconut milk, molasses, applesauce, ginger, and vanilla extract and process again until well blended. Add the wet ingredients to the dry ingredients and mix with a wooden spoon until smooth and lump-free.

4. Pour the batter into the greased pan and smooth the top with the back of the wooden spoon. Bake on the middle rack of the oven until a toothpick inserted into the center of the cake comes out clean, 50 to 55 minutes. Cool in the pan for 10 minutes before turning the cake out onto a wire rack to cool completely.

STORAGE INFORMATION _____

Gingerbread spice cake will keep in a zip-top bag for 3 days in the refrigerator or up to 1 month in the freezer.

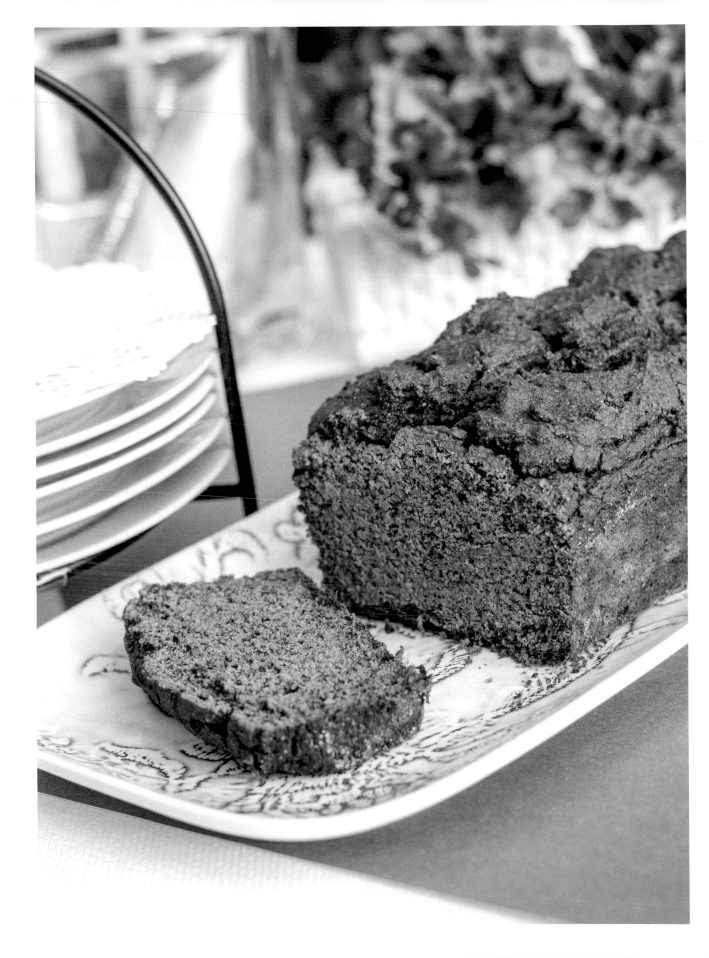

black forest ice cream

MAKES 1 pint   PREP TIME: 5 minutes, plus time to churn and freeze the ice cream

My family is really into making homemade ice cream (I'm sure it has something to do with the fact we live in South Florida!). If you have never made ice cream, it might sound like a rather elaborate process. But thanks to modern ice cream makers, it's one of the easiest desserts to make. This recipe, which borrows the classic chocolate-and-cherry flavors of a Black Forest cake, requires only a quick blend of ingredients—no cooking, hardly any mess. And then bliss…

1⅓ cups partially thawed frozen cherries, divided

1¼ cups cold coconut cream (see page 74)

¾ cup raw cashews, preferably soaked in water for 1 to 2 hours, then rinsed and drained (see Notes)

½ cup cacao powder

⅓ cup pure maple syrup

¼ cup cold water

4 medjool dates, pitted (see Notes)

2 teaspoons pure vanilla extract

Pinch of Himalayan pink salt

1 cup fresh cherries, pitted and sliced in half, for garnish (optional)

1. Put ⅓ cup of the partially thawed frozen cherries in a blender; set the remaining cup aside. Add the rest of the ingredients, except the fresh cherries, to the blender and process until smooth and creamy. Transfer the blender jar with this chocolate ice cream base to the freezer to chill while you proceed with step 2.

2. Put the reserved cup of partially thawed cherries in a food processor and pulse several times until the cherries are just barely chopped (be careful not to overprocess). Gently fold the chopped cherries into the chocolate ice cream base.

3. Pour the mixture into an ice cream maker and churn the ice cream, following the manufacturer's instructions. Transfer to a freezer-safe container and place in the freezer for about 15 minutes to firm up a bit. Serve garnished with fresh cherries, if desired.

STORAGE INFORMATION

This ice cream will keep in an airtight container in the freezer for 1 week. Once it's frozen solid, set the ice cream on the counter to soften for 10 or 15 minutes before serving.

NOTES

For best results, regardless of the type of blender you're using, the cashews should be soaked before using.

If you're using a conventional blender rather than a high-powered one and your dates are on the dry side, soak them in water for 15 to 30 minutes to soften them before pureeing (very moist, succulent medjool dates do not require soaking).

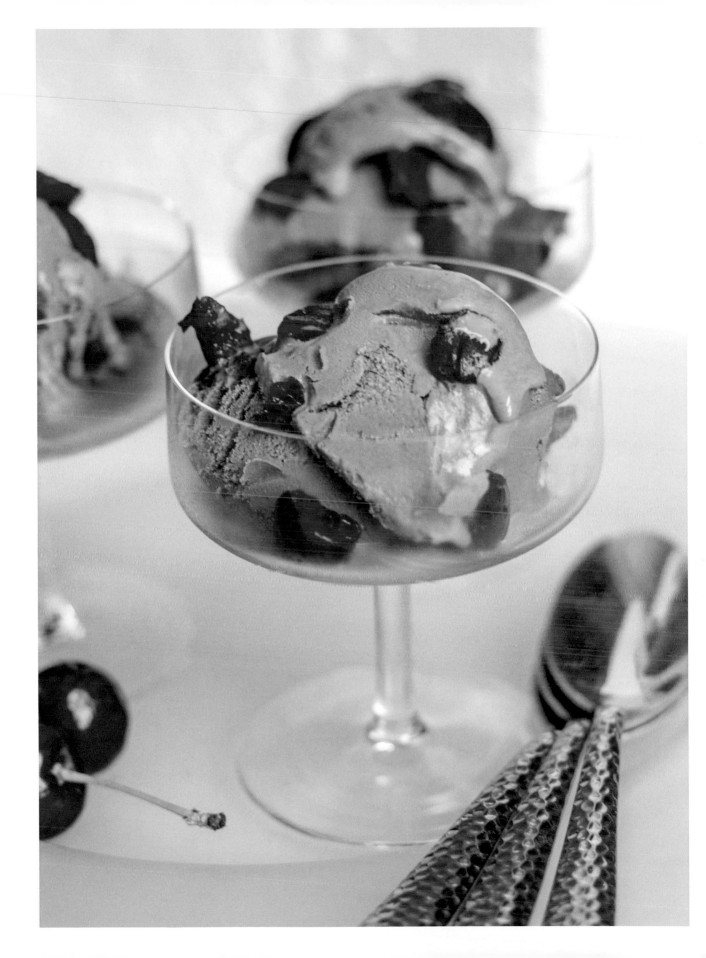

key lime pie ice cream

MAKES 2 pints   PREP TIME: 5 minutes, plus time to chill and time to churn the ice cream

My husband loves Key lime pie so much we even served it at our wedding! It is his absolute favorite dessert of all time, so I wanted to find a way to get the flavors of Key lime pie in ice cream. I came up with this recipe as a way to use up the abundance of avocados from our backyard tree. Our backyard avocados are the Florida variety, but I also tested the recipe with Hass avocados, and it is every bit as tasty! As with the oatmeal raisin cookie recipe on page 336, it's important here to use very ripe avocados so that they will puree nicely and disappear into the dish.

1¼ cups mashed, very ripe avocado (about 2 Florida avocados or 3 Hass avocados), chilled

¾ cup coconut cream (see page 74)

½ cup plus 2 tablespoons fresh Key lime juice (see Notes)

¼ cup pure maple syrup

5 medjool dates, pitted (see Notes)

1 teaspoon pure vanilla extract

¼ teaspoon Himalayan pink salt

1. Put all of the ingredients in a blender and process until smooth and creamy. Transfer the blender jar with the ice cream base to the freezer to chill for 30 minutes.

2. Pour the mixture into an ice cream maker and churn the ice cream, following the manufacturer's instructions. Serve immediately for soft-serve consistency or transfer the ice cream to a freezer-safe container and freeze until hardened, about 2 hours.

STORAGE INFORMATION
This ice cream will keep in an airtight container in the freezer for 1 week. Once it's frozen solid, set the ice cream on the counter to soften for 10 or 15 minutes before serving.

NOTES
You really do need to use real Key lime juice for the best results with this recipe. Standard lime juice simply will not give you the tart and tangy taste of a Key lime pie. If you don't have access to fresh Key limes, look for a bottle of Nellie & Joe's Famous Key West Lime Juice. It is sold nationwide at most supermarkets, but you can also buy it online.

If you're using a conventional blender rather than a high-powered one and your dates are on the dry side, soak them in water for 15 to 30 minutes to soften them before pureeing (very moist, succulent medjool dates do not require soaking).

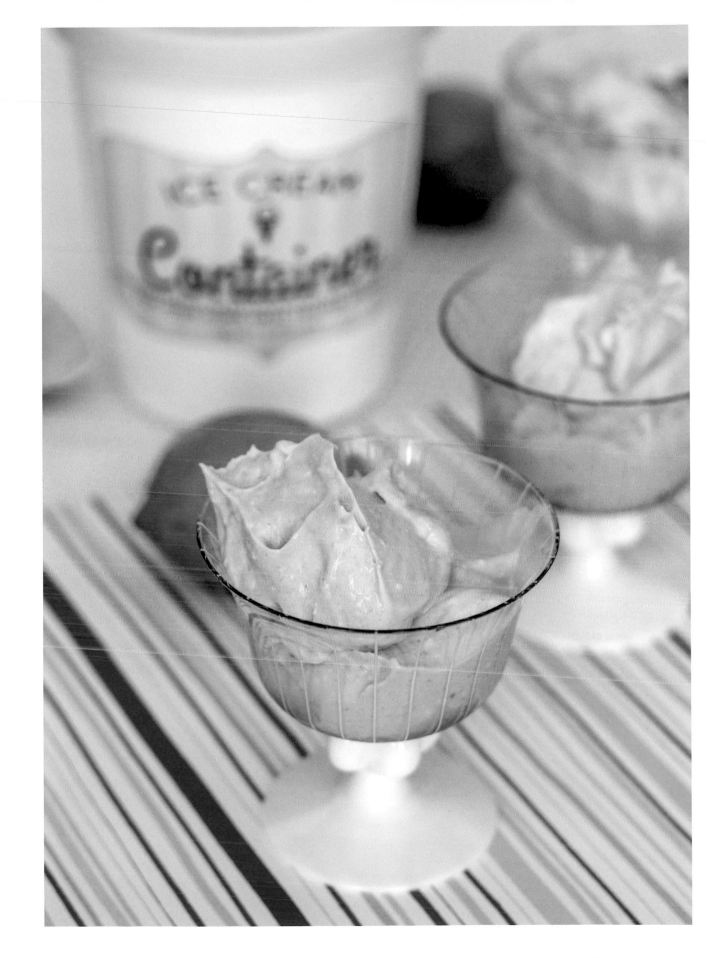

oatmeal raisin cookies

MAKES about 16 cookies   PREP TIME: 20 minutes   COOK TIME: 15 minutes

I'll admit, baking butter-free cookies that taste amazing can be a bit of a challenge. Baking butter-free cookies that are also free of refined sugar and gluten takes the challenge up a notch. Believe it or not, though, the combination of avocado and coconut oil makes a wonderful substitute for butter. If you have been disappointed with gluten-free cookie recipes in the past, don't worry—you won't be with this one!

2 cups gluten-free old-fashioned rolled oats

1 cup blanched almond flour

1 cup cassava flour (or sprouted spelt flour if not gluten- or grain-free)

1 teaspoon ground cinnamon

½ teaspoon baking powder

½ cup plus 2 tablespoons pure maple syrup

½ cup plus 1 tablespoon extra-virgin coconut oil, softened

¼ cup mashed very ripe Hass avocado (about ⅓ avocado)

1 tablespoon pure vanilla extract

½ teaspoon Himalayan pink salt

1¼ cups raisins

2 cups boiling water

¾ cup chopped raw walnuts (optional)

1. Preheat the oven to 350°F. Line 2 baking sheets with parchment paper.

2. In a large bowl, whisk together the oats, almond flour, cassava flour, cinnamon, and baking powder.

3. In another bowl, combine the maple syrup, coconut oil, avocado, vanilla, and salt; whisk until well mixed. Pour the mixture into the dry ingredients and stir well. Set aside.

4. Place the raisins in a medium-sized bowl, add the boiling water, and soak for 10 minutes. Pour through a fine-mesh strainer and pat the raisins dry with paper towels to remove as much moisture as possible. Add the raisins and walnuts (if using) to the cookie dough and mix until combined.

5. Using a lightly oiled ¼-cup measuring cup, scoop the cookie dough onto the prepared baking sheets, spaced ½ inch apart. Flatten the mounds of dough slightly and bake for 15 minutes, or until golden around the edges. Using a spatula, carefully transfer the cookies to a wire rack to cool. The cookies will be crumbly and very soft when you first remove them from the oven, but they will harden as they cool.

STORAGE INFORMATION _____

These cookies are best stored in a covered container in the freezer. They will keep for up to 4 weeks.

MAKE IT NUT-FREE _____
Omit the walnuts.

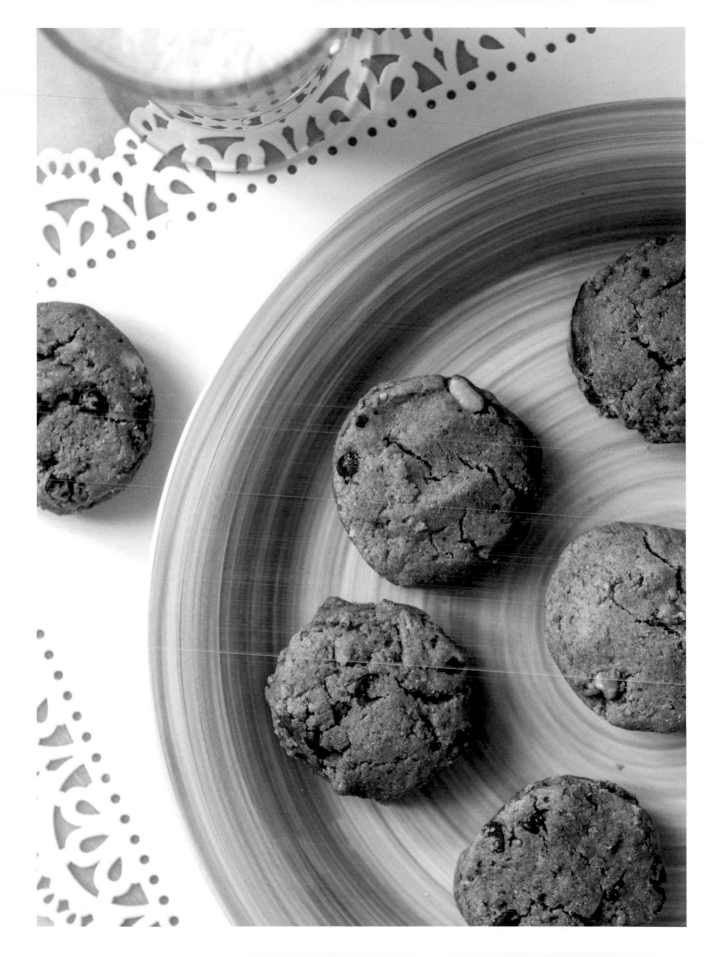

mint chocolate cupcakes
with mint chocolate frosting

MAKES 1 dozen cupcakes   PREP TIME: 30 minutes   COOK TIME: 20 minutes

I initially created this recipe as a three-layer cake for my dad's eighty-ninth birthday several years ago. It's to-die-for delicious, if I do say so myself. If I were ever to compete on *Cupcake Wars*, this is the recipe I would make! It's impossible to tell that it is dairy-free and gluten-free and has no refined sugar.

For the cupcakes:

¾ cup cassava flour (or sprouted spelt flour if not gluten- or grain-free)

⅓ cup cacao powder

¼ cup plus 2 tablespoons gluten-free oat flour

½ teaspoon baking powder

½ teaspoon baking soda

¼ teaspoon Himalayan pink salt

1 cup almond milk, homemade (page 368) or store-bought, or hemp milk

⅓ packed cup fresh mint leaves

¼ cup plus 2 tablespoons coconut sugar

¼ cup pure maple syrup

3 tablespoons melted extra-virgin coconut oil

1 teaspoon pure peppermint extract

1 large egg

For the frosting:

¾ cup raw cashews, preferably soaked for 1 to 2 hours, then rinsed and drained (see Note)

¼ packed cup fresh mint leaves

3 tablespoons cacao powder

3 tablespoons pure maple syrup

2 tablespoons coconut butter or coconut manna, softened

2 tablespoons water

½ teaspoon pure peppermint extract

Pinch of Himalayan pink salt

For garnish (optional):

12 fresh mint leaves

TO MAKE THE CUPCAKES:

1. Preheat the oven to 350°F. Line a standard-size 12-well muffin tin with paper liners.

2. In a medium-sized bowl, whisk together the cassava flour, cacao powder, oat flour, baking powder, baking soda, and salt. Set aside.

3. Put the almond milk, mint, coconut sugar, maple syrup, coconut oil, peppermint extract, and egg in a blender. Process on high speed until the ingredients are well blended, about 1 full minute.

4. Add the wet ingredients to the dry ingredients and mix well until thoroughly blended.

5. Divide the batter among the muffin wells, filling each about three-quarters full. Bake until a toothpick inserted in the center of a cupcake comes out clean, about 20 minutes. Transfer the cupcakes to a wire rack. Allow to cool completely before frosting.

TO MAKE THE FROSTING: Place all the frosting ingredients in a blender or food processor and process until smooth and creamy. (Note: You will likely need to stop the blender or food processor several times and scrape down the sides with a rubber spatula.) If the frosting seems too thick to spread easily, add up to 1 tablespoon more of water. Top the cooled cupcakes with the frosting and garnish each with a fresh mint leaf, if desired.

For best results, regardless of the type of blender you're using, the cashews should be soaked before using.

STORAGE INFORMATION _____

These cupcakes will keep in a covered container in the refrigerator for up to 2 days.

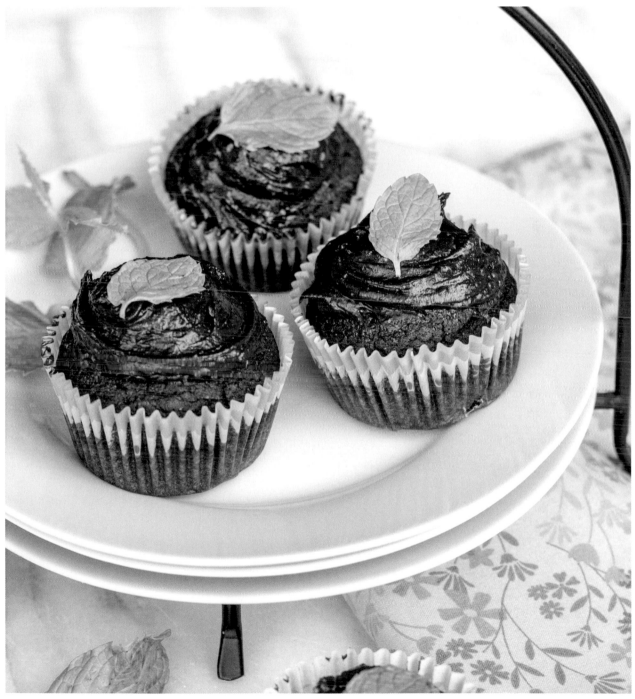

pineapple upside-down cake

MAKES one single-layer 9-inch cake   PREP TIME: 20 minutes, plus time to chill the cake
COOK TIME: 1 hour 5 minutes

A conventional recipe for pineapple upside-down cake calls for about 1 cup of refined sugar. This one uses just 3 tablespoons of unrefined coconut sugar. But don't worry, it's still every bit as desirably sticky-sweet as the real deal! I originally made this recipe with sprouted spelt flour, and it was absolutely delicious. But everyone in the family prefers this gluten-free version. The spelt version is fluffier and lighter, but somehow with pineapple upside-down cake, the denser, gluten-free version just seems to work better. If you are not gluten-free, you can always use 1½ cups sprouted spelt flour (standard spelt flour would also work) instead of the sorghum and cassava flour.

---

2 (20-ounce) cans unsweetened pineapple rings, drained

3 tablespoons coconut sugar

1 cup sorghum flour

½ cup cassava flour (or sprouted spelt flour if not gluten- or grain-free)

2 teaspoons baking powder

1 teaspoon ground cardamom

¼ teaspoon Himalayan pink salt

8 medjool dates, pitted (see Note)

¾ cup almond milk, homemade (page 368) or store-bought, or ½ cup coconut milk plus ¼ cup water

½ cup extra-virgin coconut oil, softened, plus more for the pan

½ cup pineapple puree (made from about ¾ cup chopped fresh or frozen pineapple)

3 tablespoons dark rum, divided

1 tablespoon pure vanilla extract

2 large eggs

4 to 6 fresh cherries, pitted and sliced in half

1. Preheat the oven to 350°F.

2. Gently press the liquid out of the pineapple rings using a paper towel. Set the pineapple aside.

3. Generously grease a 9-inch springform pan with about 1 tablespoon of coconut oil, using your hands to distribute the oil evenly on the bottom and sides of the pan. Sprinkle the coconut sugar on the bottom of the pan. Arrange two layers of pineapple rings on top of the sugar. Set the pan aside.

4. In a medium-sized mixing bowl, whisk together the sorghum flour, cassava flour, baking powder, cardamom, and salt. Make a well in the center of the dry ingredients. Set aside.

5. Place the dates, almond milk, coconut oil, pineapple puree, 1 tablespoon of the rum, vanilla extract, and eggs in a blender. Process on high speed until the mixture is smooth and creamy. Pour the mixture into the well in the dry ingredients. Whisk the ingredients together thoroughly but briefly, until just combined; do not overmix the batter.

6. Pour the batter on top of the pineapple rings. Bake for 1 hour 5 minutes, or until a knife inserted in the middle comes out clean.

7. Remove the cake from the oven and transfer to a cooling rack. Once the cake is at room temperature, transfer it to the refrigerator to chill for 30 minutes (this will firm up the cake).

8. To unpan the cake, invert a plate over the springform pan, keeping the plate and pan firmly pressed together. Flip the plate and pan over so the plate is on the bottom and remove the outer ring of the pan and then the bottom. Drizzle the remaining 2 tablespoons of rum over the cake. Add the cherry halves to the center of each pineapple ring for decoration. Slice and serve!

NOTE _____
*If you're using a conventional blender rather than a high-powered one and
your dates are on the dry side, soak them in water for 15 to 30 minutes to
soften them before pureeing (very moist, succulent medjool dates do not
require soaking).*

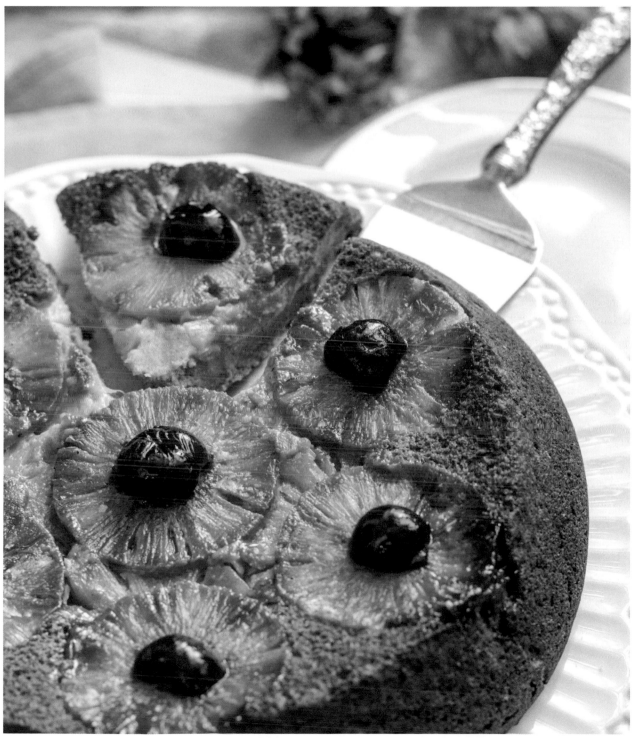

pumpkin custard

SERVES 4   PREP TIME: 15 minutes, plus time to chill the custards   COOK TIME: 50 to 55 minutes

Sometimes it is hard to re-create a favorite childhood recipe when you grow up. Lucky for me, Libby's Famous Pumpkin Pie recipe is still printed on the back of their canned pumpkin puree—so I knew where to start in making a clean version of the pumpkin pie of my childhood memories. This custard is a super-clean, quick, and easy way to satisfy a pumpkin pie craving. It's a much better choice than what I tried when I decided to eat "healthy" for Thanksgiving when I was about fourteen years old. I ate just the store-bought frozen crust of Grandma's pumpkin pie: it wasn't sweet, so I thought it must be the healthiest part. (I didn't know the refined flour and partially hydrogenated oil in store-bought pie crust is every bit as unhealthy as sugar!) Luckily, my teenage "health kick" didn't last longer than Thanksgiving dinner that year!

---

3 tablespoons hemp seeds

1 cup water

11 Deglet Noor dates, or 8 medjool dates, pitted (see Note)

¾ cup unsweetened pumpkin puree

⅓ cup raw walnuts

1 teaspoon pure vanilla extract

1 teaspoon grated fresh ginger

3 large eggs

1½ teaspoons ground cinnamon

¼ teaspoon ground allspice

⅛ teaspoon ground cloves

⅛ teaspoon Himalayan pink salt

½ teaspoon turmeric powder

For garnish (optional):

Whipped coconut cream (see page 346)

Chopped raw walnuts

1. Preheat the oven to 350°F. Lightly oil the bottom and sides of four 4-ounce ramekins. Fill a roasting pan with ¼ inch of water and place the ramekins in the water.

2. Put all of the ingredients in a blender in the order given in the ingredients list. Process on high speed until smooth and creamy, about 1 minute.

3. Pour the pumpkin mixture into the prepared ramekins, filling each about three-quarters full. Bake for 50 to 55 minutes, until set. Let cool to room temperature, then refrigerate for at least 45 minutes before serving. If desired, unmold into pretty serving dishes. Top with whipped coconut cream and/or chopped walnuts, if desired.

NOTE

If you're using a conventional blender rather than a high-powered one and you're using Deglet Noor dates or your medjool dates are on the dry side, soak them in water for 15 to 30 minutes to soften them before pureeing (very moist, succulent medjool dates do not require soaking).

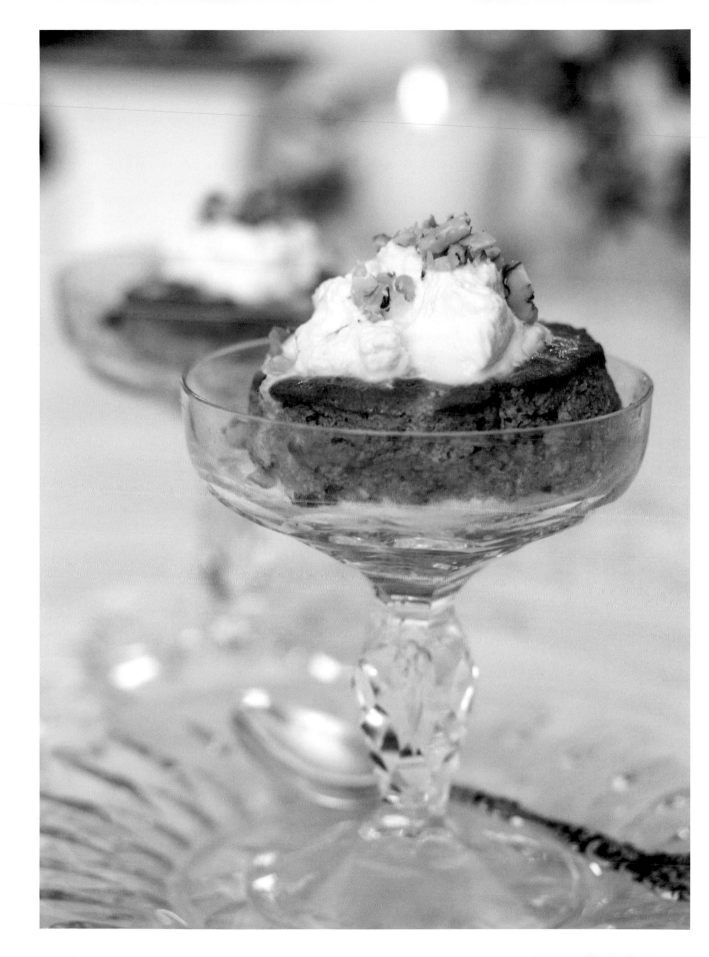

best brownies ever

MAKES 1 dozen brownies   PREP TIME: 15 minutes   COOK TIME: 33 to 35 minutes

If you are a chocolate fanatic (like me!), then you have to stop whatever you are doing and make these brownies right this minute. Seriously. The fact that they are gluten-free, grain-free, dairy-free, made with an unrefined vegetable-based flour, and have no refined sugar is beside the point. I truly think they could very well be the very best brownies you have ever had. Ever.

⅓ cup plus 1 tablespoon cacao powder

⅓ cup cassava flour (or sprouted spelt flour if not gluten- or grain-free)

⅛ teaspoon Himalayan pink salt

3 large eggs

½ cup plus 2 tablespoons pure maple syrup

½ cup extra-virgin coconut oil, softened, plus more for the pan

¼ cup unsweetened applesauce

10 medjool dates, pitted (see Note)

1 tablespoon pure vanilla extract

1 cup chopped raw pecans or walnuts

1. Preheat the oven to 325°F. Lightly oil the sides of an 8-inch square baking dish and line the bottom with parchment paper.

2. In a medium-sized mixing bowl, whisk together the cacao powder, cassava flour, and salt. Set the mixture aside.

3. Put the eggs, maple syrup, coconut oil, applesauce, dates, and vanilla extract in a high-powered blender or food processor. Process on high speed until smooth and creamy.

4. Add the wet ingredients to the dry and mix well with a wooden spoon. Stir in the nuts.

5. Pour the batter into the prepared baking dish and bake for 33 to 35 minutes, until a toothpick inserted in the middle comes out clean. Remove from the oven and allow to cool slightly. Cut into 12 squares and serve warm.

STORAGE INFORMATION

Brownies can be stored in a covered container in the refrigerator for up to 5 days or in the freezer for up to 3 weeks. For the best-tasting results, warm refrigerated or thawed brownies in the microwave for 1 minute on high before serving.

NOTE

If you're using a food processor and your dates are on the dry side, soak them in water for 15 to 30 minutes to soften them before pureeing (very moist, succulent medjool dates do not require soaking).

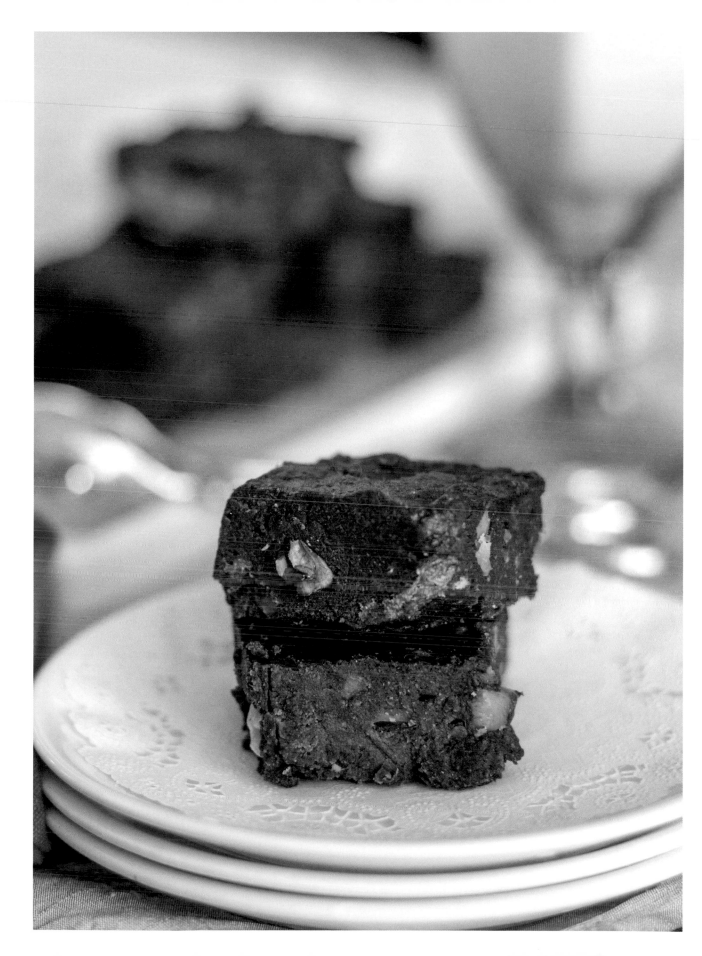

strawberry shortcake

SERVES 10   PREP TIME: 40 minutes   COOK TIME: 33 to 35 minutes

It's hard to go wrong serving strawberry shortcake. As American as apple pie, it's the perfect summer treat for just about any occasion. The first time I made this recipe was for a Memorial Day barbecue at our house. It overshadowed everything else on the menu! If you have never made strawberry shortcake, you will be surprised by how easy it is. As with all recipes, though, I suggest you read the instructions carefully before you begin. And no, the hard-boiled egg yolks are not a misprint! Pulsing hard-boiled egg yolks in with the flour is an old Northern European baker's secret that delivers incredibly tender baked goods.

For the shortcakes:

2 hard-boiled egg yolks

¾ cup cassava flour (or sprouted spelt flour if not gluten- or grain-free)

½ cup plus 1 tablespoon gluten-free oat flour

¼ cup masa harina corn flour

3 tablespoons coconut sugar, plus more for sprinkling

1 tablespoon baking powder

¼ teaspoon Himalayan pink salt

¼ cup plus 2 tablespoons cold extra-virgin coconut oil

⅔ cup plus 2 tablespoons coconut cream (see page 74), divided

For the whipped coconut cream:
(Makes about ⅔ cup)

½ cup cold coconut cream (see page 74)

1 tablespoon coconut sugar, plus more to taste (optional)

½ teaspoon pure vanilla extract

Pinch of Himalayan pink salt

1. Preheat the oven to 350°F. Line a baking sheet with parchment paper. Place a mixing bowl and beaters or whisk attachment for an electric mixer in the freezer for making the whipped coconut cream.

2. To make the shortcakes, place the egg yolks, cassava flour, oat flour, masa harina, coconut sugar, baking powder, and salt in a food processor and pulse to combine. Add the coconut oil and pulse just until the coconut oil is well incorporated into the flour (no portion of the flour should be dry); do not overmix. Add ⅔ cup of the coconut cream, then pulse two or three times to barely incorporate. Transfer the dough to a lightly floured work surface and gently knead several times just to ensure the oil is thoroughly blended.

3. Use a 2-ounce ice cream scoop to make 10 small balls and place them on the lined baking sheet about ½ inch apart. Do not flatten. (Note: If you do not have an ice cream scoop, you can measure out 2 heaping tablespoons of dough instead.) Cover and place in the freezer until cold, about 15 minutes.

4. Meanwhile, make the whipped coconut cream: Remove the chilled bowl and beaters or whisk attachment from the freezer. Put the ½ cup of cold coconut cream in the bowl and beat with an electric mixer on the highest speed until soft peaks form. Add the coconut sugar (if using), vanilla extract, and salt and continue beating for a couple more minutes, until soft peaks form. Set the whipped coconut cream in the refrigerator.

5. Remove the shortcakes from the freezer, brush the tops with the remaining 2 tablespoons of coconut cream, and sprinkle a little coconut sugar on top of each. Bake until golden and the sides are firm to the touch, 33 to 35 minutes. When the shortcakes are done, remove them from the oven and let them cool on a cooling rack for at least 15 minutes.

For the strawberry topping:

2 pounds fresh strawberries, hulled and halved or quartered if large

¼ cup coconut sugar

1 teaspoon grated lemon zest

Pinch of Himalayan pink salt

2 tablespoons water

1 tablespoon arrowroot

1 tablespoon fresh lemon juice

Fresh mint leaves, for garnish (optional)

STORAGE INFORMATION

This dessert does not store well after it has been assembled. However, the shortcakes can be made up to 2 days in advance and stored in the refrigerator in a covered container. The strawberry sauce can be made up to 5 days in advance and stored in a covered container in the refrigerator.

6. While the shortcakes are baking, make the strawberry topping: Put the strawberries, coconut sugar, lemon zest, and salt in a medium-sized bowl and gently toss to combine. Transfer half of the strawberries to a large saucepan and add the water. Cook the strawberries over medium-low heat, stirring frequently, for about 15 minutes, until they start to break down and become jammy. Remove from the heat.

7. In a small bowl, whisk together the arrowroot and lemon juice. Pour the lemon-arrowroot mixture into the cooked strawberries and mix well to combine. Add the cooked strawberries to the bowl with the uncooked strawberries and gently toss to combine. Set aside.

8. To assemble, slice the shortcakes in half horizontally and assemble as you would a sandwich, placing one layer of shortcake on the bottom of a serving dish, ladling the strawberry filling on top, and topping with another layer of shortcake and then the whipped coconut cream. Alternatively, for a lighter dessert, ladle the strawberries on the bottom of a serving dish and top with one of the shortcake slices and then the whipped cream. Garnish with fresh mint leaves, if desired, and serve at once.

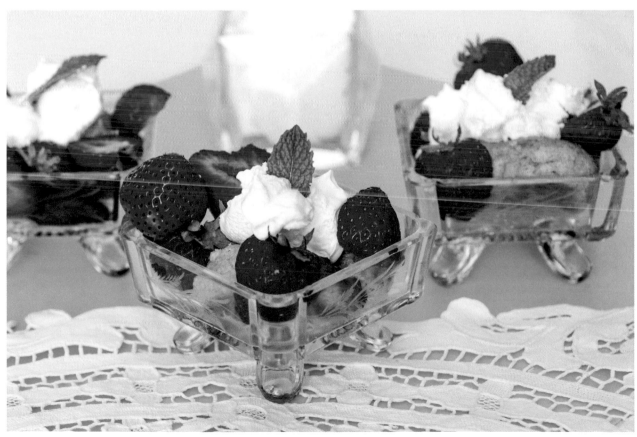

chocolate-covered frozen bananas

MAKES 6 frozen bananas   PREP TIME: 15 minutes, plus time to freeze the bananas
COOK TIME: 5 minutes

When I was growing up, Disney World was the place every kid wanted to go for family vacation. (I suppose it still is!) And when you went, you just had to get a chocolate-covered banana! I grew up eating this treat, and I've been making this clean version for my son for years. The Disney version always had peanuts, but I like using omega-3-rich walnuts instead. But really, you can use any chopped nut (or even crushed cereal) that you like.

3 large bananas, peeled and cut in half crosswise

¼ cup plus 1 tablespoon extra-virgin coconut oil

½ cup cacao powder

¼ cup pure maple syrup

2 teaspoons pure vanilla extract

Pinch of Himalayan pink salt

½ cup finely chopped raw walnuts

¼ cup mini dairy-free dark chocolate chips (optional)

1. Line a rimmed baking sheet or large plate with parchment paper. Insert a popsicle stick into the cut side of each banana half. Place all the bananas on the lined baking sheet or plate and transfer to the freezer. Freeze for at least 2 to 3 hours, or overnight.

2. In a small saucepan, heat the coconut oil over low heat for about 1 minute, or until the oil is melted. Slowly stir in the cacao powder, maple syrup, and vanilla extract. Mix to combine well and stir until the cacao powder has completely dissolved. Stir in the salt. Transfer the melted chocolate to a narrow glass.

3. Sprinkle the walnuts and chocolate chips (if using) on the parchment-lined baking sheet around the bananas. Dip a frozen banana half into the chocolate. Allow the excess chocolate to drip off, then place the dipped banana back on the parchment paper and immediately roll it in the walnuts so that all sides of the banana are equally coated (use your hands to gently press the walnut pieces onto the banana to help them stick). Roll the banana in the chocolate chips (if using). Repeat with the remaining bananas.

4. Return the bananas to the freezer for 30 to 60 minutes to harden.

STORAGE INFORMATION _____
Store in an airtight zip-top bag in the freezer for up to a week.

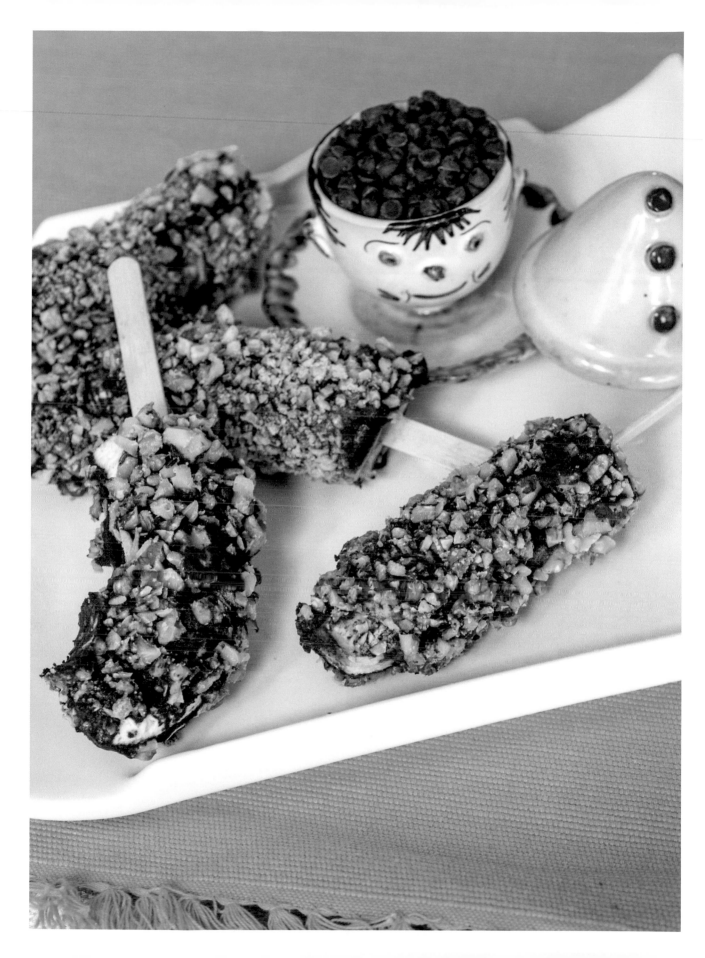

mom's individual blackberry cobblers

MAKES 6 individual cobblers   PREP TIME: 20 minutes   COOK TIME: 35 minutes

Fruit cobbler was one of the dessert recipes my mom made most frequently. Mom's cobblers were always perfect. They also were not very sweet; Mom always thought super-sweet cobblers masked the delicious flavor of the fruit. She was right: you really don't need much sugar at all for a great cobbler. However, Mom's cobbler was neither gluten-free nor dairy-free, and it was no easy task to get this recipe right without wheat flour or butter. Mom helped me with this one, and after remaking it five times, we finally got it right! PS: If you want to make it super decadent, try serving it with coconut milk vanilla ice cream.

For the filling:

4 cups blackberries

2 tablespoons pure maple syrup

1 tablespoon arrowroot

1 teaspoon ground cinnamon

For the topping:

1½ cups gluten-free old-fashioned rolled oats

½ cup brown rice flour

1 teaspoon ground cinnamon

¼ teaspoon Himalayan pink salt

½ cup extra-virgin coconut oil, softened

¼ cup pure maple syrup

¾ cup finely chopped raw pecans

1. Preheat the oven to 350°F. Lightly oil the bottom and sides of four 8-ounce ramekins.

2. To make the filling: Place the blackberries in a large mixing bowl. Pour the maple syrup over the blackberries and sprinkle with the arrowroot and cinnamon. Carefully toss to coat the berries, but be careful not to smash them. Set aside.

3. To make the topping: In a large mixing bowl, combine the oats, brown rice flour, cinnamon, and salt and mix together with a wooden spoon. Add the coconut oil and maple syrup and stir until just combined. Stir in the chopped pecans. The mixture will be crumbly.

4. Divide the blackberry filling among the ramekins. Spoon the crumbly topping evenly over the blackberries. Transfer the ramekins to a large baking sheet and bake for 35 minutes, or until the topping is lightly browned.

STORAGE INFORMATION _____

Cobbler will keep in a covered container in the refrigerator for up to 3 days. For best results, reheat each portion in the microwave for 1 minute on high before serving.

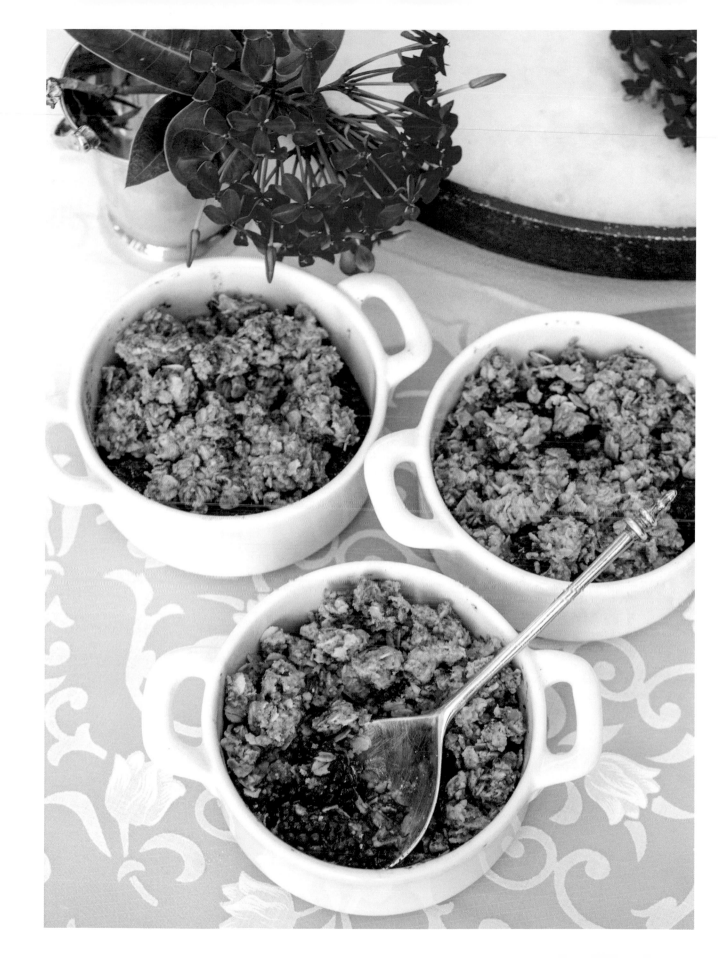

apple-blackberry-cranberry pie

MAKES one 9-inch pie   PREP TIME: 25 minutes   COOK TIME: 30 to 35 minutes

For years and years, apple pie was my favorite dessert of all time. I never would have thought the combination of apples, blackberries, and cranberries could beat good old apple pie, but this recipe proved me wrong! My son, Blake, created this recipe himself on Christmas morning when he got the whim to bake an apple pie. We only had two apples in the house and none of the stores were open, so he dug up what fruit he could. Voilà—my new favorite fruit pie was born.

For the filling:

2 apples, chopped (leave the skins on)

4 cups fresh blackberries

1 cup frozen cranberries

2 tablespoons coconut sugar

1 tablespoon arrowroot

1 tablespoon fresh lemon juice

1 teaspoon ground cinnamon

For the crust:

1 par-baked Speedy Sweet Pie Crust (page 362)

For the topping:

1 cup gluten-free old-fashioned rolled oats

½ cup cassava flour (or sprouted spelt flour if not gluten- or grain-free)

½ cup raw pecans

⅓ cup coconut sugar

¼ cup extra-virgin coconut oil, softened

⅛ teaspoon Himalayan pink salt

1. Preheat the oven to 350°F.

2. To make the filling, gently toss together all of the filling ingredients in a large mixing bowl. Add the filling to the par-baked pie crust.

3. To make the topping, put the topping ingredients in the same bowl you used to make the filling. Mix the ingredients with your fingers or a pastry cutter until crumbly, then sprinkle the topping evenly over the fruit.

4. Bake for 30 to 35 minutes, until the fruit is soft and the topping is slightly browned. Let rest for 30 minutes before slicing.

STORAGE INFORMATION ───────────────────────

This pie will keep in a covered container in the refrigerator for up to 3 days.

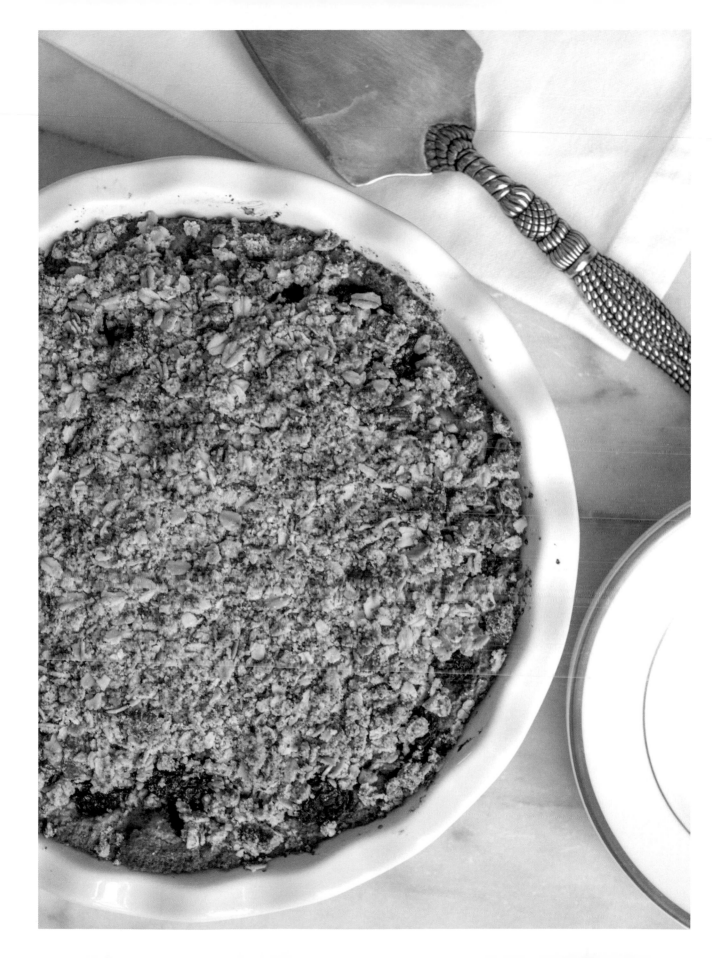

benji's blondie bars

MAKES 16 bars   PREP TIME: 15 minutes   COOK TIME: 20 minutes

Fourteen-year-old Benji Gans created this recipe. If you follow our blog, you have surely heard me share Benji's incredible story of overcoming many of the challenges of autism. I have known Benji and his mom, Debby, for over ten years, and as optimistic as I always like to be, when I first met Benji I didn't have much hope that he would ever be able to function normally. But his mother knew better, and she never gave up on her son. Benji and his family tackled autism from multiple directions, through diet changes, occupational and speech therapy, lots of loving support, and more. Cleaning up his diet absolutely played a role in Benji's remarkable success (especially eliminating refined sugar and gluten), but he would be the first to tell you it wasn't the only factor. You can read more about Benji on his website, BenjiTalks.com, and his TEDx Talk can be seen on YouTube. This is one kid who never stops amazing me. Note: Benji's original recipe called for dried cranberries rather than goji berries and mini chocolate chips instead of cacao nibs (and twice the amount of chocolate, too!). I have to admit, Benji's original version is more decadent, but this version is still super delicious!

Extra-virgin coconut oil, for greasing the pan

½ cup unsalted, unsweetened smooth raw almond butter

¼ cup coconut cream (see page 74)

1 large egg

3 tablespoons pure maple syrup

1 tablespoon pure vanilla extract

1 cup cassava flour (or sprouted spelt flour if not gluten- or grain-free)

½ cup coconut sugar

1 teaspoon baking soda

¼ teaspoon Himalayan pink salt

½ cup dried goji berries or dried cranberries

¾ cup cacao nibs (for less-sweet bars) or dairy-free mini chocolate chips

1. Preheat the oven to 350°F. Generously grease the bottom and sides of an 8-inch square baking dish.

2. In a medium-sized bowl, use a wooden spoon to mix together the almond butter, coconut cream, egg, maple syrup, and vanilla extract.

3. In a large bowl, whisk together the flour, coconut sugar, baking soda, and salt until blended.

4. Add the wet ingredients to the dry and mix well with a wooden spoon. Fold in the goji berries and cacao nibs.

5. Transfer the batter to the prepared baking dish and bake for 20 minutes, or until a toothpick inserted in the middle comes out clean. Allow to cool to room temperature and then slice and serve.

STORAGE INFORMATION

Blondies will keep in a covered container in the refrigerator for up to 5 days or in the freezer for up to 3 weeks.

My life can be challenging at times, but it can also be simple. For example, I primarily behave similar to most fourteen-year-olds, except not. In my early years, I was a true example of someone on the autism spectrum. I said my first word, "Mommy," at age four after many hours of therapy; neurotypical kids attain the ability to verbalize at a much earlier age.

When I was younger, all I had the ability to do was go to therapy. After some hard work, I started in a mainstream school in December 2009. After more therapies, I started to get more comfortable with it. Yet I had a very different experience from most kids, such as attending class with accommodations, which I still do to this day. In the category of social skills, I always used to sit alone, but I am getting better at hanging out with my friends. I am getting to bond with my class a little more and I do have a couple of friends. I have been on a few sleepovers and go to playdates occasionally. Ironically, I talk with grown-ups better than I do with kids. My memory for random details is superb. I can memorize flight details from last month, but I can forget little stuff—like ensuring that I do my math homework correctly!

Not only did therapy help shape me into the person I am today, modifying my diet played a major role as well. For example, removing wheat and barley helped me behave better and think more clearly. Cleaning up my diet and removing junk foods has also helped my body perform better. Ivy has taught me the importance of eating more fruits and vegetables, and so I try to do that as best I can. Ivy also taught me how to sweeten my desserts (like my blondie recipe) using dates and unrefined sugar. I notice that, on the whole, I just feel better the better I eat. Ivy's recipes help me feel better, and I'm just so glad they taste good too!

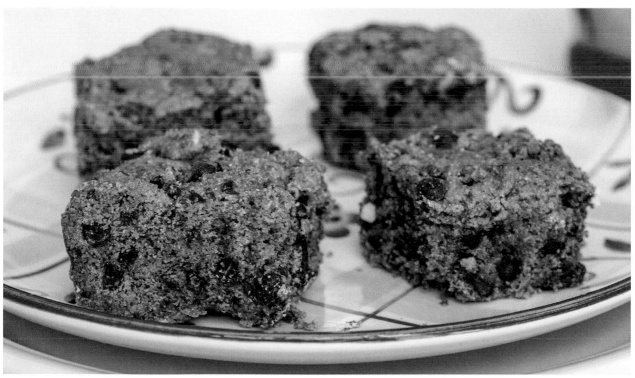

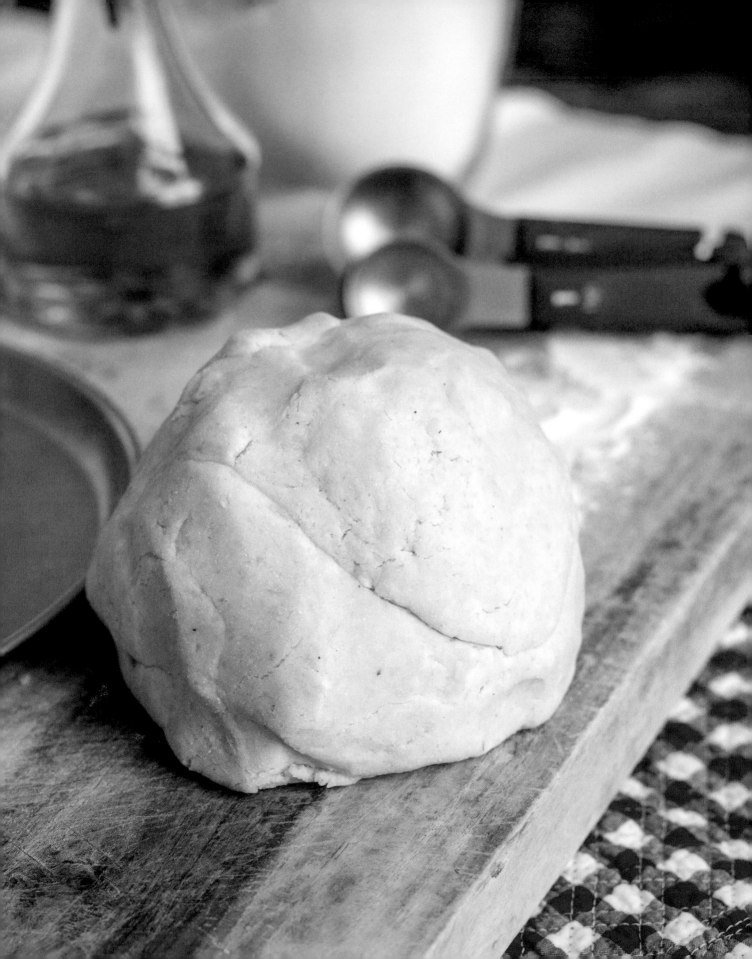

CHAPTER 18

clean cuisine basics

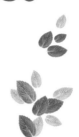

garlic herbed croutons

MAKES about 7 cups   PREP TIME: 10 minutes   COOK TIME: 20 minutes

Before I was into clean eating, I was one of those people who would buy croutons with no intention of ever making a salad. And if I went to a salad bar, the lettuce-to-crouton ratio would be about 1:1. I haven't lost my love of croutons, but I have learned to make clean ones at home. I've also learned that once you try homemade croutons, there is just no going back to store-bought. These are so tasty you could eat them as a snack. I sometimes still do!

½ cup extra-virgin olive oil

4 large cloves garlic, cut lengthwise into thin slices

1 teaspoon dried oregano leaves

1 teaspoon dried basil leaves

¾ teaspoon Himalayan pink salt, divided

½ teaspoon ground black pepper

7 slices gluten-free bread, crusts removed and cut into ¾-inch pieces (about 7 cups)

1. Preheat the oven to 350°F. Place a rack in the middle position in the oven.

2. In a small saucepan, combine the oil, garlic, oregano, basil, ½ teaspoon of the salt, and the pepper. Simmer for 5 minutes over low heat. Discard the garlic.

3. In a large mixing bowl, toss the pieces of bread with the herbed oil mixture, then spread them out on a rimmed baking sheet. Bake the croutons on the middle rack of the oven for 8 minutes. Remove from the oven, toss, and bake for another 7 to 8 minutes, until golden. Sprinkle the croutons with the remaining ¼ teaspoon of salt and let them cool before using.

STORAGE INFORMATION

Store croutons in an airtight container in the pantry for up to 2 days.

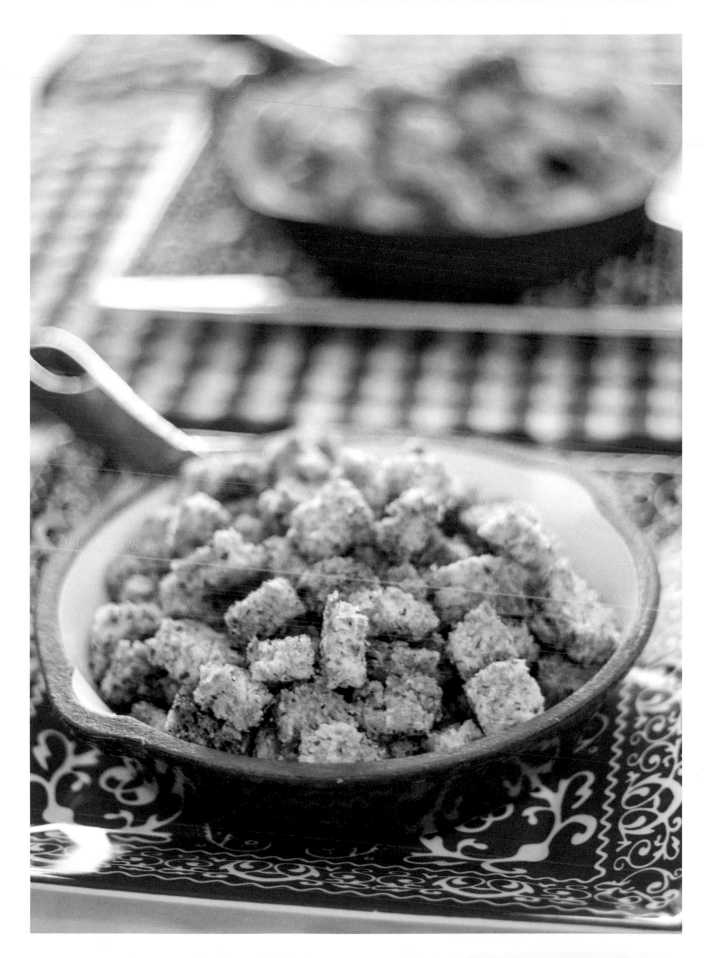

savory crust

MAKES one 9-inch deep-dish pie crust or 12-inch tart crust
PREP TIME: 15 minutes, plus time to chill the dough   COOK TIME: 10 or 15 minutes

Perfect for quiche (like the Spinach & Artichoke Quiche on page 234) and not-too-sweet fruity desserts, this savory pie crust recipe is incredibly easy to make. I even managed to sneak in a full ¼ cup of chia seeds. Not only do the chia seeds boost omega-3s, fiber, and overall nutrition, but they serve a culinary purpose, too: they help the crust bind together.

---

1 cup brown rice flour, plus more for the work surface

½ cup blanched almond flour

½ cup millet flour

¼ cup chia seeds

2 tablespoons medium-grind cornmeal

½ teaspoon Himalayan pink salt

¼ cup plus 2 tablespoons extra-virgin coconut oil, softened

1 large egg

2 to 5 tablespoons cold water

1 large egg white, for brushing the crust

1. In a food processor, mix together the brown rice flour, almond flour, millet flour, chia seeds, cornmeal, and salt. Add the extra-virgin coconut oil, 1 tablespoon at a time, and mix on medium speed until crumbles form. Add the whole egg and continue to mix until the egg is well blended into the flour mixture. Keeping the mixer on, add 2 tablespoons of cold water and then add up to 3 additional tablespoons of cold water, 1 tablespoon at a time, until the dough detaches from the bowl.

2. Gather the dough into a ball, flatten it into a disc, and wrap it in a cheesecloth. (Note: I use cheesecloth as a safer alternative to plastic wrap.) Refrigerate for at least 1 hour and up to 2 hours.

3. Preheat the oven to 400°F.

4. Clear a large work surface and lightly dust it with brown rice flour. Roll out the dough to an 11-inch circle and then fit it into a 9-inch pie plate. Use your fingertips to press the dough into the pie plate and use a fork to poke small holes all over the bottom. Cover the dough with parchment paper and top it with pie weights or a small saucepan (the weight will prevent the crust from puffing up).

5. *To par-bake the crust,* place it in the oven for 10 minutes. Remove it from the oven, then remove the parchment paper and weights. Allow the crust to cool before filling.

   To prebake the crust (for pies that do not require additional baking), follow the instructions for par-baking. After removing the parchment paper and weights, brush the par-baked crust with the egg white, return the crust to the oven, and bake for another 5 minutes, or until lightly browned. Remove the crust from the oven and allow it to cool before filling.

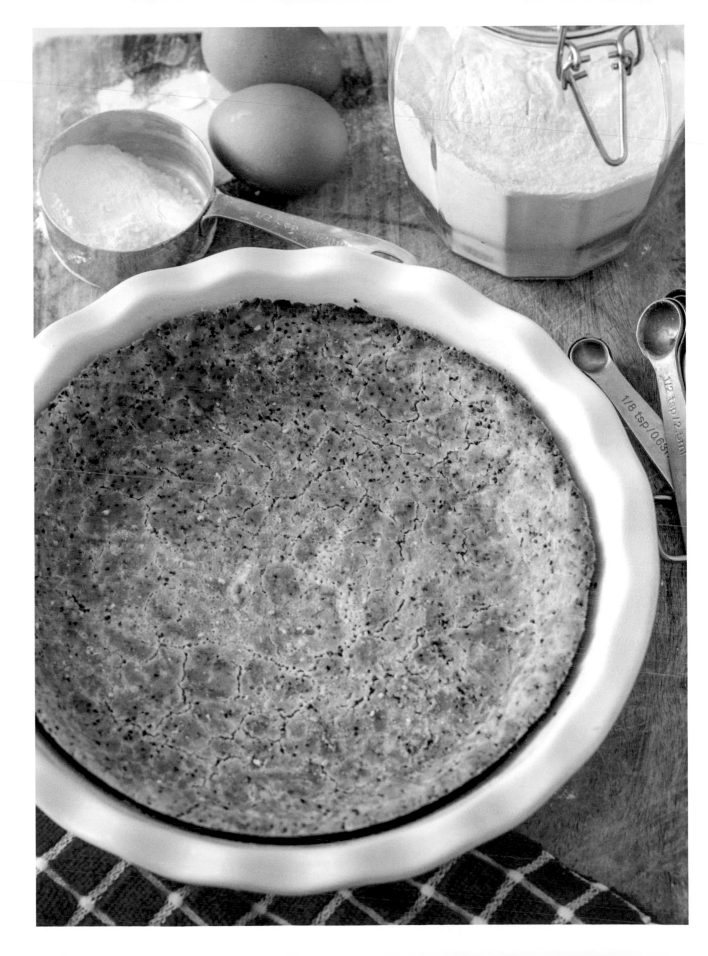

speedy sweet pie crust

MAKES one 9-inch deep-dish pie crust or 12-inch tart crust   PREP TIME: 15 minutes
COOK TIME: 5 or 20 minutes

A basic pie crust recipe is one of those staples once passed down from generation to generation. Of course, traditionally it wouldn't be a gluten-free pie crust recipe, nor would it be nutritious in any way, but it most certainly would be foolproof. And tasty. Nowadays most people just grab some factory-made crust from the frozen food section. But if you are craving the taste of a real-deal homemade pie crust that is also nutritious (yes! such a thing does exist), this is the perfect solution! This recipe will save you from falling into the frozen-pie-crust trap and also keep you from spending all day in the kitchen. You won't even need to dig up your rolling pin!

⅔ cup cassava flour (or sprouted spelt flour if not gluten- and grain-free)

⅓ cup brown rice flour

⅓ cup oat flour

1½ teaspoons arrowroot

½ teaspoon Himalayan pink salt

½ cup cold extra-virgin coconut oil (see Note)

¼ cup pure maple syrup

1½ teaspoons pure vanilla extract

1 large egg

3 tablespoons water

NOTE _____

It is important for the coconut oil to be cold (and hard) before you add it to the flour. The fastest way to harden coconut oil is to put it in the freezer for at least 30 minutes.

1. Preheat the oven to 350°F. Generously grease the bottom and sides of a 9-inch pie plate.

2. Put the cassava flour, brown rice flour, oat flour, arrowroot, and salt in a food processor and process briefly, until the ingredients are well mixed.

3. Add the coconut oil, maple syrup, and vanilla extract and process until crumbles form. Add the egg and process until the egg is well incorporated. With the food processor on, gradually add the water, 1 tablespoon at a time. Continue mixing until the dough is soft and moist and sticks together.

4. Transfer the dough to the pie plate. Use your fingertips to press the dough into the bottom and up the sides of the pie plate and use a fork to poke small holes all over the bottom. Cover the dough with parchment paper and top it with pie weights or a small saucepan (the weight will prevent the crust from puffing up). To prevent the edges from burning, cover them with a crust shield or aluminum foil.

5. *To par-bake the crust,* place it in the oven and bake for 5 minutes. Remove it from the oven, then remove the parchment paper and weights. Allow the crust to cool before filling.

   To prebake the crust (for pies that do not require additional baking), follow the instructions for par-baking. After removing the parchment paper and weights, return the crust to the oven and bake for another 15 minutes, or until lightly browned. Remove the crust from the oven and allow it to cool completely before adding the filling.

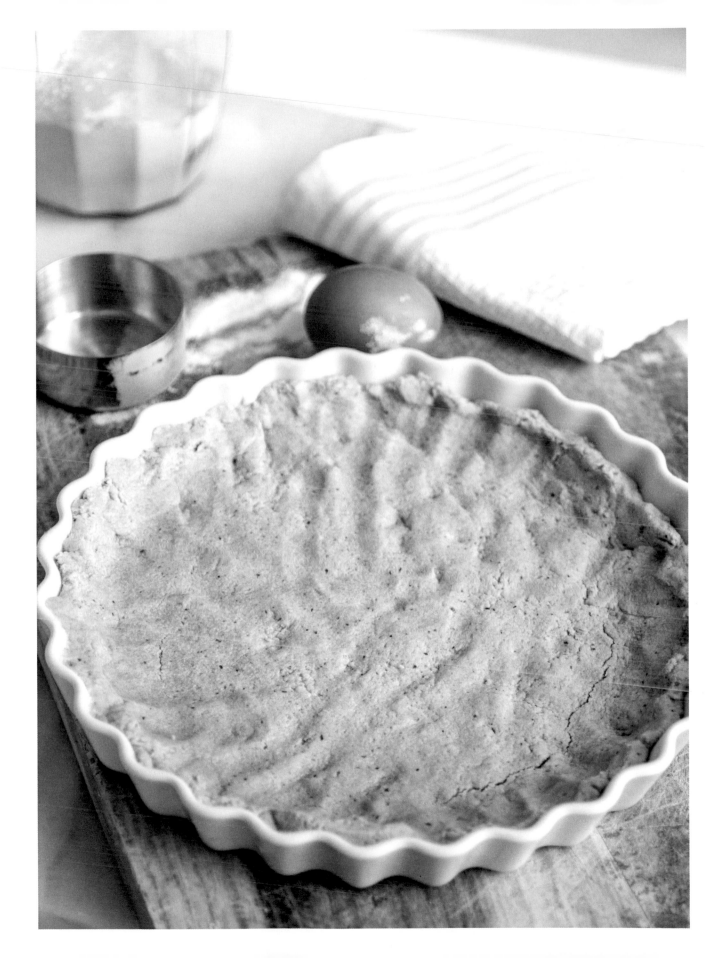

super-easy mini pizza crusts

MAKES 4 personal-sized crusts   PREP TIME: 20 minutes, plus time for the dough to rise
COOK TIME: 14 to 20 minutes, depending on the thickness of the crust

Nobody ever complains about dinner on pizza night! And when it comes to pizza, nothing beats home-cooked. I know it might seem like a hassle to make your own pizza crust, but it's so much easier than it sounds. And there's just something magical about making a whole pizza from scratch. You can use these mini crusts to make the Roman Pizza on page 254, the Personal-Size White Pizzas with Garlic & Mushrooms on page 252, or any pizza you wish!

1¼ cups hot water

2 teaspoons fast-acting instant yeast

2 teaspoons Himalayan pink salt

1½ cups cassava flour (or sprouted spelt flour if not gluten- or grain-free), plus more for the work surface

1 cup blanched almond flour

2 tablespoons extra-virgin olive oil

1. Pour the water into a medium-sized mixing bowl. Add the yeast and salt and stir until the yeast particles are dissolved. Add the cassava flour and almond flour and stir with a wooden spoon until the dough forms a ball. Drizzle in the oil and then transfer the dough to a floured work surface.

2. Knead the dough for about 1 minute, until there are no dry spots in the dough and it feels soft and moist. Transfer the dough back to the mixing bowl and cover with plastic wrap. Let the dough sit in a warm place for 1 hour, or until it rises slightly.

3. Place an oven rack in the top position and preheat the oven to 475°F. Generously oil 2 baking sheets (or 4 personal-sized pizza stones).

4. Place the dough onto a lightly floured work surface. Using your hands, knead the dough until it's soft and workable. Divide the dough into 4 equal portions and then use your hands to roll each dough portion into a ball. *For thick-crust pizza:* Use your hands to flatten the dough balls into 5-inch pizza crusts that are about ½ inch thick. *For thin-crust pizza:* Use your hands to flatten the dough balls into 8-inch pizza crusts that are about ¼ inch thick. Transfer the crusts to the oiled baking pans (or pizza stones) and add toppings of your choice.

5. *For thick-crust pizza:* Bake the pizzas for 18 to 20 minutes, until the crusts are crispy on the outside and soft on the inside. *For thin-crust pizza:* Bake the pizzas for 14 to 16 minutes, until the crusts are crispy on the outside. Remove the pizzas from the oven and let sit at least 5 minutes before serving. Serve at once.

NOTE _____

Make sure you use plenty of oil on the baking sheets! Otherwise the crust can stick during baking and make a big mess.

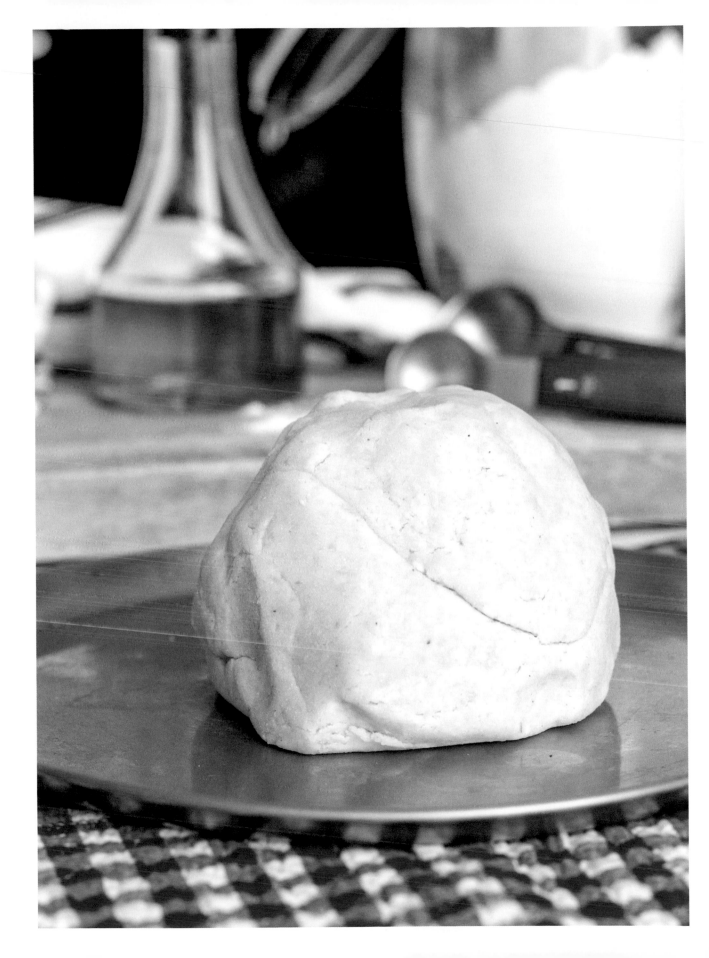

tortillas

MAKES ten 6-inch tortillas   PREP TIME: 15 minutes   COOK TIME: 10 minutes

It can be hard to keep up with a child's or teenager's appetite while also trying to raise them on a clean diet. But if you have a stack of tortillas, you can make healthy (and filling!) meals in minutes. Pretty much anything goes in or on top of a tortilla. Blake is especially fond of Refried Black Bean Tostadas (page 238). But we also fill these tortillas with eggs, chicken, hummus, sautéed veggies, and even fruit! One of his absolute favorite after-school snacks has always been a tortilla spread with almond butter or peanut butter and topped with sliced fruit (apples, nectarines, pears, and bananas are especially good).

1 cup cassava flour (or sprouted spelt flour if not gluten- or grain-free)

¾ cup blanched almond flour

½ teaspoon Himalayan pink salt

2 tablespoons extra-virgin coconut oil, softened, plus more for the pan

1 cup warm water

1. In a medium-sized bowl, whisk together the cassava flour, almond flour, and salt. Add the oil and use your hands to combine the oil-and-flour mixture until the ingredients are well blended and the mixture is very soft. Add the water and knead until the dough is nice and smooth. The dough should not be too dry or too wet and sticky. If the dough is too dry (i.e., it's crumbly and not forming into a ball), add warm water 1 teaspoon at a time. If the dough is too sticky (i.e., it's sticking to your finger when you touch it), add cassava flour 1 teaspoon at a time.

2. Divide the dough into 10 equal-size portions (each portion should be about 2 heaping tablespoons). Using your hands, roll each piece of dough into a ball.

3. Place a dough ball between 2 pieces of parchment paper, put a thin cutting board or other firm, flat object on top of the parchment paper, and use your hands to press down until the ball flattens into a ¼-inch-thick tortilla. Repeat with the rest of the dough balls.

4. Place a 10- or 12-inch lightly oiled cast-iron skillet over medium-high heat and let it preheat for several minutes. Once the skillet is hot, cook the tortillas in batches of 2 or 3 at a time for about 1 minute, until bubbles start to form. Flip and cook on the other side for another minute or so, until both sides are ever so lightly browned. Serve warm.

STORAGE INFORMATION

Store these tortillas in a plastic bag in the refrigerator for up to 3 days or in the freezer for up to 4 weeks. To reheat, microwave on high for about 45 seconds, until soft.

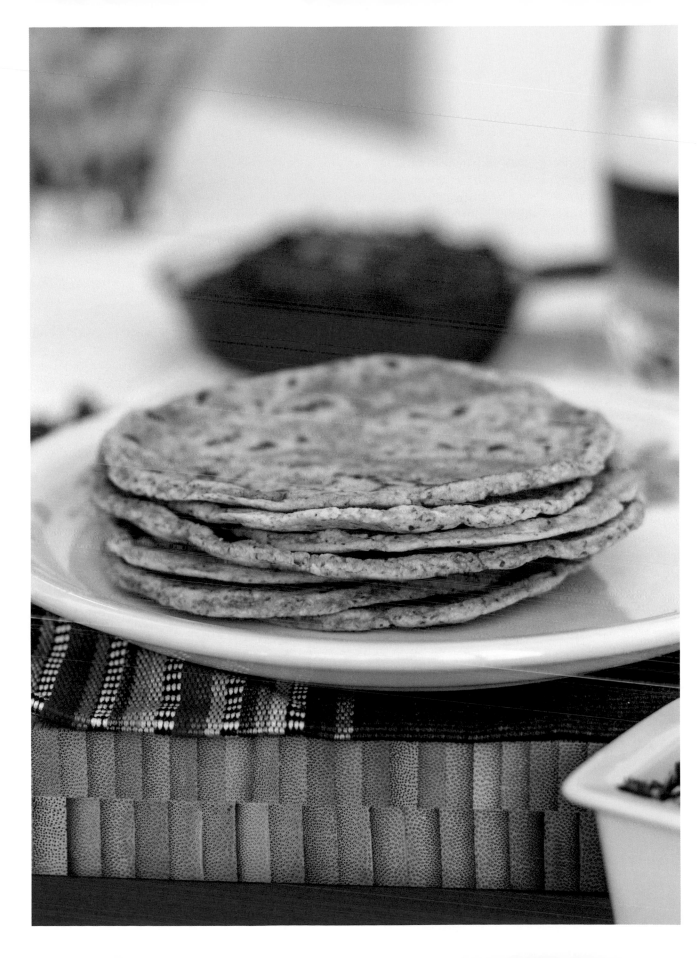

whole almond milk

MAKES 2½ cups   PREP TIME: 5 minutes

Unlike my husband and me, who grew up on cow's milk, our son has been raised on whole almond milk—not the highly refined kind often sold in supermarkets. The problem with most almond milk brands is that they contain less than 5 percent almonds; the rest of the "milk" consists of water with some emulsifiers and added synthetic nutrients. The other important difference is that in whole almond milk, the ground nut meal isn't strained from the milk. Straining the almond meal removes a significant amount of the nutrients! If you're not quite convinced, please see the post on our blog called "Health Benefits of Almond Milk + Why 'Whole' Almond Milk Is Best."

There are a few brands of whole almond milk available in stores (see Resources, page 403), but I like to make it from scratch. It's a quick recipe, especially if you have a high-powered blender, and I promise you that you'll never go back to watery store-bought options or homemade recipes that call for straining the milk.

½ cup raw almonds, preferably soaked for 4 to 8 hours, then rinsed and drained (see Notes)

2 medjool dates, pitted (see Notes)

¼ teaspoon pure vanilla extract

2½ cups cold filtered water

⅛ teaspoon Himalayan pink salt

Put all of the ingredients in a blender in the order given in the ingredients list. Process on high speed for 1 full minute, or until the mixture is smooth and creamy. Refrigerate and serve cold. Shake well before serving (the milk tends to separate while sitting).

STORAGE INFORMATION _____

Almond milk will keep in a covered container in the refrigerator for up to 4 days.

NOTES _____

If you're using a high-powered blender, soaking the almonds is optional, but it does create a creamier milk. If you're using a conventional blender instead of a high-powered one, soaking the almonds is necessary to get the right texture.

If you're using a conventional blender rather than a high-powered one and your dates are on the dry side, soak them in water for 15 to 30 minutes to soften them before using (very moist, succulent medjool dates do not require soaking).

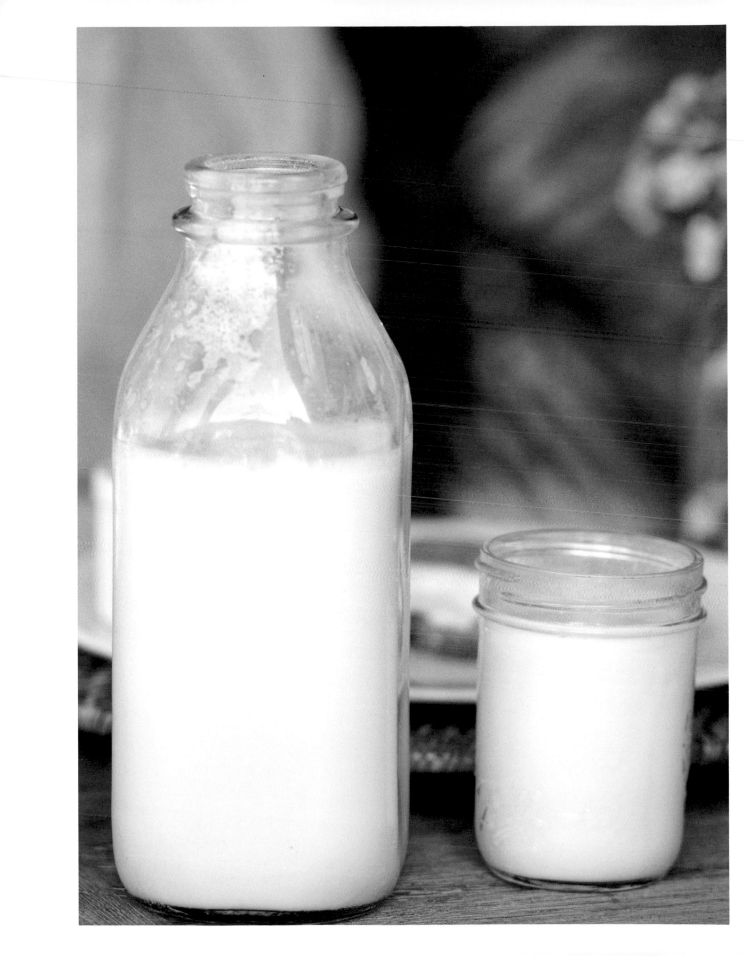

parmesan nut "cheese"

MAKES 1 cup   PREP TIME: 5 minutes   COOK TIME: 35 minutes

If going to the trouble of making a plant-based nut "cheese" sounds even less enticing than giving up cheese altogether, trust me, I totally get it. Before I start making any recipe, I try to factor in the time-to-taste ratio—in other words, the more time I spend making a recipe, the better I expect it to taste! But not only does this nut "cheese" recipe take less than ten minutes of hands-on time to prepare, it seriously tastes good. Better than good, actually; it's downright delicious. And unlike most other homemade dairy-free cheeses, it doesn't require a dehydrator. My family is crazy for this stuff: we sprinkle it on everything from pizza (see pages 230, 252, and 254) to roasted vegetables, salads, grain bowls, baked potatoes, and anything else you might put Parmesan on.

---

1 cup pine nuts

2 teaspoons unfortified nutritional yeast

½ teaspoon fresh lemon juice

¼ teaspoon Himalayan pink salt

¼ teaspoon onion powder

1. Preheat the oven to 200°F and line a rimmed baking sheet with parchment paper.

2. Place all the ingredients in a mini food processor and process until well combined.

3. Using your hands, crumble the mixture onto the parchment paper, then bake for 30 to 35 minutes, until lightly toasted.

SPECIAL TOOLS _____
Mini food processor

STORAGE INFORMATION _____
This "cheese" will keep in a covered container in the refrigerator for up to a week.

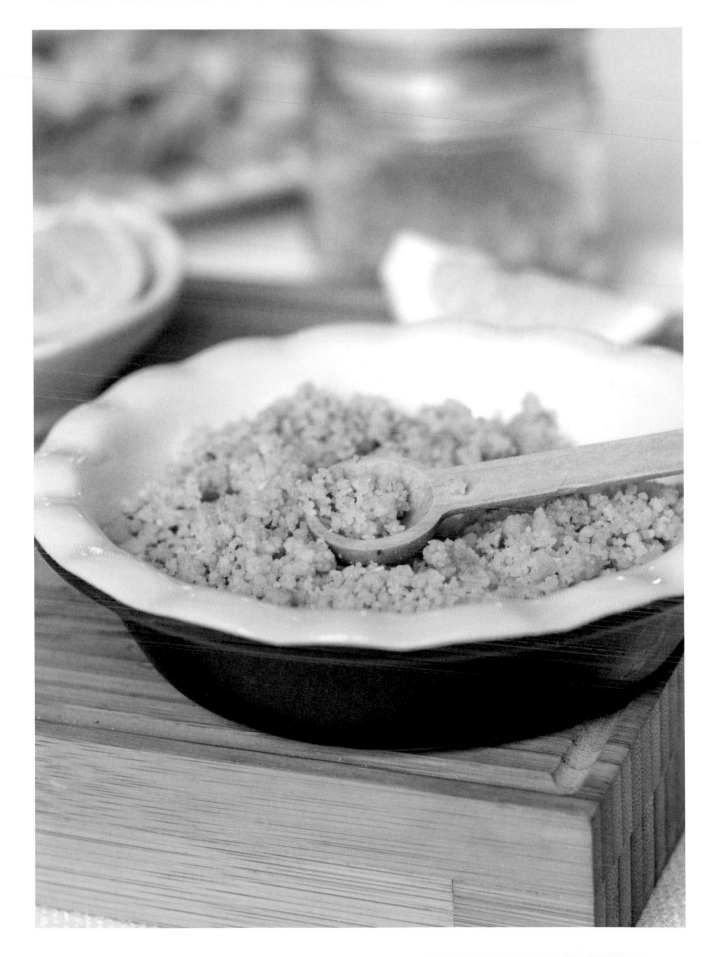

clean cuisine sour cream

MAKES 1¾ cups   PREP TIME: 10 minutes

Sour cream was a very difficult food for me to give up when I first started eating clean in the late nineties. I have yet to find a store-bought dairy-free version that is clean and also tastes good. But in the last few years, I realized I could make my own, and it is so easy! Rich, decadently creamy, and incredibly smooth, this homespun sour cream recipe can be used just like conventional sour cream. There's just one slight difference: this dairy-free version melts more easily when put on top of hot foods. I love it on my Slow Cooker Beef Stroganoff (page 216), on chili (page 240) and baked potatoes, mixed into pureed vegetable soups, as a base for salad dressings, and so much more! And for a special treat—and always on New Year's—my husband and I treat ourselves to caviar toast appetizers (toasted sprouted whole-grain bread spread with sour cream and topped with a dollop of caviar—shown in the photo), which just aren't the same without sour cream. (I know, caviar can be very pricey, but pink salmon caviar is about half the price of black caviar, and they even sell it at Costco!)

1 cup water

½ cup extra-virgin olive oil

¾ teaspoon manuka honey or other raw honey

¼ cup plus 1 tablespoon fresh lemon juice

2 cups raw macadamia nuts or cashews, preferably soaked for 1 to 2 hours, then rinsed and drained (see Note)

1¼ teaspoons Himalayan pink salt

Place all the ingredients in a blender or food processor in the order given in the ingredients list. Process on high speed until smooth and creamy.

STORAGE INFORMATION

This sour cream will keep in a jar in the refrigerator for up to a week.

NOTE

If you're using a high-powered blender, soaking the nuts is optional, but it does create a creamier texture. If you're using a conventional blender instead of a high-powered one, soaking the nuts is necessary to get the right texture.

MAKE IT VEGAN

Omit the honey.

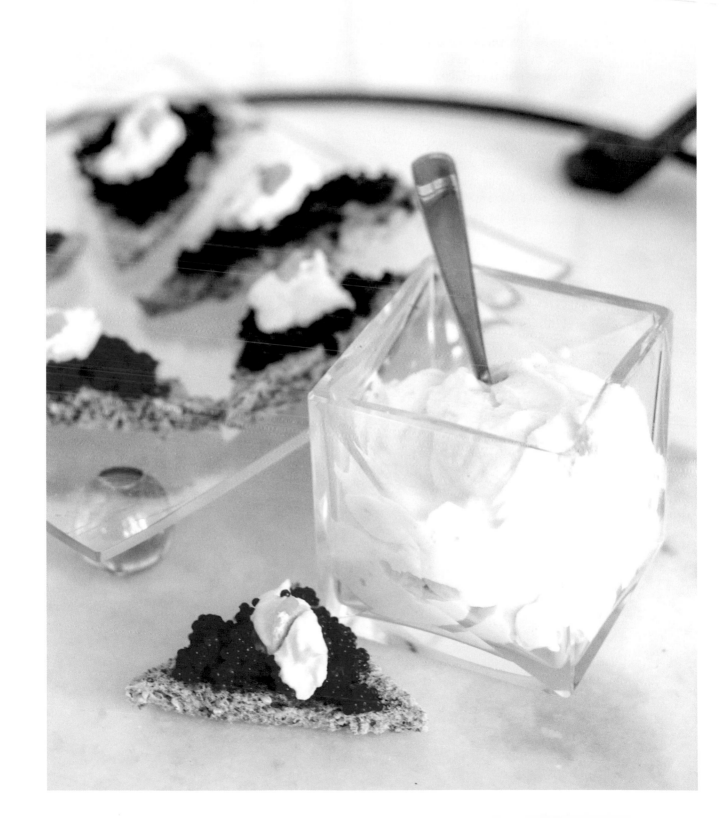

pineapple teriyaki sauce

MAKES 1¼ cups   PREP TIME: 5 minutes

I love pretty much anything teriyaki. Salmon Teriyaki (page 180). Chicken teriyaki rice bowls. Teriyaki meatballs. As far as I'm concerned, teriyaki sauce is good on just about any protein. Of course, you can't make teriyaki anything without a sweet, tasty teriyaki sauce. Unfortunately, conventional store-bought teriyaki sauce is filled to the brim with refined sugar. The good news is, you can make your own in less than ten minutes. Once you try homemade teriyaki sauce, you'll never go back to store-bought again.

---

11 medjool dates, pitted (see Note)

3 cloves garlic, coarsely chopped

1 (¼-inch) piece fresh ginger, peeled and coarsely chopped

½ cup plus 2 tablespoons water

½ cup chopped fresh or frozen pineapple

¼ cup plus 3 tablespoons gluten-free tamari (or unpasteurized soy sauce, if not gluten-free)

1 tablespoon manuka honey or other raw honey

Place all the ingredients in a blender and process on high until smooth and creamy. Transfer to a mason jar and refrigerate until ready to use.

NOTE _____

If you're using a conventional blender rather than a high-powered one and your dates are on the dry side, soak them in water for 15 to 30 minutes to soften them before pureeing (very moist, succulent medjool dates do not require soaking).

STORAGE INFORMATION _____

This sauce will keep in a jar in the refrigerator for up to a week.

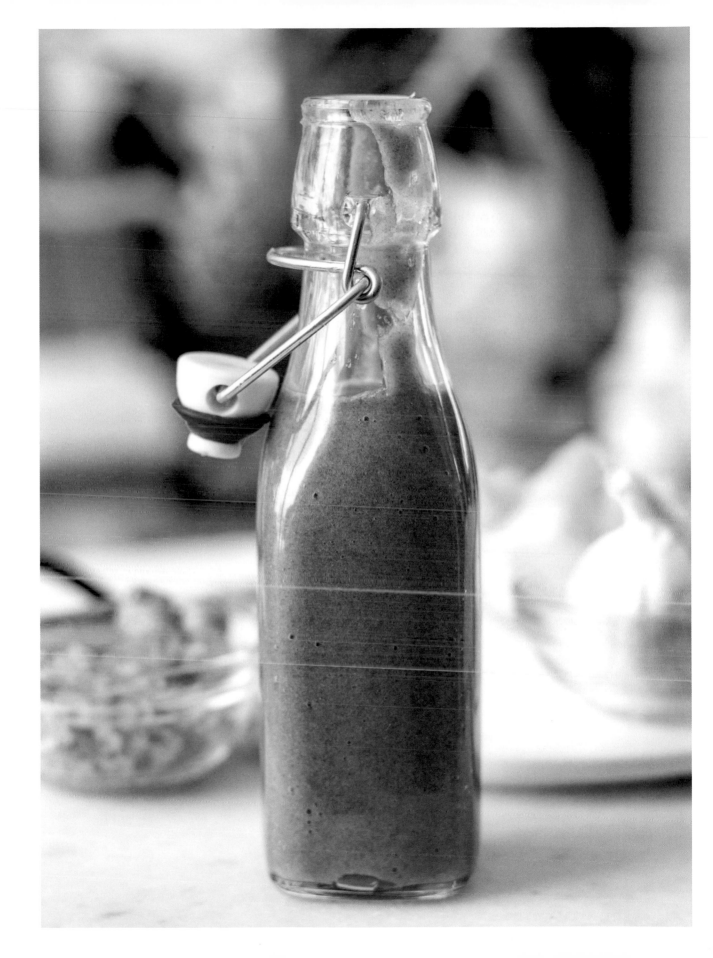

jonn & julia's almond asian sauce

MAKES about 1¼ cups   PREP TIME: 10 minutes

Whenever my husband and I have a barbecue and invite our friends Dr. Jonn and Julia Mc-Clellan, they bring this rich, creamy, savory sauce. Not only is Jonn our family chiropractor, but Andy and I have known him since grade school, and he's one of the most health-conscious and nutritionally savvy people we know. Whatever he's eating, you know it's got to be one of the healthiest foods on the planet! So it's no surprise that since almond butter has more vitamins, minerals, and healthy monounsaturated fats than peanut butter, Jonn prefers using almond butter for a recipe that conventionally uses peanut butter. Jonn and Julia have been bringing this sauce for years, and each time it's a little bit different. Sometimes they substitute coconut milk for the water to give it a more distinct Thai flavor, and other times they add extra lime or swirl in some cilantro for a green almond Asian sauce. The measurements don't need to be exact!

As for how to use it, you can slather or drizzle it on just about anything you happen to be grilling—chicken, shrimp, corn, potatoes—and even use it as a veggie dip. It's also incredibly good with noodles; I especially love to mix it with a combination of zucchini noodles and 100 percent buckwheat soba noodles and top it all with cilantro. So good!

⅓ cup water

4 medjool dates, pitted (see Note)

1 (1-inch) piece fresh ginger, peeled and coarsely chopped (see Note)

2 large cloves garlic, peeled (see Note)

½ cup plus 2 tablespoons unsalted, unsweetened smooth raw almond butter

3 tablespoons gluten-free tamari (or unpasteurized soy sauce, if not gluten-free)

2 tablespoons fresh lime juice

½ teaspoon crushed red pepper

½ teaspoon fish sauce

Place all the ingredients in a blender or food processor in the order given in the ingredients list. Process on high speed for 1 full minute, or until the mixture is smooth and creamy.

NOTE _____

If you're using a conventional blender rather than a high-powered one or a food processor and your dates are on the dry side, soak them in water for 15 to 30 minutes to soften them before pureeing (very moist, succulent medjool dates do not require soaking). Also, for best results, grate the ginger and finely chop the garlic before using.

STORAGE INFORMATION _____

This sauce will keep in a jar in the refrigerator for up to a week.

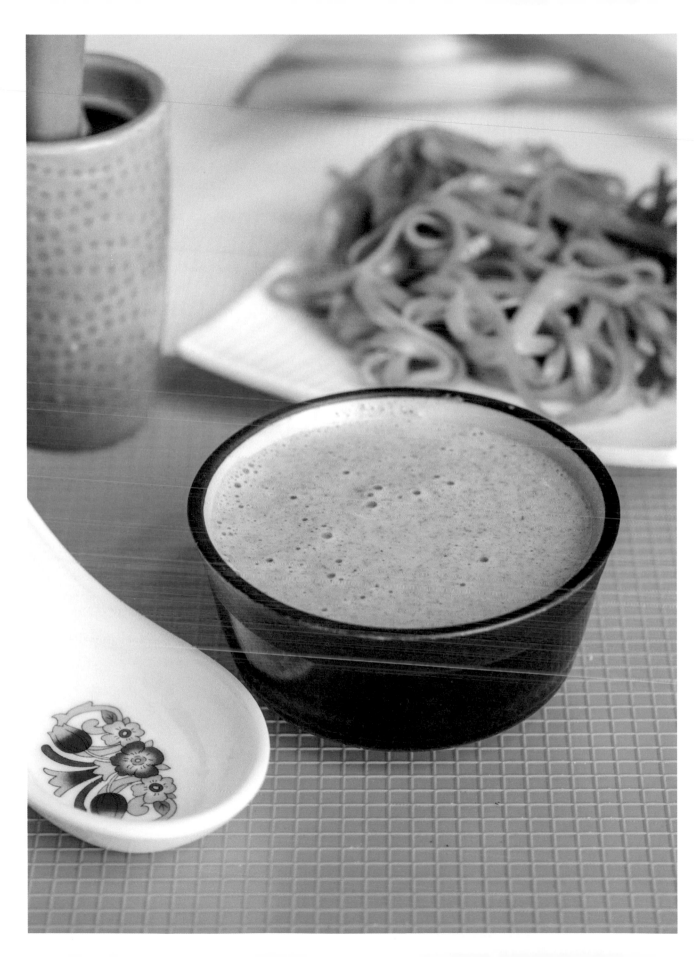

hidden veggie marinara

MAKES about 6 cups   PREP TIME: 20 minutes   COOK TIME: 50 minutes

If you are trying to get your family to eat more vegetables, this sauce is the way to go! In fact, a number of my friends say their little ones prefer this sauce to conventional marinara sauce, probably because it is less acidic and has a milder, mellower flavor. And speaking of kids, I promise they will not be able to tell the sauce is hiding eight different vegetables. Use it just as you would any marinara sauce. It's delicious on top of whole-grain pasta and veggie noodles, as a pizza topping, over baked potatoes, and as a topping for polenta on eggs. Oh, and it freezes beautifully!

¼ cup extra-virgin olive oil

1 medium onion, chopped

4 medium carrots, peeled and chopped

3 stalks celery, chopped

8 cloves garlic, minced

1 cup shiitake mushrooms, stemmed and chopped

1 medium zucchini, chopped

1 cup frozen cubed butternut squash, or ⅔ cup butternut squash puree

1 (28-ounce) can diced tomatoes

½ cup vegetable broth

¼ cup tomato paste

2 tablespoons coconut sugar

1 tablespoon dried oregano leaves

¼ teaspoon Himalayan pink salt

1 bay leaf

1 (12-ounce) jar roasted red peppers, rinsed and drained

1. Heat the oil in a large saucepan over medium heat. Add the onion, carrots, and celery and sauté for 5 to 6 minutes, until the vegetables are soft. Add the garlic and sauté for an additional minute.

2. Add the mushrooms and sauté until soft, 4 to 5 minutes. Add the zucchini and sauté until soft, 2 to 3 minutes. Add the butternut squash cubes and sauté until thawed, 2 to 3 minutes (if using the puree, simply stir it in until it's combined with the vegetables).

3. Stir in the diced tomatoes, vegetable broth, tomato paste, coconut sugar, oregano, and salt. Add the bay leaf. Simmer, uncovered, for 30 minutes, or until thickened and fragrant.

4. Remove the bay leaf. Add the roasted red peppers. Using a handheld stick blender, process until smooth, or blend it in small batches in a jar blender. Taste and adjust seasoning if needed. Serve warm.

STORAGE INFORMATION _____

This sauce will keep in a covered container in the refrigerator for up to 5 days or in the freezer for up to a month.

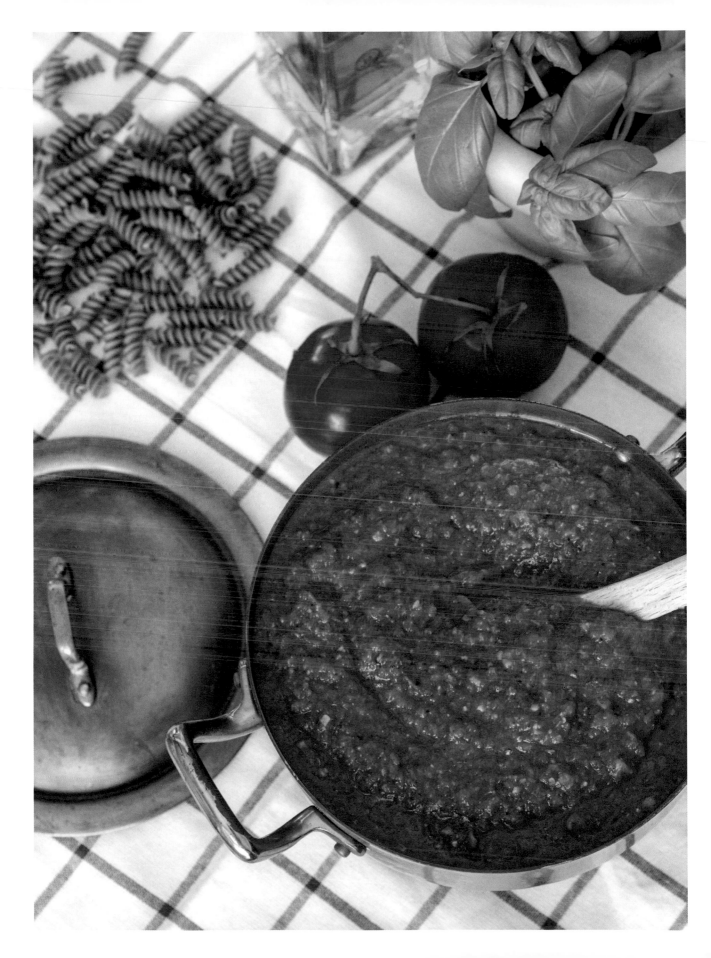

tomato sauce with garlic & italian herbs

MAKES about 7 cups   PREP TIME: 15 minutes   COOK TIME: 1 hour 10 minutes

I admit, many times I use a store-bought tomato sauce for my everyday cooking. But as with most things, nothing beats homemade. Over the years I have tried numerous different tomato sauce recipes, and I've finally come up with one that we are all just crazy for. The three big secrets are: (1) use triple the amount of garlic called for in conventional sauces, (2) use an equal amount of two different types of canned tomatoes—crushed Italian plum tomatoes and whole peeled San Marzano tomatoes, and (3) use a handheld stick blender to puree everything at the very end (it saves the trouble of transferring everything to a blender). It takes about 15 minutes of hands-on work to make this sauce from scratch, but trust me, you won't be disappointed!

½ cup extra-virgin olive oil

¾ cup finely chopped onions

1 stalk celery, finely chopped

1 medium carrot, peeled and finely chopped

8 cloves garlic, finely chopped

1½ teaspoons Italian seasoning

1 teaspoon Himalayan pink salt

½ teaspoon ground black pepper

1 (28-ounce) can crushed tomatoes (preferably crushed Italian plum tomatoes; see Note)

1 (28-ounce) can whole peeled San Marzano tomatoes, with juices (see Note)

1. Heat the oil in a large saucepan over medium heat. Add the onions, celery, and carrot and sauté for about 6 to 7 minutes, until the vegetables are very soft. Add the garlic and sauté for another minute. Add the Italian seasoning, salt, and pepper.

2. Lower the heat to medium-low and add the tomatoes. Simmer the sauce, uncovered, for 1 hour, until thickened and fragrant.

3. Use a handheld stick blender to puree everything together. Let the tomato sauce sit for at least 30 minutes before serving for the flavors to fully develop. Taste and adjust the seasoning as needed.

STORAGE INFORMATION _____
Leftover sauce can be stored in an airtight container in the refrigerator for up to a week or in the freezer for up to a month.

NOTE _____
The flavor of canned tomatoes can vary tremendously, so it is important to buy the absolute best quality for the best results. For whole peeled tomatoes and crushed tomatoes, I prefer Cento brand organic because it does not include calcium chloride as a preservative. While any type of whole tomatoes can be used, I prefer to use the San Marzano variety for its superior flavor (see Notes, page 250).

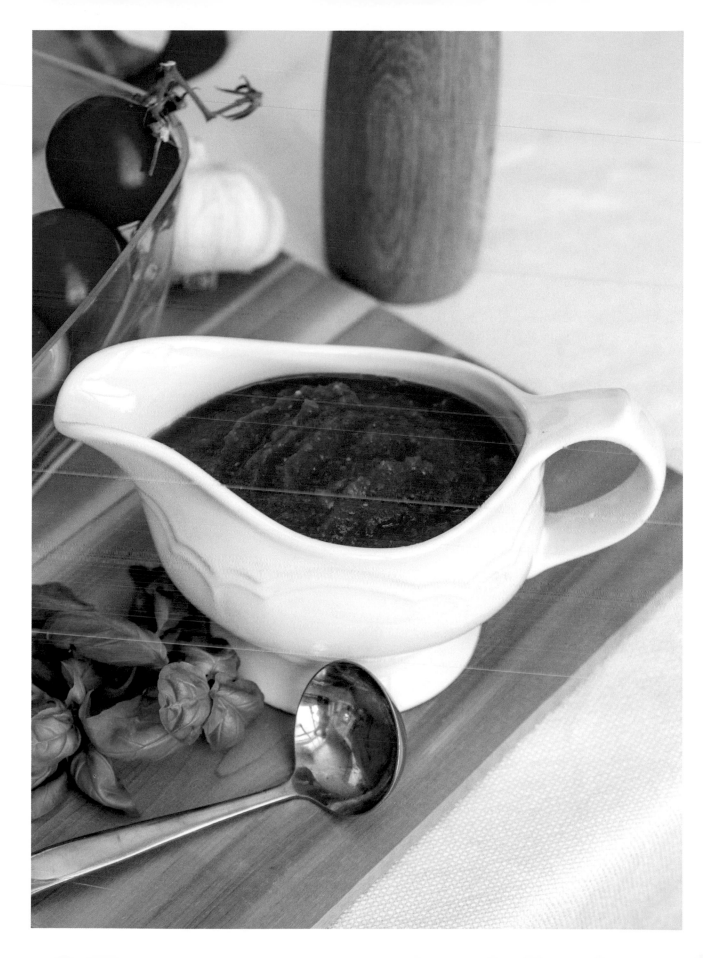

alfredo sauce

MAKES about 1¼ cups   PREP TIME: 5 minutes   COOK TIME: 10 minutes

Yes, it is definitely possible to make Alfredo sauce without butter, cream, or cheese! I promise you it's out of this world, too. In less than fifteen minutes, you'll whip up a cream sauce that is every bit as decadent as the real deal. You can use Alfredo sauce on pasta or zoodles, as a sauce for baking chicken, on baked potatoes, and more. And be sure to check out the Personal-Size White Pizzas with Garlic & Mushrooms recipe on page 252, which uses this Alfredo sauce.

1 tablespoon extra-virgin olive oil

½ cup chopped shallots

⅛ teaspoon Himalayan pink salt

1 cup raw cashews, preferably soaked for 1 to 2 hours, then rinsed and drained (see Note)

1 cup water

2 teaspoons fresh lemon juice

1 teaspoon unfortified nutritional yeast

⅛ teaspoon ground white pepper

3 pinches ground nutmeg

2 cloves garlic, peeled

1. Heat the oil in a small saucepan over medium-low heat. Add the shallots and cook for 4 to 5 minutes, until softened, then season with the salt.

2. Transfer the shallots to a blender and add the cashews, water, lemon juice, nutritional yeast, white pepper, nutmeg, and garlic. Process on high speed for 1 full minute, or until the mixture is smooth and creamy.

3. Pour the mixture into the same saucepan you used to cook the shallots and heat over low heat for about 2 minutes, or until warmed through, stirring constantly. Add more water and salt, if necessary, to adjust the consistency and seasoning. Serve warm.

NOTE

If you're using a high-powered blender, soaking the cashews is optional, but it does create a creamier texture. If you're using a conventional blender instead of a high-powered one, soaking the cashews is necessary to get the right texture.

STORAGE INFORMATION

This sauce will keep in a covered container in the refrigerator for up to 3 days.

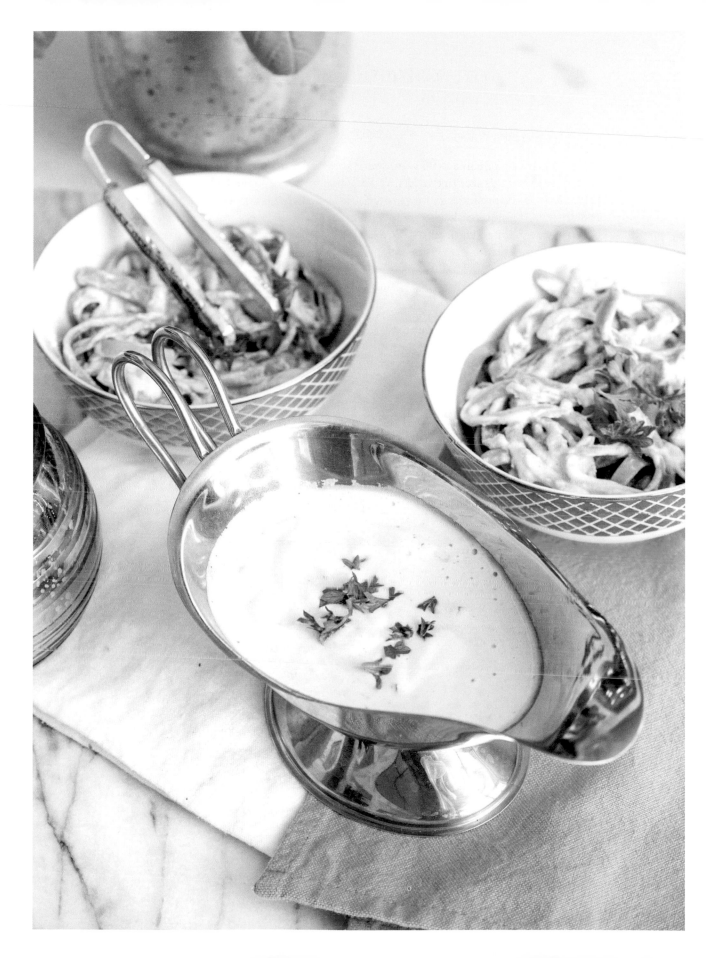

fresh strawberry sauce

MAKES about 1½ cups   PREP TIME: 10 minutes   COOK TIME: 25 minutes

Summer food at its finest and simplest, fresh strawberry sauce requires just four ingredients (well, five if you count water) and very little hands-on prep time. Plus, it has zero added sugar (unlike most strawberry sauce recipes, which call for about ½ cup of sugar!). This one is definitely a summertime staple at our house, and I am always amazed at how creatively everyone uses it. Waffles (page 106) are always a great match. My son likes to spread store-bought almond cream cheese (see Resources, page 403, for brands) on whole-grain rice cakes and then top it off with a spoonful of strawberry sauce. My husband puts it on his wild salmon. It makes the perfect oatmeal stir-in, it's to die for when mixed with whipped coconut cream, and it's the ideal sauce for a dairy-free yogurt parfait. But without a doubt, the crepes on page 118 are my personal favorite food to pair with this sauce!

¼ cup water

5 medjool dates, pitted (see Note)

2 tablespoons fresh lemon juice

1 pound fresh strawberries, hulled, and sliced

1½ teaspoons arrowroot

1. Put the water, dates, and lemon juice in a blender and process on high speed until smooth.

2. Transfer the date mixture to a small saucepan and add the strawberries. Bring to a boil, then turn the heat down to medium-low and cook until the strawberries are very, very soft, about 20 minutes.

3. Remove the saucepan from the heat. Transfer ⅓ cup of the liquid to a small mixing bowl and allow it to cool to room temperature. Stir the arrowroot into the cooled liquid in the mixing bowl and mix well, then pour the arrowroot mixture back into the saucepan.

4. Let the sauce sit for about 20 minutes to thicken before serving. Serve warm or cold.

NOTE _____

If you're using a conventional blender rather than a high-powered one and your dates are on the dry side, soak them in water for 15 to 30 minutes to soften them before using (very moist, succulent medjool dates do not require soaking).

STORAGE INFORMATION _____

This sauce will keep in a covered container in the refrigerator for up to 4 days or in the freezer for up to 3 weeks. To thaw frozen sauce, heat it in a saucepan over medium heat.

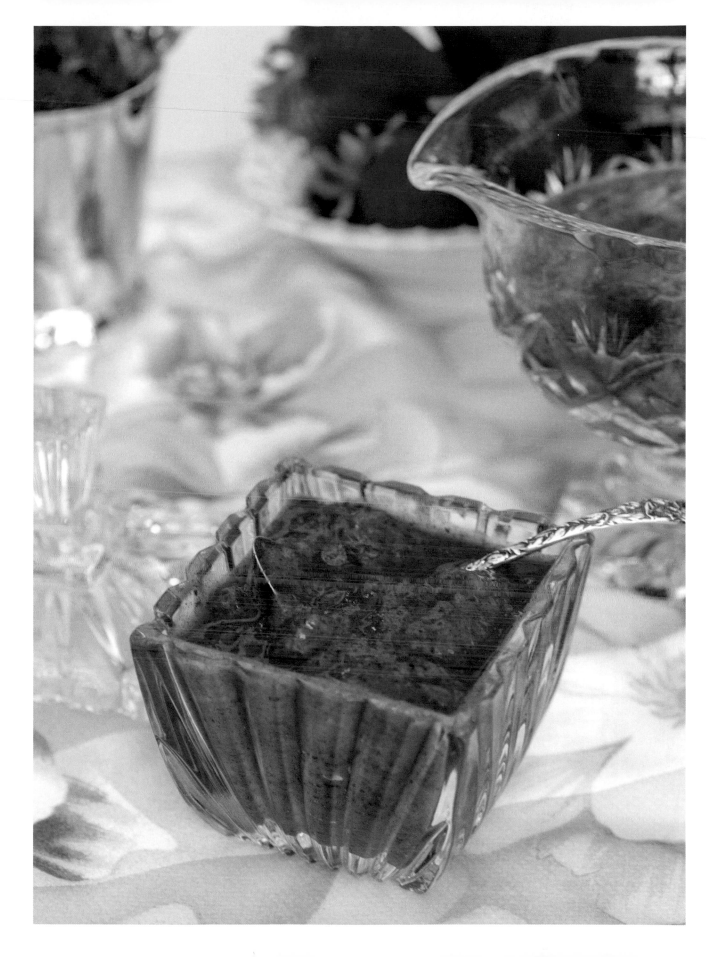

barbecue sauce

MAKES 1¼ cups   PREP TIME: 10 minutes   COOK TIME: 15 minutes

I know a lot of people take their barbecue sauce very seriously. Just ask the contestants of Saucekers, the ultimate barbecue competition (it's basically the Oscars for barbecue sauce). To me, if a barbecue sauce is not sweet, then it's not really barbecue sauce. Even without refined sugar, this one is plenty sweet. But it's also a touch vinegary, a smidgen savory, a little bit tangy, and a tiny bit tart, too. In other words, it is complex enough to be interesting. And it makes the best finger-licking Oven-Style Barbecue Chicken (page 184) ever!

3 tablespoons extra-virgin olive oil

1 cup chopped onions

4 small cloves garlic, chopped

⅛ teaspoon Himalayan pink salt

1 (8-ounce) can unflavored tomato sauce

2 tablespoons manuka honey or other raw honey

2 tablespoons raw apple cider vinegar

2 teaspoons Dijon mustard

2 teaspoons gluten-free Worcestershire sauce

5 medjool dates, pitted (see Note)

1 teaspoon chili powder

1 teaspoon paprika

1. Heat the oil in a small saucepan over medium heat. Add the onions and garlic to the pan and sauté for 6 to 7 minutes, until the onions soften. Add the salt and tomato sauce and simmer for 5 to 6 minutes. Remove from the heat and set aside to cool.

2. Transfer the cooled sauce to a high-powered blender or food processor and add the rest of the ingredients. Process on high speed for about a minute, or until all the ingredients are well blended and the mixture is smooth. Adjust the seasonings as desired. If the sauce is too thick for your taste, thin it out by adding 1 tablespoon of water at a time.

STORAGE INFORMATION _____

Barbecue sauce will keep in a sealed jar in the refrigerator for up to a week.

NOTE _____

If you're using a food processor and your dates are on the dry side, soak them in water for 15 to 30 minutes to soften them before pureeing (very moist, succulent medjool dates do not require soaking).

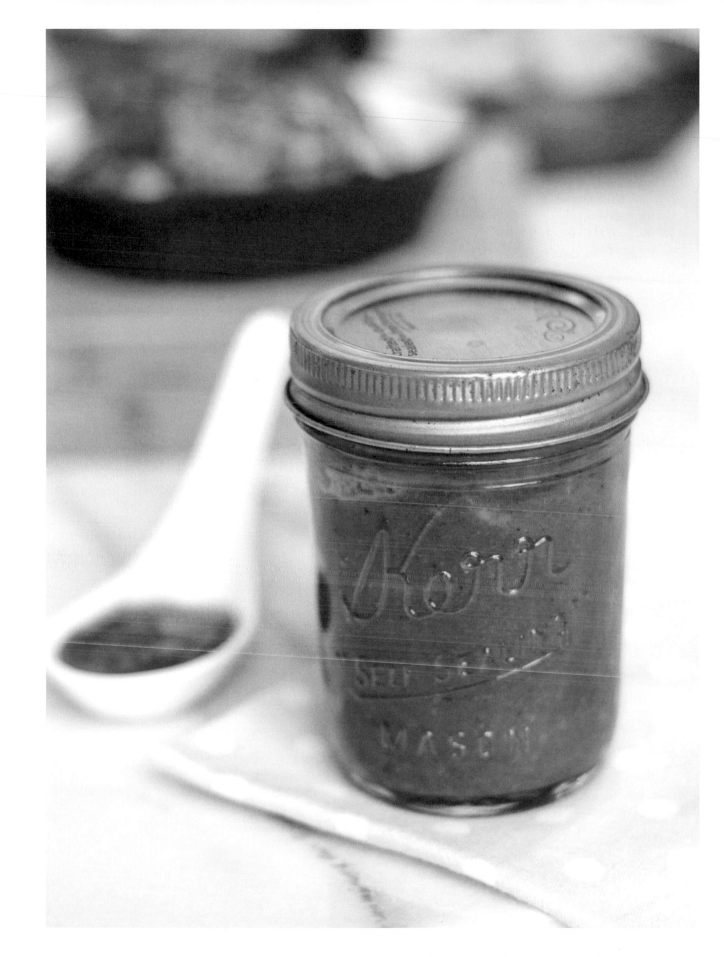

honey mustard sauce

MAKES ½ cup   PREP TIME: 5 minutes

Honey mustard sauce is one of those "back in the day" condiments I stopped eating when I cleaned up my diet two decades ago. The kind of honey mustard sauce I loved was nothing fancy—it was the rich, creamy, and sweet kind you might find at Outback Steakhouse. When my son was fourteen years old, he asked me to make healthy chicken nuggets with honey mustard sauce (the nugget recipe is on the blog, by the way), and I came up with a clean version of that sauce I'd always loved. I initially made it using just Dijon mustard, but one day when I was short of Dijon I had to add some yellow mustard. I thought it was good before, but adding yellow mustard made it so much better. I guess some things just happen for a reason.

⅓ cup plus 1 tablespoon water

½ cup raw cashews, preferably soaked for 1 to 2 hours, then rinsed and drained (see Notes)

7 Deglet Noor dates, pitted (see Notes)

2 tablespoons Dijon mustard

1 tablespoon plus 2 teaspoons prepared yellow mustard

2 teaspoons manuka honey or other raw honey (see Notes)

1 teaspoon fresh thyme leaves (optional)

⅛ teaspoon Himalayan pink salt

Put all the ingredients in a blender or food processor in the order given in the ingredients list. Process on high speed until smooth and creamy, stopping the machine as necessary to scrape down the sides. Add more water, 1 tablespoon at a time, if the sauce is too thick.

STORAGE INFORMATION _____

This sauce will keep in a jar in the refrigerator for up to a week.

NOTES _____

If you're using a high-powered blender, soaking the cashews is optional, but it does create a creamier texture. If you're using a conventional blender instead of a high-powered one, soaking the cashews is necessary to get the right texture.

If you're not using a high-powered blender, soak the dates in water for 15 to 30 minutes to soften them before pureeing.

One of my favorite uses for this sauce is Honey Mustard Sheet Pan Chicken Dinner (page 212). If you plan to use this sauce for that recipe—or any recipe that requires cooking—do not use manuka honey; it's quite expensive, and its amazing health benefits are destroyed when the honey is heated.

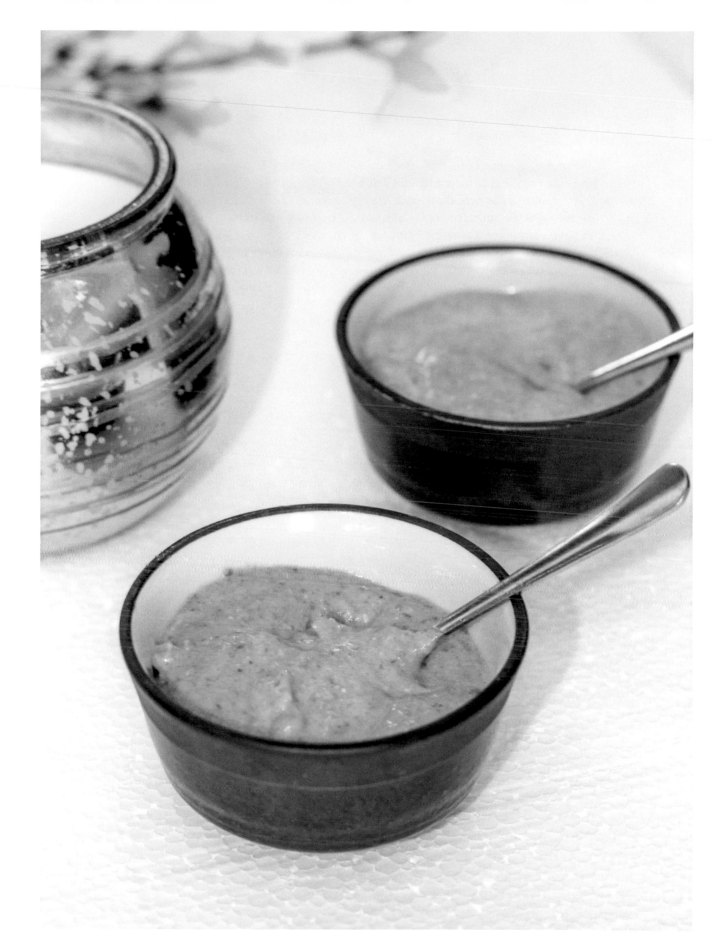

ketchup

MAKES 1¼ cups   PREP TIME: 10 minutes   COOK TIME: 1 hour

"Ketchup ketchup in a bottle, none will come and then a lot'll"—it's a little rhyme my dad would always say when I would (unsuccessfully) try to get lots of ketchup on my food as a kid. I was one of those kids who put ketchup on just about everything—eggs, toast, burgers, steak, french fries, baked potatoes, and even mac and cheese… Now that I am all grown up, I have not outgrown my love for ketchup. To this day, my husband cringes when we are at a fancy restaurant and I ask the waiter to please bring the ketchup bottle for my fish. Even though I know commercial ketchup is complete junk, I just love it so much I have to have just a little. When at home, though, I make my own clean ketchup from healthy and nourishing ingredients. If you are a big ketchup lover, you will probably want to make a double batch!

---

1 pint cherry tomatoes

2 teaspoons extra-virgin olive oil

½ cup chopped onions

2 cloves garlic, peeled

2 tablespoons tomato paste

1 tablespoon raw apple cider vinegar

½ teaspoon gluten-free Worcestershire sauce

¼ teaspoon Himalayan pink salt

8 medjool dates, pitted (see Note)

1. Preheat the oven to 400°F.

2. Place the tomatoes on a rimmed baking sheet, then drizzle with the oil and toss to coat. Roast for 40 minutes, or until soft. Remove the baking sheet from the oven, add the onions, and roast for another 20 to 25 minutes, until the tomatoes and onions are both very soft. Remove from the oven and set aside to cool.

3. Transfer the cooled tomatoes and onions to a blender or food processor and add the remaining ingredients. Process until the ketchup is smooth and lump-free.

STORAGE INFORMATION _____
Ketchup will keep in a sealed glass bottle in the refrigerator for 2 weeks.

NOTE _____
If you're using a conventional blender rather than a high-powered one and your dates are on the dry side, soak them in water for 15 to 30 minutes to soften them before pureeing (very moist, succulent medjool dates do not require soaking).

MAKE IT VEGAN AND VEGETARIAN _____
Use a vegan Worcestershire sauce.

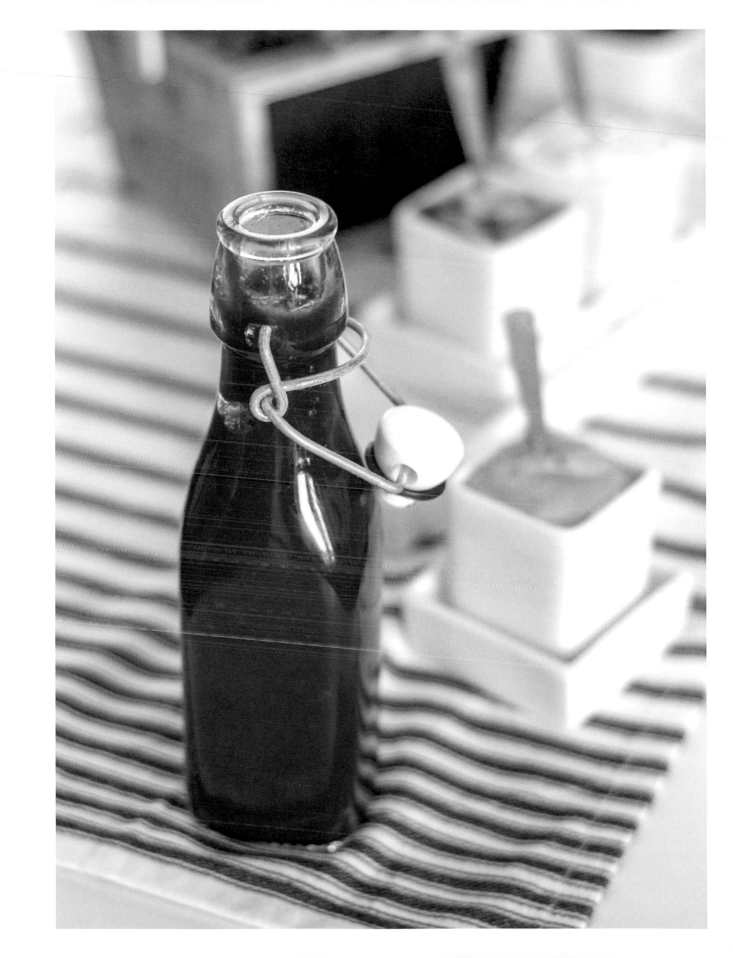

egg-free mayonnaise

MAKES 1¼ cups   PREP TIME: 12 minutes, plus time soak the nuts

I worked very hard on getting this recipe just right. All the work was worth it, though, because it is definitely a staple condiment in our house. I originally made this recipe using extra-virgin olive oil, and it did taste good—but with avocado oil, it tastes so much better. If you are wondering why I don't just use store-bought mayonnaise, it's because the eggs have to be pasteurized (which can deplete important nutrients) in order to have a long shelf life, and with the exception of one brand (Primal Kitchen), store-bought mayonnaise contains refined oils. The low-fat versions are even worse because they taste terrible and the ingredients are highly refined. Also, I made this recipe egg-free because even though I have nothing against eggs (assuming they are pasture-raised), I still can't bring myself to use raw eggs, which is what most homemade mayo recipes call for. So there you have it, that's the long-winded explanation of why I made this recipe in the first place. But I promise you will not miss the refined oil or eggs one bit!

¼ cup plus 2 tablespoons water

¼ cup plus 1 tablespoon fresh lemon juice

¼ cup unrefined avocado oil

1 cup raw macadamia nuts, preferably soaked in water for 1 to 2 hours, then rinsed and drained (see Notes)

1 medjool date, pitted

½ teaspoon Himalayan pink salt

½ teaspoon Dijon mustard

1 teaspoon raw apple cider vinegar

⅛ teaspoon dry mustard

Put all the ingredients in a blender in the order given in the ingredients list. Process on high speed for 1 full minute, or until the ingredients are thoroughly blended and the mixture is smooth and creamy.

STORAGE INFORMATION

Mayonnaise will keep in a jar in the refrigerator for up to a week.

NOTES

For best results, regardless of the type of blender you're using, the nuts should be soaked before using. However, if you're using a conventional blender instead of a high-powered one, the results still won't be quite as good as with a high-powered blender.

If you don't have a high-powered blender, another option is to use a NutriBullet: soak the nuts as instructed, then blend the nuts and water in the NutriBullet until smooth. Transfer the mixture to a regular blender, add the remaining ingredients, and process on high speed until the mixture is smooth and creamy.

If you're using a conventional blender rather than a high-powered one and your date is on the dry side, soak it in water for 15 to 30 minutes to soften it before using (very moist, succulent medjool dates do not require soaking).

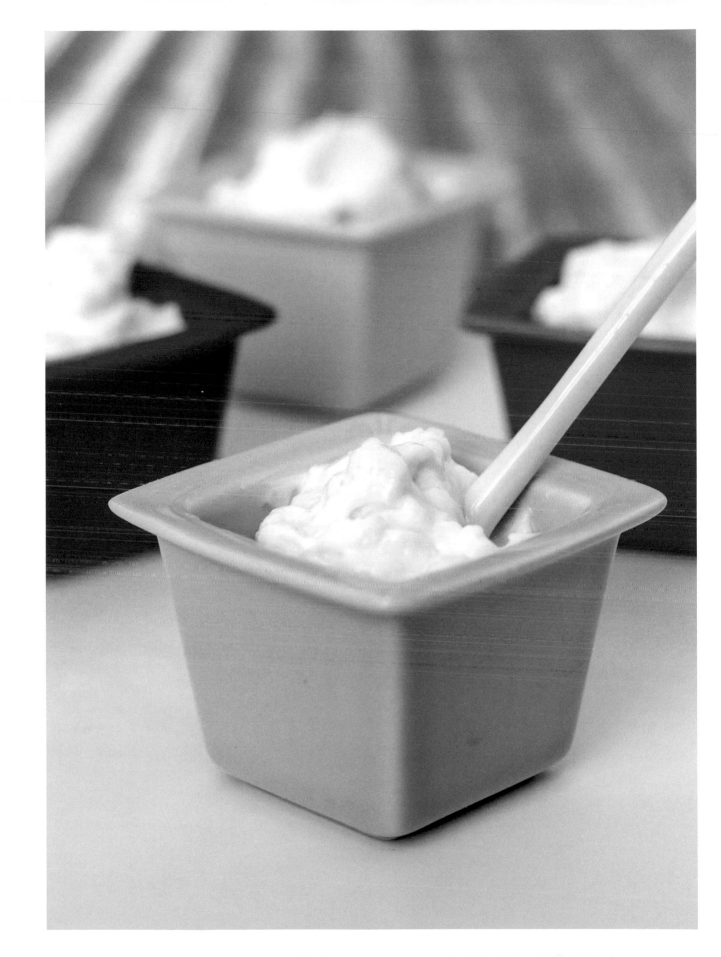

green goddess dressing/dip

MAKES about 1¼ cups   PREP TIME: 10 minutes

There are lots of variations of this California classic. I make mine without oils, and I use pureed cashews and hemp seeds for a full-bodied texture. Not only does it make a delicious salad dressing (be sure to try it on my Southern Cobb Salad, page 172), but I also often serve it as a dip for crudités. The dressing is definitely thick, but it can be thinned with water if you prefer.

1½ cups plus 2 tablespoons water

¾ cup raw cashews, preferably soaked in water for 1 to 2 hours, then rinsed and drained (see Notes)

¼ cup chopped fresh parsley

3 tablespoons fresh lemon juice

3 tablespoons hemp seeds

2 tablespoons chopped fresh chives

2 tablespoons chopped fresh dill

2 teaspoons manuka honey or other raw honey

2 cloves garlic, peeled (see Notes)

1 teaspoon gluten-free Worcestershire sauce

½ teaspoon onion powder

¼ teaspoon Himalayan pink salt

¼ teaspoon ground black pepper

Put all the ingredients in a blender or food processor and process until smooth and creamy. Taste and add more salt and pepper if desired. The mixture will be pretty thick; if you want to thin it out, add 1 tablespoon of water at a time until you have the desired consistency.

NOTES

If you're using a high-powered blender, soaking the cashews is optional, but it does create a creamier texture. If you're using a conventional blender instead of a high-powered one, soaking the cashews is necessary to get the right texture.

If you're using a conventional blender, be sure to coarsely chop the garlic before using.

STORAGE INFORMATION

This dressing will keep in a jar in the refrigerator for up to 5 days.

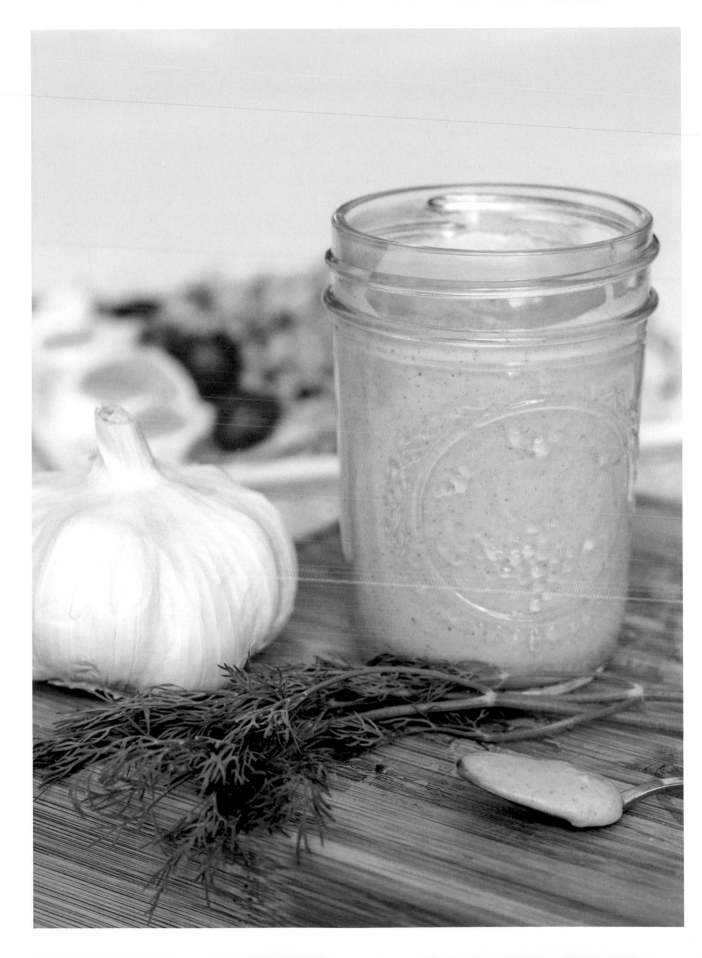

thank you

This book has been twenty years in the making—it contains everything we've learned since we started eating clean in 1998. And if it were not for all of the people mentioned below, it just wouldn't be the same. In fact, the book probably wouldn't even exist at all, because pulling everything together truly took a village.

First, our biggest thank-you goes to Ivy's mom, Gail Ingram. Although we have published books in the past, we had no idea what we were getting into with our first cookbook, and we simply could not have done it without Gail's help. She was our food stylist and food photographer, but Gail's role extended far beyond making the food look good. Without her attention to detail, creativity, and artistic flair, this book would look very different (and not in a good way!). It would take far more than a full page to list everything Gail has done over the years to help us, but we want to extend our deepest and most sincere appreciation for the countless hours she has dedicated to this particular book. We love you, Mom.

To Karen Herrera, our recipe tester and dear friend: What would we ever do without you?! You have become far more than a friend. You are part of the family, and you have become like a sister to Ivy. There is no doubt our life paths crossed for a reason. Beyond the countless hours you have spent working on this book, you have helped us all so much more than you may realize. We hope you know how much we appreciate everything you do— and always with a smile! We love you (and of course Antonio, Kaitlin, and Ashley, too)! You have been a true blessing to us all.

To our longtime family friend, Debby Gans: Thank you for being far more than our photographer. Not only do you make the people you photograph look amazing, but you make them feel even better. As the saying goes, people will forget what you say and they will forget what you do, but they will never forget how you make them feel, and you have the gift of making people feel special and loved. We will always love you for that.

To David Scarola: Thank you for being the easiest guy on earth to work with. We mean that. With Debby out of town, we would not have been able to meet the deadline for the last photos if you had not stepped up to the plate in the final hour. We know your job was not easy, and we greatly appreciate your being such a team player. And, of course, the photos are amazing!

A great big thank-you to our entire publishing team at Victory Belt. We had no idea what it would take to pull a cookbook together, and we couldn't have asked for a more passionate or dedicated team to help guide us. To our publisher, Erich Krauss: We can't thank you enough for believing in us and giving us the space and flexibility to create the cookbook of our dreams. To Lance Freimuth: We so much appreciated your guidance (and patience!) through every step … and there sure were a lot of steps! To our three editors (and yes, it took *three* editors to get the job done), Erin Granville, Holly Jennings, and Pam Mourouzis: Thank you all for your impeccable attention to detail. It took an incredible amount of work, tremendous organization, and many, many long hours to pull this all together. We greatly appreciate your dedication to making this the best book possible. And to Susan Lloyd: We don't know how you do it, but with ten different balls in the air at all times, you somehow always manage to catch them all! You not only kept us on track and on time, you kept Ivy calm, and that's a job all by itself (wink). Truly, from the bottom of our hearts, we couldn't ask for a better group of people to work with. To everyone at Victory Belt, thank you ALL.

Always behind the scenes of just about everything we do and one of Ivy's closest friends, our Clean Cuisine health coach Cherie Fromson is always pitching in to help us out one way or another. Cherie spent countless hours pulling together the resources section, not to mention helping Ivy stay organized. She even pitched in to help taste-test the Palm Beach Pineapple Sangria recipe on page 300 (wink). We love you, Cherie.

To Ivy's longtime friend, the hugely talented Erin Lodeesen of Rhizome Content: Your ongoing support and enthusiasm for Clean Cuisine has always meant so much to us. And you always manage to bring something brilliant to the table, in this case the cover design. Thank you for making it—and everything you do—perfect.

We can't write a book without also thanking Peter Vegso, Allison Janse, and Kim Weiss for helping us get off the ground. We will always be grateful.

To our very young friends, Mia Fromson, Emery Fromson, Carly Gans, Benji Gans, Cami Kresser, and Elle Kresser: Each and every one of you is so very special to our family. Thank you for the many hours you spent cheerfully smiling so we could get the pictures perfect. You each bring so much joy to us all, and we are so happy to have you be a part of our book.

To Andy's parents, Ken and Elaine Larson: The older we get, the more we appreciate and recognize the importance of the solid foundation you provided for Andy in his life … and in all of ours.

To Ivy's dad, Norman Ingram: Ivy has learned more from you than from anyone else in her life. This book wouldn't be the same without you because Ivy wouldn't be the same.

And to our dear son, Blake: Raising you has always felt like the most important job in our lives. Feeding you well has played a very big role in that job, and so without you, the time and effort that went into creating the recipes in this book would not have been invested. Neither the book nor anything else in our lives would be the same without you. We love you.

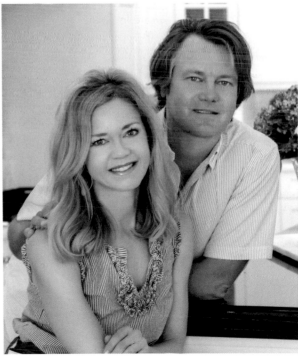

resources

FLOURS
Bob's Red Mill
King Arthur Flour
Nuts.com

Cassava flour
Anthony's
Otto's
Terrasoul Superfoods

Gluten-free oat flour
Arrowhead Mills
Bob's Red Mill
King Arthur Flour

Sprouted spelt flour (contains gluten)
Bob's Red Mill
One Degree Organics

BEANS & LEGUMES
Eden Organics
Fig Food Co.
Pomi

Canned beans (BPA-free)
365 Organics

Dried heirloom beans
Rancho Gordo

GLUTEN-FREE WHOLE GRAINS
Arrowhead Mills
Bob's Red Mill
Lundberg
truRoots

Black rice
Lotus Foods
Lundberg

Buckwheat
Bob's Red Mill
Eden Foods

Quinoa (white and red)
Rancho Gordo
truRoots

Sprouted brown rice
Floating Leaf
truRoots

Gluten-free crackers
Mary's Gone Crackers

Puffed brown rice cereal
One Degree Organics

BREADS & TORTILLAS
Almond tortillas
Siete

Gluten-free whole-grain bread
Canyon Bakehouse

Sprouted corn tortillas
Food for Life

Sprouted whole-grain bread (contains gluten)
Food for Life
Manna Organic Bakery

Sprouted whole-grain hamburger buns (contains gluten)
Ezekiel 4:9

UNREFINED OILS
La Tourangelle
Nutiva

Unrefined avocado oil
365 Everyday Value
La Tourangelle
Primal Kitchen

Unrefined extra-virgin coconut oil
Barleans
La Tourangelle
Nutiva

Unrefined extra-virgin olive oil
365 Everyday Value 100% California Unfiltered
California Olive Ranch
Kirkland
Lucini Premium
McEvoy Ranch
Trader Joe's California Estate

Unrefined flax oil
Barleans

Unrefined hemp oil
Nutiva
Tempt

Unrefined macadamia nut oil
Brookfarm
NOW Foods

Unrefined toasted sesame oil
Eden Foods
Spectrum Organics

Unrefined walnut oil
Flora
La Tourangelle
Roland

DRIED FRUITS (buy in bulk)
Made in Nature
Nuts.com
Sincerely Nuts

Dried cabernet grapes
Ray Zyn

Goji berries
Himalania
Navitas Organics
Nuts.com
Sincerely Nuts

Mulberries
Navitas Organics
Nuts.com
Sincerely Nuts

Raisins (golden and black)
365 Everyday Value
Nuts.com
Sincerely Nuts

SUPERFOOD POWDERS
Navitas Organics

GRASS-FED GELATIN
Vital Proteins Beef Gelatin

NATURAL SWEETENERS

Blackstrap molasses
Wholesome

Dates (medjool and Deglet Noor)
Nuts.com
Sincerely Nuts

Manuka honey
Wedderspoon

**Organic coconut palm sugar
(coconut crystals)**
Big Tree Farms
Navitas Organics
Wholesome

Pure maple syrup
Shady Maple Farms

Raw honey
Really Raw Honey
White Gold Honey

Stevia
Organic Sweetleaf

CUPBOARD CONDIMENTS & CANNED ITEMS

Canned artichokes
Native Forest
365 Everyday Value

Canned & boxed tomatoes
365 Everyday Value
Muir Glen
Pomi

Canned hearts of palm
365 Everyday Value
Native Forest
Palmini

Coconut butter / coconut manna
Nikki's Coconut Butter
Nutiva

Dairy-free chocolate chips
Enjoy Life
Lily's Dark Chocolate
Pascha

Full-fat coconut milk
365 Everyday Value
Thai Kitchen

Marinara sauce
Amy's
Monte Bene
Rao's Marinara

Organic broth (vegetable, chicken & beef)
Imagine Foods
Pacific Naturals

Organic roasted red peppers
365 Everyday Value
Mediterranean Organic

Organic Worcestershire sauce
Annie's Naturals
The Wizard's

Raw unsweetened cacao nibs
Navitas Organics

Tomato paste
365 Everyday Value
Muir Glen

Unsweetened cacao powder
Navitas Organics

NUT & SEED BUTTERS

Freshly ground peanut butter
MaraNatha
Santa Cruz Organic

Macadamia butter
Wilderness Poets

Pistachio butter
Wilderness Poets

Raw or roasted almond butter
Artisana Organics
MaraNatha

Tahini
Artisana Organics

TEAS

Ito En
Mighty Leaf
Pique Tea
The Republic of Tea
Tazo
Traditional Medicinals

Lemon balm
Nuts.com
The Republic of Tea
Traditional Medicinals

Peppermint
Ito En
Nuts.com
The Republic of Tea
Traditional Medicinals

Yerba mate
Guayaki

SALT, SPICES, VINEGARS & CONDIMENTS

Frontier Co-Op
Organicville
Simply Organic

Himalayan pink salt
Himalania

Other salts & seasonings
Maldon Sea Salt
Old Bay Seasoning

Balsamic vinegar
Acetaia Malpighi Balsamo of
    Modena

Barbecue sauce
Organicville
Tessemae's

Fish sauce
Thai Kitchen

Food-grade/therapeutic lemon essential oil
Ancient Apothecary
doTerra
Young Living

Gluten-free tamari
San-J

Ketchup
Organicville
Sir Kensington's
Tessemae's

Liquid aminos
Bragg

Mayonnaise
Primal Kitchen
Sir Kensington's

Organic hot sauce
Hot Winter Original

Peppermint extract or peppermint essential oil
Ancient Apothecary
doTerra
Simply Organic
Young Living

Prepared horseradish
Bubbies

Red and green curry paste
Thai Kitchen

Rice vinegar (no sodium, no sugar, gluten-free)
Nakano Rice Vinegar

Sriracha sauce
Organicville
Wildbrine

Sun-dried tomatoes
365 Everyday Value

Ume plum vinegar
Eden Foods

Unfortified nutritional yeast
Sari Foods

CANNED SEAFOOD

Bar Harbor
Crown Prince
Wild Planet

MISCELLANEOUS ITEMS

Aluminum-free baking powder
Bob's Red Mill

Baking soda
365 Everyday Value
Bob's Red Mill

Unsweetened applesauce
Natural Nectar
Santa Cruz Organic

PASTAS & NOODLES
Brown rice noodles
Annie Chun's

Brown rice pasta
Lundberg

Buckwheat soba noodles
Eden Foods

Chickpea pasta
Banza

Quinoa pasta
Ancient Harvest

NUTS & SEEDS
Now Foods
Nuts.com
Organic Fruits & Nuts
Sincerely Nuts

Raw cashews
Navitas Organics
Nuts
Organic Fruits & Nuts
Sincerely Nuts

Chia seeds
Barleans
Nutiva
Organic Fruits & Nuts

Flax seeds
Arrowhead Mills
Barleans
Organic Fruits & Nuts

Hemp seeds
Navitas Organics
Nutiva
Organic Fruits & Nuts

Sunflower seeds
Bob's Red Mill
Nuts.com
Organic Fruits & Nuts

FROZEN FRUITS & VEGETABLES
365 Everyday Value
Cascadian Farm
Woodstock

Frozen cherries
365 Everyday Value
Wyman's

Frozen wild blueberries
Wyman's

Unsweetened acai packets
Sambazon

Veggie burgers
Dr. Praeger's
Engine 2
Hilary's

PLANT-BASED DAIRY ALTERNATIVES
Almond-based yogurt and cream cheese
Kite Hill

Coconut-based ice cream
Nada Moo

Hemp milk (without carrageenan)
Hemp Bliss

Nut cheese
Dr-Cow
Miyokos

Whole, unsweetened almond milk
Elmhurst
Malk Organics
New Barn

PLANT-BASED PROTEINS
Extra-firm organic tofu
Nasoya

Organic tempeh
Lightlife

FERMENTED FAVORITES
Chickpea miso
Miso Master

Fermented probiotic beverages
Farmhouse Culture

Fermented vegetables
Farmhouse Culture
Wildbrine

Kimchi
Sunja's

Kombucha
GT's Living Foods

Pickles
Bubbies
Grillos Pickles

Sauerkraut
Farmhouse Culture
Wildbrine

PASTURE-RAISED EGGS & CHICKEN

Eggs

Vital Farms

Poultry

US Wellness Meats

CLEAN SEAFOOD & MEATS

Fresh wild seafood

Cod & Capers

Grass-fed ground beef

US Wellness Meats

DRINKS & ALCOHOL

Coconut water

Harmless Harvest

Organic natural wine

Any of the brands sold at
Dry Farm Wines

**Silver/blanco tequila
(100% agave-based)**

123 Certified Organic Tequila

Casamigos Tequila Blanco

Patrón

Sparkling water

Perrier

San Pellegrino

Vodka

Devotion Vodka

NUTRITIONAL ENHANCEMENTS & SUPPLEMENTS

Brain boosters

Amare MentaFocus, a supplement
that supports focus, mental
sharpness, clarity, creativity, and
cognitive functioning

Amare MentaSync, a supplement
that supports communication in
the gut-brain axis

**Green drink powders
(phytonutrient/antioxidant
boosters)**

Amazing Grass

Green Vibrance

Multivitamins

GOOP Wellness Supplements (our
favorite is High School Genes)

Hardy Nutritionals Daily
Essentials

Omega-3s

Amare OmMEGA

Nordic Naturals Ultimate Omega
2X

Probiotics and prebiotics

Amare Fundamentals, probiotics
and prebiotics that support a
healthy gut-brain axis

Amare MentaBiotics, probiotics
and prebiotics that support
mental wellness

Dr. Ohhira's Probiotics, a probiotic
and prebiotic supplement
designed to support overall
wellness and a healthy immune
system

allergen index

recipe	page	🌰	🥛	🥚	🌾	🌽	🥜	P	🐟	🌿	🍃
banana oat muffins	104	✓	✓		✓				✓		✓
weekend waffles	106	✓	✓		✓				✓		✓
dutch apple pancakes	108	✓	✓		✓		○		✓		✓
baked oatmeal with wild blueberries & crunchy almond topping	110	✓	✓		✓				✓		✓
donuts two ways	112	✓	✓		✓	✓	○	✓	✓		✓
lemon-blueberry scones	114	✓	✓		✓		✓		✓		✓
nut butter granola	116	✓	✓		✓				✓		✓
sweet crepes	118	✓	✓		✓		✓		✓		✓
cinnamon "butter"	120	✓	✓	✓	✓	✓	✓	✓	✓		✓
the world's easiest & healthiest blackberry jam	122	✓	✓		✓	✓	✓	✓	✓		
cornbread muffins with kale	124	✓	✓		✓				✓		✓
chocolate hazelnut spread	128	✓	✓	✓	✓	✓		✓	✓	✓	✓
kim's spiced party chickpeas	130		✓	✓	✓				✓	✓	✓
sweet & savory party nuts	132	✓			✓	✓		✓	✓	✓	
deviled eggs	134	✓			✓	✓			✓	✓	✓
smoked salmon dip	136	✓	✓	○	✓	✓			✓	✓	
strawberry-banana chia pops	138	✓	✓	✓	✓	✓	✓		✓	✓	✓
spinach & artichoke dip	140	✓	✓		✓	✓			✓	✓	✓
chocolate popcorn	142	✓	✓	✓	✓		✓		✓	✓	✓
carrot hummus	144	✓	✓	✓	✓	✓	✓	✓	✓	✓	✓
cream (or no cream) of tomato soup	148	✓	✓		✓	○	○	○	✓	○	✓
cream of mushroom soup	150	○	✓		✓	✓		○	✓	✓	✓
japanese restaurant–style salad with ginger dressing	152		✓		✓	✓					✓
red curry butternut squash soup	154	✓	✓		✓	✓	✓	✓		✓	✓
salmon niçoise salad with lemon tarragon dressing	156	✓	✓		✓	✓	✓	✓			
classic-style caesar salad	158	✓	✓	✓	✓	○	✓	○	✓	○	○
manhattan clam chowder	160	✓	✓	✓	✓	✓	✓	✓	✓		
vegetable chowder	162	✓	✓	✓	✓				✓	✓	✓
seven-layer salad	164		✓		✓		✓		✓		✓
cream of broccoli soup	166	✓	✓	✓	✓	✓			✓	✓	○	✓
waldorf salad	168	✓	✓	○	✓	✓			✓	✓	○	✓
dad's chopped salad with garlic dressing	170	✓	✓	✓	✓		✓		✓	✓	✓
southern cobb salad	172		✓		✓				✓		✓
chunky (or creamy!) vegetable soup with basil pesto	174	✓	✓		✓	✓		✓		○	○
tomato-watermelon gazpacho with cilantro pesto	176	✓	✓		✓	✓	✓	P	✓	✓	✓
salmon teriyaki	180	✓	✓		✓	✓	✓	✓			
hidden veggie meatloaf	182	✓	✓		✓		✓		✓		
oven-style barbecue chicken	184	✓	✓		✓	✓	✓	✓	✓		
chicken cacciatore	186	✓	✓		✓	✓	✓	✓	✓		
the blake burger	188				✓	✓	✓	✓	✓		
better-than-takeout cashew chicken	190	✓			✓			✓			
blake's bouillabaisse	192	✓	✓		✓	✓	✓	✓	✓		
linguine with clam sauce	194	✓	✓		✓	○	✓	○	✓		
chicken tikka masala	196	○	✓		✓	✓		○	✓		
crab cakes	198	✓	✓		✓		✓		✓		
chinese takeout chicken lo mein	200	✓	✓	✓	✓		✓				

allergen index

recipe	page	1	2	3	4	5	6	P	8	9	10
dawn's italian meatballs	202		✓	✓	✓	✓	✓	✓	✓		
shrimp & grits	204	✓	✓	✓	✓				✓		
macadamia-crusted baked fish	206	✓	✓	O	✓	✓		✓	✓		
dinner party stuffed cornish hens	208	✓	✓	✓	✓				✓		
honey mustard sheet pan chicken dinner	212	✓	✓	✓	✓	✓		✓	✓		
salmon noodle casserole	214	✓	✓	✓	✓	O			✓		
slow cooker beef stroganoff	216	✓	✓	✓	✓	O		O	✓		
lemony chicken & dumplings	218	✓	✓		✓		✓		✓		
turkey shepherd's pie with whipped sweet potatoes	220	✓	✓	✓	✓	O		O	✓		
skillet meat & bean casserole with cornbread topping	222		✓		✓						
slow cooker bolognese	224	✓	✓	✓	✓	✓		O			
slow cooker chicken & vegetable thai curry	226	O	✓	✓	✓	✓	✓	O	O		
polenta pizza with white sauce & mushrooms	230	✓	✓	✓	✓				✓	✓	✓
roasted vegetable lasagna	232	✓	✓		✓						✓
spinach & artichoke quiche	234	✓	✓	✓					✓		✓
risotto with asparagus & shiitake mushrooms	236	✓	✓	✓	✓				✓	✓	✓
refried black bean tostadas	238		✓	✓	✓	✓			✓	O	✓
live to 100 vegetable chili	240		✓	✓	✓	✓	✓		✓	✓	✓
black bean burgers	242		✓	✓	✓				✓	✓	✓
the legienza veggie burger	244		✓		✓				✓		✓
sweet potato & chickpea curry	246		✓	✓	✓	✓	✓		✓	✓	✓
easy pad thai	248		✓	✓	✓					O	O
pasta alla vodka	250	✓	✓	✓	✓	O			✓	✓	✓
personal-size white pizzas with garlic & mushrooms	252	✓	✓	✓	✓	✓		✓	✓	✓	✓
roman pizza	254	✓	✓	✓	✓	✓		✓	✓	✓	✓
baked beans	258		✓	✓	✓	✓	✓		✓	O	O
chinese-style cauliflower fried rice	260	✓	✓		✓	✓	✓	✓	✓	✓	✓
wild rice pilaf	262	✓	✓		✓	O		O	✓	✓	✓
thanksgiving day green bean casserole	264	✓	✓	✓	✓	✓			✓	✓	✓
mac and cheese	266		✓	✓	✓	O			✓	O	✓
joe's perfect broccoli rabe	268	✓	✓	✓	✓	✓	✓	✓	✓	✓	✓
an easier ratatouille	270	✓	✓	✓	✓	✓	✓	✓	✓	✓	✓
karen's easy refried beans	272		✓	✓	✓	✓	✓		✓	✓	✓
sweet potato chili fries	274	✓	✓	✓	✓		✓	✓	✓	✓	✓
zucchini boats	276	✓	✓	✓	✓				✓	✓	✓
stuffed tomatoes	278	✓	✓	✓	✓	O		O	✓	✓	✓
three-bean salad	280		✓	✓	✓	✓	✓		✓	O	O
picnic-style potato salad	282	✓	✓	✓	✓	✓		✓	✓	O	✓
detoxifying green juice	286	✓	✓	✓	✓	✓	✓	✓	✓	✓	✓
whole watermelon juice	288	✓	✓	✓	✓	✓	✓	✓	✓	✓	✓
golden chai	290	✓	✓	✓	✓	✓	✓	✓	✓	✓	✓
frozen avocado margaritas	292	✓	✓	✓	✓	✓	✓	✓	✓	✓	✓
bloody marys for a crowd	294	✓	✓	✓	✓	✓	✓	✓	✓	O	O
lemon-lime dateorade	296	✓	✓	✓	✓	✓	✓	✓	✓	✓	✓
frozen raspberry-mango daiquiris	298	✓	✓	✓	✓	✓	✓	✓	✓	✓	✓

allergen index

recipe	page	🌀	🥛	💧	🌿	🌾	🍃	P	🐟	🌱	🖌️
palm beach pineapple sangria	300	✓	✓	✓	✓	✓	✓	✓	✓		✓
turmeric lemon toddy	302	✓	✓	✓	✓	✓	✓	✓	✓		✓
the best strawberry no-milk shake	306	✓	✓	✓	✓	✓			✓	✓	✓
chocolate no-milk shake	308	✓	✓	✓	✓				✓	✓	✓
blackberry-lemon cobbler no-milk shake	310	✓	✓	✓	✓				✓	✓	✓
mint chocolate chip no-milk shake	312	✓	✓	✓	✓	✓	✓	✓	✓	✓	✓
red velvet no-milk shake	314	✓	✓	✓	✓	○	✓	✓	✓		✓
orange cream no-milk shake	316	✓	✓	✓	✓		✓	✓	✓		✓
roasted peach cobbler no-milk shake	318	✓	✓	✓	✓				✓	✓	✓
hot cinnamon apple no-milk shake	320	✓	✓	✓	✓	✓			✓	✓	✓
egg nog no-milk shake	322	✓	✓	✓	✓				✓	✓	✓
cherry almond no-milk shake	324	✓	✓	✓	✓				✓	✓	
raspberry-lemon panna cotta	328	✓	✓	✓	✓	✓	✓	✓			
gingerbread spice cake	330	✓	✓		✓			✓		✓	✓
black forest ice cream	332	✓	✓		✓			✓	✓	✓	✓
key lime pie ice cream	334	✓	✓		✓		✓	✓	✓	✓	✓
oatmeal raisin cookies	336	✓	✓	✓	✓				✓	✓	✓
mint chocolate cupcakes with mint chocolate frosting	338	✓	✓		✓				✓		✓
pineapple upside-down cake	340	✓	✓		✓				✓		✓
pumpkin custard	342	✓	✓		✓		✓		✓		✓
best brownies ever	344	✓	✓		✓		✓		✓		✓
strawberry shortcake	346	✓	✓		✓		✓		✓		✓
chocolate-covered frozen bananas	348	✓	✓	✓	✓	✓		✓	✓	✓	✓
mom's individual blackberry cobblers	350	✓	✓	✓	✓				✓	✓	✓
apple-blackberry-cranberry pie	352	✓	✓		✓				✓		✓
benji's blondie bars	354	✓	✓		✓	✓		✓	✓		✓
garlic herbed croutons	358	✓	✓	✓	✓		✓		✓	✓	✓
savory crust	360	✓	✓		✓				✓		✓
speedy sweet pie crust	362	✓	✓		✓		✓		✓		✓
super-easy mini pizza crusts	364	✓	✓	✓	✓	✓		✓	✓	✓	✓
tortillas	366	✓	✓	✓	✓	✓		✓	✓	✓	✓
whole almond milk	368	✓	✓	✓	✓	✓		✓	✓	✓	✓
parmesan nut "cheese"	370	✓	✓	✓	✓	✓		✓	✓	✓	✓
clean cuisine sour cream	372	✓	✓	✓	✓	✓		✓	✓	○	✓
pineapple teriyaki sauce	374	✓	✓	✓	✓	✓	✓	✓			✓
jonn & julia's almond asian sauce	376	✓	✓	✓	✓	✓		✓			
hidden veggie marinara	378	✓	✓	✓	✓	✓	✓	✓	✓	✓	✓
tomato sauce with garlic & italian herbs	380	✓	✓	✓	✓	✓	✓	✓	✓	✓	✓
alfredo sauce	382	✓	✓	✓	✓	✓		✓	✓	✓	✓
fresh strawberry sauce	384	✓	✓	✓	✓	✓	✓	✓	✓	✓	✓
barbecue sauce	386	✓	✓	✓	✓	✓	✓	✓	✓		✓
honey mustard sauce	388	✓	✓	✓	✓			✓	✓		✓
ketchup	390	✓	✓	✓	✓	✓	✓	✓	✓	○	○
egg-free mayonnaise	392	✓	✓	✓	✓	✓		✓	✓	✓	✓
green goddess dressing/dip	394	✓	✓	✓	✓	✓		✓	✓		✓

general index